"*Counseling for Peripartum Depression* is a must read for counseling professionals. It is a well-written and addictive work on the critical topic of maternal mental health. Highly recommended!"

Shannon L. Karl, PhD, *professor, Department of Counseling, Nova Southeastern University*

"This is the first book that recognizes that women are at risk for depression throughout pregnancy as well as after. The text takes a multi-faceted approach to understanding the causes and treatment of this particular form of depression. It promotes a strength-based approach and addresses critical topics such as cultural issues, couple dynamics, and diagnosis. It is a resource that every clinician needs, because anyone who works with parents will certainly encounter this issue and need evidence-based, best practices to help their clients."

Mark E. Young, PhD, *professor emeritus, University of Central Florida*

Counseling for Peripartum Depression

Counseling for Peripartum Depression provides counselors and other mental health professionals with a comprehensive understanding of peripartum depression (PPD) and related disorders during pregnancy and after birth. The book offers diagnostic criteria and screening tools that clinicians can use in session, and focuses on holistic wellness as well as current research on the etiology and risk factors for PPD. In particular, the simple and practical STRENGTHS model can help clinicians address various social and cultural factors related to the experience of pregnancy, giving birth, taking care of children, becoming parents, and the stigma associated with maternal mental health conditions. Using case studies and stories of women who have experienced PPD, chapters explore the individual, societal, and cultural factors associated with the development of PPD, and they also present clinicians with best practices and suggestions for preventative efforts and complementary approaches to treatment.

Isabel A. Thompson, PhD, is a licensed mental health counselor in the state of Florida and an associate professor teaching and supervising graduate students in the Department of Counseling at Nova Southeastern University.

Vanessa Beatriz Teixeira, EdD, is a licensed mental health counselor in the state of Florida and an assistant professor in the Department of Counseling at Nova Southeastern University.

Eric S. Thompson, PhD, is a certified school counselor and registered mental health counselor intern in the state of Florida and an associate professor in the Department of Counseling at Nova Southeastern University.

Counseling for Peripartum Depression

A Strengths-Based Approach to Conceptualization and Treatment

Isabel A. Thompson,
Vanessa Beatriz Teixeira, and
Eric S. Thompson

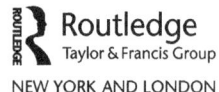

Designed cover image: © Getty Images

First published 2024
by Routledge
605 Third Avenue, New York, NY 10158

and by Routledge
4 Park Square, Milton Park, Abingdon, Oxon, OX14 4RN

Routledge is an imprint of the Taylor & Francis Group, an informa business

© 2024 Isabel A. Thompson, Vanessa Beatriz Teixeira, and Eric S. Thompson

The right of Isabel A. Thompson, Vanessa Beatriz Teixeira, and Eric S. Thompson to be identified as authors of this work has been asserted in accordance with sections 77 and 78 of the Copyright, Designs and Patents Act 1988.

All rights reserved. No part of this book may be reprinted or reproduced or utilised in any form or by any electronic, mechanical, or other means, now known or hereafter invented, including photocopying and recording, or in any information storage or retrieval system, without permission in writing from the publishers.

Trademark notice: Product or corporate names may be trademarks or registered trademarks, and are used only for identification and explanation without intent to infringe.

Library of Congress Cataloging-in-Publication Data
Names: Thompson, Isabel A., author. | Teixeira, Vanessa Beatriz, author. | Thompson, Eric S., author.
Title: Counseling for peripartum depression : a strengths-based approach to conceptualization and treatment / Isabel A. Thompson, Vanessa Beatriz Teixeira, and Eric S. Thompson.
Description: New York, NY : Routledge, 2024. |
Includes bibliographical references and index.
Identifiers: LCCN 2023018460 (print) | LCCN 2023018461 (ebook) |
ISBN 9781138320741 (hardback) | ISBN 9781138320758 (paperback) |
ISBN 9780429440892 (ebook)
Subjects: LCSH: Postpartum depression. | Pregnancy–Psychological aspects. | Childbirth–Psychological aspects. | Mental illness in pregnancy.
Classification: LCC RG852 .T44 2024 (print) | LCC RG852 (ebook) |
DDC 618.7/6–dc23/eng/20230724
LC record available at https://lccn.loc.gov/2023018460
LC ebook record available at https://lccn.loc.gov/2023018461

ISBN: 9781138320741 (hbk)
ISBN: 9781138320758 (pbk)
ISBN: 9780429440892 (ebk)

DOI: 10.4324/9780429440892

Typeset in Minion
by Newgen Publishing UK

To my father, Graham C. Thompson, Jr.
Isabel A. Thompson

I dedicate and honor this book to my stepfather, Thomas, who always supported and encouraged me in my professional and personal dreams.
Vanessa Beatriz Teixeira

For the benefit of everyone.
Eric S. Thompson

Contents

Acknowledgments	xviii
About the Authors	xx
About the Contributors	xxi

1 Understanding Peripartum Depression   1
Isabel A. Thompson

Advocating for Maternal Mental Health Needs	4
Diagnosis of Peripartum Depression	5
The "Baby Blues" and Other Mood Disorders	6
The Scope of the Problem	7
Common Stressors during the Peripartum Period	8
Impacts of Peripartum Depression	11
An Overview of Screening and Preventative Approaches	12
Impact of the COVID-19 Pandemic	13
Theoretical Perspectives	14
Conclusion	14

2 A Strengths-Based Approach to Case Conceptualization   19
Vanessa Beatriz Teixeira

Significant Individual, Infant, Family, Societal, and Cultural Factors	19
Treatment Barriers	22
Risk Factors	23
Enlisting Support from Family, the Community, and Medical Professionals	24
Noticeable Symptoms, Severity, and DSM-5-TR Diagnosis OR Needs Identified by Family and Treatment Team	26
Goals Identified by Family	28
Treatment Recommendations	30
Helpful, Protective, and Resilience Factors	31
Self-Care & Wellness	32
Applying the STRENGTHS Model—The Case of Leila	35
Significant Individual, Infant, Family, Societal, and Cultural Factors	35
Treatment Barriers	36
Risk Factors	36
Enlisting Support from Family, the Community, and Medical Professionals	36
Noticeable Symptoms, Severity, & DSM-5-TR Diagnosis/Needs Identified by Family & Treatment Team	37
Goals Identified by Family	37

	Treatment Recommendations	38
	Helpful, Protective, and Resilience Factors	38
	Self-Care & Wellness	38

3 Social and Cultural Factors Associated with Peripartum Depression and Maternal Stress — 42
Isabel A. Thompson

Social and Cultural Factors	43
Understanding the Role Expectations Related to Motherhood	43
Socio-Cultural Values and Lack of Maternity, Paternity, and Parental Leave	44
Cultural Norms of Support after Childbirth	45
Racial and Ethnic Maternal Health Disparities	46
Maternal Mental Health Disparities	47
Working with Mothers from Marginalized Racial and Ethnic Backgrounds	47
Multicultural and Social Justice Counseling Competencies	48
Pregnancy and Disability	51
Spirituality and Religious Diversity	53
Applying the *Competencies for Addressing Spiritual and Religious Issue in Counseling*	55
Working with LGBTGEQIAP+ Communities	57
Applying the *Competencies for Counseling with Lesbian, Gay, Bisexual, Queer, Questioning, Intersex, and Ally Individuals*	58
Applying the *Competencies for Counseling with Transgender Clients*	59
Working with Military Service Members, Veterans, and Their Families	60
Multiple Perspectives: Father/Partner	60
Ethical and Legal Considerations	61
Impact of the COVID-19 Pandemic	61
Conclusion	61
Applying the STRENGTHS Model—The Case of Cristina	63
Significant Individual, Infant, Family, Societal, and Cultural Factors	63
Treatment Barriers	63
Risk Factors	63
Enlisting Support from Family, the Community, and Medical Professionals	64
Noticeable Symptoms, Severity, & DSM-5-TR Diagnosis OR Needs Identified by Family & Treatment Team	64
Goals Identified by Family	64
Treatment Recommendations	64
Helpful, Protective, and Resilience Factors	64
Self-Care & Wellness	65

4 Assessing Risk Factors for Peripartum Depression and Enhancing Protective Factors to Support Wellbeing — 70
Isabel A. Thompson with contributor Jamie Hildebrandt Jerome

Risk Factors for the Development of PPD	72

The Significance of Partner Support	73
Lack of Societal Support	73
Societal Judgment	74
Judgment Related to Breastfeeding Decisions	74
Personal History of Depression	75
Peripartum Suicidality	75
Risk Factors Associated with Maternal Suicide Attempts	76
Risk Factors for Postpartum Psychosis	76
Maternal Age	76
Teenage Mothers	77
Mothers Who Are Pregnant Over Age 35	77
Psychosocial Risk Factors	77
Enhancing Protective Factors	78
Bonding between Mother and Baby	78
Breastfeeding and Bonding	78
Establishing a Self-Care Routine	79
The Power of Social Support	80
Multiple Perspectives: Father/Partner, Family, Relationships	81
Multicultural Considerations	81
Applications to Counseling	82
Addressing Self-care and Wellness in Treatment	83
Enhancing Partner and Social Support in Treatment	83
Support Related to Feeding/Breastfeeding	84
Biopsychosocial Theoretical Model	84
Ethical Considerations	85
Barriers to Treatment	85
COVID-19 and Online Support	86
Looking Forward: Enhanced Screening During Prenatal and Pediatrician Visits	86
Conclusion	87
Applying the STRENGTHS Model—The Case of Juliette	89
Significant Individual, Infant, Family, Societal, and Cultural Factors	89
Treatment Barriers	90
Risk Factors	90
Enlisting Support from Family, the Community, and Medical Professionals	90
Noticeable Symptoms, Severity, & DSM-5-TR Diagnosis OR Needs Identified by Family & Treatment Team	90
Goals Identified by Family	90
Treatment Recommendations	90
Helpful, Protective, and Resilience Factors	91
Self-Care & Wellness	91
Applying the STRENGTHS Model—The Case of Jaelyn	91
Significant Individual, Infant, Family, Societal, and Cultural Factors	91
Treatment Barriers	91
Risk Factors	91
Enlisting Support from Family, the Community, and Medical Professionals	92

Noticeable Symptoms, Severity, & DSM-5-TR Diagnosis OR Needs Identified by Family & Treatment Team	92
Goals Identified by Family	92
Treatment Recommendations	92
Helpful, Protective, and Resilience Factors	92
Self-Care & Wellness	92

5 Conception, Pregnancy, and Birth 97
Isabel A. Thompson

Conception	100
Infertility	100
Assessing Conception-Related Risk Factors	101
The Adjustments of Pregnancy	101
Understanding the Impact of Medical Complications of Pregnancy	102
Changing Bodies, Body Image, and Self-Acceptance	104
Birth	104
The Process of Birth	105
Birth Culture	106
Healthcare and Birth Attendants	107
Birth Trauma and Obstetrical Complications	108
Preterm Birth and Neonatal Intensive Care	109
C-Section	109
Postpartum Hemorrhage	109
Maternal Mortality	109
Challenges of the Immediate and Early Postpartum	110
Multiple Perspectives: Father/Partner and Family Relationships	111
Multicultural Considerations	112
Conception and Pregnancy for LGBTQ+ Couples	113
Applications to Counseling	114
Addressing Conception, Pregnancy, and Birth in Treatment	114
Birth Narratives: What Is Your Birth Story?	115
Assessing Substance Use During Pregnancy	115
Assessing History of Sexual Abuse and/or Sexual Assault	116
Assessing Intimate Partner Violence During Pregnancy	116
Biopsychosocial Theoretical Model	116
Ethical and Legal Considerations	117
Barriers to Treatment	117
Impact of the COVID-19 Pandemic	119
Looking Forward: Improving Screening and Intervention During Pregnancy	119
Conclusion	120
Applying the STRENGTHS Model—The Case of Jesse	120
Significant Individual, Infant, Family, Societal, and Cultural Factors	120
Treatment Barriers	120
Risk Factors	120
Enlisting Support from Family, the Community, and Medical Professionals	120

Noticeable Symptoms, Severity, & DSM-5-TR Diagnosis OR Needs Identified by Family & Treatment Team	120
Goals Identified by Family	121
Treatment Recommendations	121
Helpful, Protective, and Resilience Factors	121
Self-Care & Wellness	121

6 Screening and Diagnosis of Peripartum Depression and Related Disorders — 125
Vanessa Beatriz Teixeira

Screening and Suicide Prevention	126
Diagnosis of Peripartum Depression and Related Disorders	128
Postadoption Depression (PAD)	131
Perinatal Loss	132
Multiple Perspectives: Paternal PPD	134
Perinatal Death—Family Members and Siblings	134
Multicultural Considerations: Perinatal Loss	135
Applications to Counseling	136
Treating Paternal Peripartum Depression	138
Ethical and Legal Considerations	139
Barriers to Treatment	140
Impact of the COVID-19 Pandemic	140
Conclusion	140
Applying the STRENGTHS Model—The Case of Johanna	141
Significant Individual, Infant, Family, Societal, and Cultural Factors	141
Treatment Barriers	142
Risk Factors	142
Enlisting Support from Family, the Community, and Medical Professionals	142
Noticeable Symptoms, Severity, & DSM-5-TR Diagnosis OR Needs Identified by Family & Treatment Team	142
Goals Identified by Family	142
Treatment Recommendations	143
Helpful, Protective, and Resilience Factors	143
Self-Care & Wellness	143

7 Multiple Routes to Motherhood: Role and Identity Changes and Clinical Implications — 149
Isabel A. Thompson with contributor Carly Paro-Tompkins

The Adjustment to Motherhood	150
First-Time Biological Mothers	151
PPD and First-Time Mothers	151
Surrogacy	152
Mothers of Multiples	152
Non-biological Mothers	153
Adoptive Mothers	154

Stepmothers	155
Lesbian Non-biological Mothers	157
Family Dynamics	157
Changes in Friendships	158
Multiple Perspectives: Father/Partner and Extended Family Relationships	159
First-time Fathers	159
Multicultural Considerations	160
Applications to Counseling	160
Promoting Emotional Wellness	161
Addressing Couple and Family Relationships in Counseling	161
Individual Counseling: The Journey of Motherhood	162
Ethical and Legal Considerations	163
Barriers to Treatment	163
Resources for Treatment	164
Impact of the COVID-19 Pandemic	164
Applying the STRENGTHS Model—The Case of Ceci	167
Significant Individual, Infant, Family, Societal, and Cultural Factors	167
Treatment Barriers	167
Risk Factors	167
Enlisting Support from Family, the Community, and Medical Professionals	167
Noticeable Symptoms, Severity, & DSM-5-TR Diagnosis OR Needs Identified by Family & Treatment Team	167
Goals Identified by Family	168
Treatment Recommendations	168
Helpful, Protective, and Resilience Factors	168
Self-Care & Wellness	168

8 Shift in Couple Dynamics 173
Vanessa Beatriz Teixeira with contributor Samantha Fernandez

Sexual Difficulties and Risk Factors	174
Obstetrical Violence	175
Assessment of Sexual Difficulties	176
Parental Roles and Responsibilities	177
Parenting	178
Multiple Perspectives: Father/Partner	179
Multicultural Considerations	180
Treatment of Sexual Difficulties	180
Solutions for Sharing Parenting Roles and Responsibilities	183
Imago Therapy Approaches for Addressing Parenting Responsibilities	184
Application to Couples Counseling	185
Ethical and Legal Considerations	188
Barriers to Treatment	189
Impact of the COVID-19 Pandemic	189
Conclusion	190
Applying the STRENGTHS Model—The Case of Roberta	192

	Significant Individual, Infant, Family, Societal, and Cultural Factors	192
	Treatment Barriers	192
	Risk Factors	192
	Enlisting Support from Family, the Community, and Medical Professionals	192
	Noticeable Symptoms, Severity, & DSM-5-TR Diagnosis OR Needs Identified by Family & Treatment Team	192
	Goals Identified by Family	193
	Treatment Recommendations	193
	Helpful, Protective, and Resilience Factors	193
	Self-Care & Wellness	193

9 Finding a Rhythm as a Mother and Connecting with Baby — 197
Vanessa Beatriz Teixeira with contributor Dawn Hoffman

Enhancing the Mother–Baby Bond	198
Warm and Responsive Reactions to Infant Needs	199
Cooperative and Stimulating Interaction and Play between Mother and Infant	200
Frequent Breastfeeding	201
Implications of Untreated PPD for Baby's Development	202
Coping with the Challenges of Motherhood and PPD	204
Multiple Perspectives	205
Multicultural Considerations	205
Applications to Counseling	206
Ethical and Legal Considerations	209
Barriers to Treatment	209
COVID-19 and Online Support	211
Conclusion	212
Applying the STRENGTHS Model—The Case of Kennedy	213
Significant Individual, Infant, Family, Societal, and Cultural Factors	213
Treatment Barriers	213
Risk Factors	214
Enlisting Support from Family, the Community, and Medical Professionals	214
Noticeable Symptoms, Severity, & DSM-5-TR Diagnosis OR Needs Identified by Family & Treatment Team	214
Goals Identified by Family	214
Treatment Recommendations	214
Helpful, Protective, and Resilience Factors	215
Self-Care & Wellness	215

10 Career and Identity in the Peripartum — 219
Isabel A. Thompson

Women, Identity, and Career	220
Navigating Work and Motherhood while Experiencing PPD	221
Working Mothers	222
Maternity Leave (or Lack Thereof)	222

Returning to Work after Maternity Leave	223
Breastfeeding Working Mothers	224
Benefits of Paid Employment for Working Mothers	224
Stay-at-Home Mothers	225
Work from Home Mothers	225
Navigating Maternal Roles with Professional Roles and Priorities	226
Feminism and Sexism in the Workplace and Gender Role Socialization	228
Multiple Perspectives: Fathers/Partners	229
Multicultural Considerations	230
Applications to Counseling	230
Ethical and Legal Considerations	231
Barriers to Treatment	232
Impact of the COVID-19 Pandemic	233
Conclusion	233
Applying the STRENGTHS Model—The Case of Paisley	235
Significant Individual, Infant, Family, Societal, and Cultural Factors	235
Treatment Barriers	236
Risk Factors	236
Enlisting Support from Family, the Community, and Medical Professionals	236
Noticeable Symptoms, Severity, & DSM-5-TR Diagnosis OR Needs Identified by Family & Treatment Team	236
Goals Identified by Family	236
Treatment Recommendations	237
Helpful, Protective, and Resilience Factors	237
Self-Care & Wellness	237
Applying the STRENGTHS Model—The Case of Myriel	239
Significant Individual, Infant, Family, Societal, and Cultural Factors	239
Treatment Barriers	239
Risk Factors	239
Enlisting Support from Family, the Community, and Medical Professionals	239
Noticeable Symptoms, Severity, & DSM-5-TR Diagnosis OR Needs Identified by Family & Treatment Team	240
Goals Identified by Family	240
Treatment Recommendations	240
Helpful, Protective, and Resilience Factors	240
Self-Care & Wellness	240

11 Treatment Approaches for Peripartum Depression   243
Eric S. Thompson with contributors Katlyn Bagarella and Tyler Elizabeth Hernandez

Perinatal Distress	245
Efficacy of Treatment Modalities for PPD	245
Common Existing Treatments	245
Selecting a Treatment Modality	246
Role of the Therapist	247

Cognitive Behavior Therapy	248
Therapeutic Benefits for PPD	249
Challenging Automatic Thinking	249
Automatic Thought Record	251
Integrating CBT and Motivational Interviewing for Help-Seeking Behaviors	252
Integrating Feminist Theory into Treatment	255
Interpersonal Therapy	255
Dialectical Behavioral Therapy	259
Solution-Focused Brief Therapy (SFBT) Approaches	261
Relationship in SFBT	262
Basic Assumptions	263
Supportive Approaches and Psychopharmacological Interventions	265
Complementary Treatment Modalities	266
Breastfeeding	266
Infant Massage	267
Exercise	267
Prenatal and Postnatal Yoga	267
Other Complementary and Alternative Approaches	267
Certification in Perinatal Mental Health	268
Bringing Baby Home Training	268
Multiple Perspectives: Father/Partner	268
Mindfulness-Based Interventions	269
Mindfulness of Breath	269
Self-Compassion	270
Lovingkindness	271
Conclusion	272
Applying the STRENGTHS Model—The Case of Casey	272
Significant Individual, Infant, Family, Societal, and Cultural Factors	272
Treatment Barriers	272
Risk Factors	272
Enlisting Support from Family, the Community, and Medical Professionals	272
Noticeable Symptoms, Severity, & DSM-5-TR Diagnosis OR Needs Identified by Family & Treatment Team	272
Goals Identified by Family	272
Treatment Recommendations	273
Helpful, Protective, and Resilience Factors	273
Self-Care & Wellness	273
Index	**279**

Acknowledgments

We thank all the contributors who shared their passion and expertise.

We thank the mothers who shared their narratives, whether anonymously or with their names. Your voices inspire us!

Thank you:

Katlyn Bagarella for APA style support.

Shannon Karl for reviewing drafts and providing expert feedback and collegial support.

Mark Young for his encouragement in the writing process and validation of the significance of this endeavor.

Jessica Valenzuela for reviewing the book proposal.

Tyler Hernandez for her collaboration on a presentation which helped germinate this book.

Thank you to our editor Anna Moore whose ongoing support throughout the entire process has made this book possible.

ISABEL A. THOMPSON

The ongoing support of friends and family made this book possible.

Thank you:

Vanessa Teixeira for her ongoing commitment and dedication.

Michelle Scharlop for the ongoing support and inspiration.

Amber DiPietra for believing in me and allowing me space to explore creative dimensions.

My mother, Ellen G. Thompson, for her tireless instrumental and emotional support.

My father, Graham Clark Thompson, Jr. (deceased) for knowing that I could do this even when I doubted myself.

My mother-in-law Francie Adams for the support.

My father-in-law Larry Thompson and stepmother-in-law Patricia Thompson for their support.

Thank you also to my healthcare providers and spiritual teachers.

Eric S. Thompson for your ongoing support and collaboration on this project and keeping the big picture and purpose in mind.

Our two sons Christopher and Theo have inspired me, with the intention to support clinicians and clinicians-in-training to be as effective as possible for peripartum clients.

VANESSA BEATRIZ TEIXEIRA

Writing and publishing this book has been one of the greatest accomplishments of my career. I am honored to say that I have co-authored a book on such an important topic that impacts women and families around the world. When I started writing this book, I was pregnant with my first child. Three years later, I have two wonderful kids whom I hope will be inspired by their mother's dedication, sacrifice, and work ethic in writing this book. Thank you, Skylar and Jackson, for helping me understand the many struggles and joys of becoming a parent and career-mom.

I would like to express sincere appreciation and gratitude to my own mother, Vovó, who took care of my children while I spent many days and nights researching and writing. To my husband, Christopher, thank you for believing in me and allowing me to prioritize my career for the past 14 years. I am eternally grateful for the immense support and help I have received from my family.

To all the mothers out there who may be struggling; I am cheering you on. Keep going. It does, eventually, get easier.

ERIC S. THOMPSON

I am grateful for the support from my family and colleagues during this writing endeavor. Special gratitude goes to Isabel Thompson, a colleague and my partner, who invited me to be a co-author of this book. Her spirit and dedication is a constant source of support and inspiration. My wish is that all mothers and caregivers will benefit from this book.

About the Authors

Isabel A. Thompson, PhD, is an Associate Professor at Nova Southeastern University, where she has served for over a decade teaching and supervising clinical mental health counseling students. She completed her doctoral degree at the University of Florida and her master's degree at the University of Central Florida. She is a Licensed Mental Health Counselor with five years of clinical experience in school, community, and private practice settings. Her areas of research focus include mindfulness and contemplative approaches, self-care and burnout prevention, maternal mental health, and peripartum depression (PPD). She has previously written and presented on the transition to motherhood, wellness, and counselor self-care. She and her husband Eric Thompson have two children. This is her first book.

Vanessa Beatriz Teixeira, EdD, is an Assistant Professor in the Department of Counseling at Nova Southeastern University. She is a Licensed Mental Health Counselor (LMHC) in the state of Florida, an Approved Clinical Supervisor (ACS) and a Certified Career Counselor (CCC). Dr. Teixeira's professional areas of interest include advocating for maternal mental health, LGBTQ+ and equity issues, counseling children and families with a history of trauma, promoting social justice issues, and building professional counselor development. Dr. Teixeira currently resides in Orlando, Florida with her husband and two young children and is passionate about shedding light on the importance of maternal mental health.

Eric S. Thompson, PhD, is an Associate Professor at Nova Southeastern University in the College of Psychology. He teaches in the School Counseling program and has experience working as a school counselor in middle and high school grade levels. In addition to data-driven approaches to best practices in school counseling, Eric Thompson specializes in contemplative and mindfulness practices and emotion regulation. He has maintained a personal meditation practice for over 20 years and facilitates workshops and webinars on mindfulness emotion regulation. He worked at the Family Data Center at the University of Florida linking maternal data with child outcomes and has interest in the intersection between early life stressors and later life outcomes.

About the Contributors

Katlyn Bagarella is a school psychology doctoral student at Nova Southeastern University. Her passion surrounds suicide prevention and equitable support within the school system. Much of her success is owed to the strong women in her life; the opportunity to contribute to this book is such an honor for her.

Ryanna Bobst graduated with a B.S. in psychology and is currently pursuing her M.S. in clinical mental health counseling at Nova Southeastern University. Ryanna is a proud mother with a clinical interest in helping others navigate pregnancy, motherhood, and the postpartum period.

Samantha Fernandez was born and raised in Miami, Florida. She received a B.A. in psychology from Florida International University and an M.S. in clinical mental health counseling from Nova Southeastern University. Samantha enjoys helping individuals working through trauma, anxiety, and depression through her clinical work.

Tyler Elizabeth Hernandez, PsyD, is a licensed clinical psychologist in private practice who specializes in trauma and dissociative disorders and maternal mental health. Her own transition into motherhood sparked her interest in perinatal mental health research and advocacy.

Dawn Hoffman earned a B.A. in child and family counseling from North Carolina State University and a M.S. in clinical mental health counseling from Nova Southeastern University. Dawn is passionate about mental health and enjoys using her life experience and clinical training to advocate for women.

Jamie Hildebrandt Jerome is a master's student in clinical mental health counseling at Nova Southeastern University. She is passionate about helping other women not suffer in silence and have the support and guidance they need through one of the most challenging times of their lives.

Carly Paro-Tompkins, EdD, is a licensed mental health counselor and an associate professor in the Department of Counseling at Nova Southeastern University and has 15 years of clinical experience. She is thankful and inspired by the women and families who have shared so much through their reunification and adoption experiences.

Alexandra Perez, PsyD, is an assistant professor at Emory University School of Medicine. She is a licensed psychologist who specializes in assessments and therapy for children suspected of in utero exposure to various substances. Her research and clinical interests include the impact of trauma and multicultural factors on treatment interventions and effectiveness.

1

Understanding Peripartum Depression

Isabel A. Thompson

This book is intended to support counselors, psychologists, social workers, marriage and family therapists, and other mental health professionals in their work with women, parents, and families, especially during the peripartum period. Our goal is to provide support for clinicians to bolster maternal mental health for women in the transition to motherhood as well as when families grow with the addition of a new baby, either by birth or adoption (or babies in the case of twins or multiple births). If you are reading this book, it is likely that you have some connection with this topic, whether personally, professionally, or through family or friends. Maybe you have seen someone you love experience peripartum depression and wanted to be able to offer them support or help them find effective treatment. Or perhaps you are a mental health professional working with women and families and are seeking resources to help your clients more effectively—if so, this book will provide you with a wealth of knowledge and resources. If you are a parent who is experiencing peripartum depression (PPD) or other related challenges, you will find a variety of information and resources to understand what you are experiencing, connect with mental health treatment, and access other forms of support. While this book approaches the topic from a professional perspective as a conceptualization and treatment guide for counselors and other mental health professionals, we include personal narratives from women who have experienced PPD or other challenges during pregnancy or after the birth of a child to provide a personal perspective. At times we include personal anecdotes, as all three of the authors of this book and many of the contributing authors are parents with personal experiences relevant to the topic. If you are a graduate student in counseling, psychology, or a related field, and want to work with women during the peripartum period, this book is an excellent resource, providing a broad background on pregnancy, childbirth, maternal mental health, maternal mood disorders, as well as case conceptualization and treatment approaches and information about training resources.

Our intention is to provide you with information, a background in the relevant research, new perspectives, and resources you need to help yourself or someone else navigate the delicate peripartum time with knowledge and support. In addition to information, tips, and resources offered throughout the book, we provide specific in-depth treatment options and resources in Chapter 11, which is dedicated to exploring effective and evidence-based clinical treatment for peripartum depression and other mood disorders. Moreover, Chapter 11 also explores complementary approaches that can be used in conjunction with more traditional forms of treatment.

One of the main underlying themes of this book is that there is hope for mothers experiencing PPD and other mood disorders. Moreover, there is hope for their families and loved ones. Our strengths-based perspective is intended to provide mental health professionals with a perspective that will not only help them to assist women get through PPD, but also help them enhance their resilience and build upon it to face future challenges. Strengths-based approaches are characterized by "intentional focus on the value of strengths that individuals, families, and communities inherently possess, rather than focusing on weaknesses or deficits" (Antonovsky, 1987, as cited in Lougheed, 2019, p. 337). The STRENGTHS case conceptualization model presented in Chapter 2 provides clinicians with an integrative model that includes the risk and protective factors associated with the development of PPD. Moreover, this book employs a feminist multicultural perspective in Chapter 3, which examines the impact of social and cultural factors of maternal wellbeing and mental health. From a feminist viewpoint, maternal mental health and wellbeing cannot be viewed in isolation from the social and cultural factors that impact women, their partners, and their families. Furthermore, traditional gender role expectations gain traction with the arrival of a baby, as research indicates that heterosexual couples who identify as egalitarian revert to more traditional roles after a baby's birth (Katz-Wise et al., 2010). From a multicultural perspective, mental health professional cultural competence is superordinate to their clinical competence; in other words, mental health professionals must be culturally competent to meet their clients' needs and avoid causing harm (Sue et al.,2022). Therefore, we integrate social and cultural considerations throughout the book and explore the impact of social and cultural factors in depth in Chapter 3. Applying a multicultural lens to the issues of maternal mental health, we examine differential experiences that women of color have during pregnancy and birth and health disparities as well as higher rates of infant mortality (Abu-Rish Blakeney et al., 2020; El-Sayed et al., 2015). Moreover, cultural viewpoints about what is normal during birth and pregnancy impact women and their families, and this book will explore cultural norms and expectations, encouraging mental health professionals to help women understand and explore cultural norms around pregnancy and birth (Newman & Newman, 2018).

Another underlying theme of this book is that expectations do not always match reality, especially when it comes to a major life transition such as having a baby. While expecting a baby and giving birth are generally viewed as wonderful aspects of life, pregnancy, childbirth, and caring for an infant can be enormously stressful for mothers, their partners, and their families as they adjust to this major life change (Roberts et al., 2019). Women of all cultural backgrounds experience this adjustment and the accompanying vulnerability of the peripartum period. The peripartum period is broadly defined as encompassing the period of attempting to conceive, pregnancy, birth, and postpartum time frames (Miklowitz et al., 2015). Mothers and families encounter numerous choices and new demands on their time and energy as they navigate the peripartum period, and we want to help counselors be prepared to work effectively with mothers and families, especially those experiencing challenges in the peripartum transition.

The changes associated with pregnancy are profound. This book is also intended to help readers gain greater knowledge and awareness of pregnancy and its incumbent changes. In Chapter 5 we focus on this topic in depth and explore experiences of conception, pregnancy, and birth. Pregnancy, along with creating profound physiological changes for the expectant mother, brings a mixture of emotions for the mother and the father/partner, including joyful emotions as well as challenging emotions like depression and anxious feelings (Newman & Newman, 2018). When a woman has a baby, changes in lifestyle and role are immediate. First-time mothers adjust to motherhood, while mothers who already have a child (or children) adjust to the addition of a baby (or babies) to the family (Newman & Newman, 2018). Fathers and partners adjust to parenthood or an addition to the family and children adjust to their role as a sibling (Newman & Newman, 2018). Especially in the case of first-time birth, grandparents and the entire extended family are adjusting to role shifts as they welcome the new baby into the family (Newman & Newman, 2018). In addition to common stress that accompanies these adjustments, some women may experience anxiety, depression, and other mental health concerns during the peripartum period (Roberts et al., 2019). In the case study below, a mother begins experiencing symptoms during an unexpected pregnancy.

Case Study: Lilly — *written by contributor Ryanna Bobst*

Lilly is a 20-year-old White cisgender woman and is a senior in college. She lives with her mother, stepfather, and younger brother. She is 20 weeks pregnant and reported it was unexpected. Her boyfriend is supportive of raising the child together. She is seeking counseling for the first time because she has been feeling a lot of stress and anxiety for the past two months as she tries to balance work, school, and relationships. She has difficulty sleeping, and eating well-balanced meals, has no desire to meet with friends, and is crying often. She reported worrying about her future, finishing school, childcare, and the health of herself and her baby. She has reoccurring thoughts about death and an intense fear of death.

During her first session she was very disheartened but hopes that counseling can help. During the intake process, Lilly did not disclose any previous mental health concerns or substance use. Lilly did disclose that her father physically, emotionally, and verbally abused her while she was growing up. She is experiencing frequent nightmares of her father and a fear of running into him one day. She also avoids places that she used to visit with her father. Lilly is a full-time college student and works full-time as a substitute teacher at a local middle school. She reported her support system as her mother, brother, and boyfriend.

Lilly completed the following assessments: PTSD Checklist for DSM-5 (PCL-5; Blevins et al., 2015), Patient Health Questionnaire (PHQ-9; Kroenke et al.,

1999), and the Edinburgh Postnatal Depression Scale (EPDS; Cox et al., 1987). Based on her scores on these assessments and the symptoms she was experiencing, her counselor diagnosed Lilly with F43.10 post-traumatic stress disorder (PTSD) with delayed expression, and F32.1 major depressive disorder (MDD), single episode, moderate, with anxious distress, and with peripartum onset (APA, 2022).

Reflection Questions for Clinicians

- What contextual risk and protective factors stand out to you about Lilly's case?
- What treatment approaches would you consider for Lilly, considering both the depression and post-traumatic stress symptoms?
- Are there aspects of Lilly's story that are personally triggering for you? If so, what sort of support (e.g., supervision, consultation, personal counseling for yourself) would you pursue to work effectively with Lilly?

ADVOCATING FOR MATERNAL MENTAL HEALTH NEEDS

In the case study, Lilly's symptoms began during pregnancy, and research suggests that 50 percent of cases of PPD begin during pregnancy (APA, 2022). Mental health professionals are in a unique position to advocate for maternal mental health needs, as we have a specialized training focus on prevention and screening and provide early interventions by assessing, diagnosing, and treating clients in need. Because peripartum depression (PPD) is one of the most common complications related to childbirth (Dekel et al., 2019), mental health professionals should be attuned to the symptoms, risk factors, and protective factors associated with PPD when working with women during the perinatal period. Accurate and timely assessment and diagnosis of PPD help to ensure that mothers, their babies, and families get the care they need and deserve. Effectively treating women experiencing PPD can alleviate suffering mothers, partners, and babies face during this sensitive time. Untreated or undertreated maternal depression can cause lasting detriment to children (Stuart-Parrigon & Stuart, 2014), including problems with infant–mother attachment and child development (Hübner-Liebermann et al., 2012). Further, mental health professionals must be aware of the risks of imminent harm, such as maternal suicide or infanticide (Lindahl et al., 2005). Mental health professionals must be attuned to the risk factors for suicidality among the pregnant woman or new mothers they work with. Potential suicide risk should be assessed when beginning a course of treatment with a new client (Kress & Paylo, 2019), including clients who are pregnant and new mothers. Furthermore, clinicians should be attuned to changes in behavior or mood and reassess for suicidality (Kress & Paylo, 2019). Infanticide is associated most closely with postpartum psychosis. It is crucial for mental health professionals to be trained to accurately assess these risks of harm to self or others and help families obtain the necessary level of care.

A challenge that counselors and mental health professionals face when trying to provide needed treatment for clients with severe symptoms of PPD and/or other mood disorders is that inpatient treatment facilities in the United States are not structured to keep mother and baby together. This puts mothers needing inpatient care in the difficult position of choosing between needed care and staying close to their babies to breastfeed and bond. In severe cases of imminent threat of harm, the mother will need inpatient treatment to meet her mental health needs and/or protect her life in the case of suicidality (or the life of her baby if the mother is experiencing infanticidal ideation, plan, or intent with imminent threat of harm). For mothers in the United States, this means that a new mother needing inpatient treatment is separated from her baby. While mother and baby units with joint admission (so that a baby can stay with the mother) are considered the standard of care when new mothers need psychiatric inpatient treatment in England, they are not available in the United States (Dembosky, 2021). For decades, mental health clinicians in the United States have dealt with challenges and dilemmas to effectively treat mothers' psychiatric concerns at the necessary level of care while sustaining mother–infant bonding due to the lack of such inpatient mother–baby units in the United States (Wisner et al., 1996). Attempts to create joint mother–baby units in the United States have been stymied because of challenges with healthcare structures such as insurance coverage for the baby (Dembosky, 2021). Even facilities that aim to provide mother/baby-friendly inpatient care, such as the Perinatal Psychiatry Inpatient Unit at the University of North Carolina at Chapel Hill, do not allow babies to stay overnight with their mothers (although this unit allows the baby to visit and provides many wrap-around services to enhance mother–infant bonding modeled from European mother–baby psychiatric units) (Dembosky, 2021). During an interview for an article in *Counseling Today*, I (Isabel Thompson) spoke about the need for the mother and baby to be treated as a unit, so that the bonding could proceed without interruption and the mother's mental health needs could also be met (Bray, 2019). There is an ongoing need for advocacy so that maternal mental health needs, for all kinds of treatment and especially for joint admissions for inpatient treatment, can become a reality in the United States.

DIAGNOSIS OF PERIPARTUM DEPRESSION

We would like to discuss the term "peripartum depression." Peripartum depression is a relatively new term; the term postpartum depression has been used historically in both the mental health community and by the general public. Postpartum depression, as described in the fourth edition text revision of the *Diagnostic and Statistical Manual of Mental Disorders* (4th edition, text revision; DSM-4-TR; American Psychological Association [APA], 2000), limited the onset of symptoms to the first four weeks following delivery, thereby excluding cases in which a mother's depressed mood began during pregnancy (APA, 2000). This changed with the publication of the fifth edition of the *Diagnostic and Statistical Manual of Mental Disorders* (DSM-5; APA, 2013) and continues with the fifth edition text revision *Diagnostic and Statistical Manual of Mental Disorders* (DSM-5-TR; APA, 2022), as peripartum depression is defined as onset during pregnancy or in the first four weeks following delivery, as defined in the DSM-5-TR, although it should be noted that technically clinicians would diagnose a woman with major depressive disorder with the specifier "with peripartum onset" (specifics of diagnosis are discussed in Chapter 6). Current diagnostic criteria allow for diagnosis during pregnancy, which is helpful, as 50 percent of peripartum depressive episodes begin during pregnancy (APA, 2022). The term peripartum depression will be used in this book, as it is consistent with the most recent diagnostic specifier, although clients who seek services may be more familiar with the term postpartum depression.

According to the DSM-5 and DSM-5-TR, major depressive disorder '*with peripartum onset*' (what the research literature, e.g., Dekel et al., 2019; Figueiredo et al., 2015, and our book term peripartum depression) consists of a major depressive episode, with the onset of mood symptoms during pregnancy or during the first four weeks following birth (APA, 2013; APA, 2022). The reported prevalence of PPD is approximately 1 in 8 pregnant women and new mothers (Bauman et al., 2020; Tebeka et al., 2016); however, it is likely that these rates represent under-reporting of actual incidences of PPD (O'Hara & McCabe, 2013). Some women experiencing depression in the postpartum period may not meet the DSM-5-TR criteria, if the onset of their symptoms occurs later than four weeks postpartum (Stowe et al., 2005; APA, 2022). Some psychiatric researchers have used the World Health Organization (WHO, 2010 as cited in Dekel et al., 2019) criteria that recognize PPD if a depressive episode occurs within 12 months postpartum.

THE "BABY BLUES" AND OTHER MOOD DISORDERS

Counselors and other mental health professionals should be aware that all mothers go through a pronounced shift once the baby is born; some mothers navigate this shift without experiencing marked mood symptoms, many experience the "baby blues," and some develop peripartum depression and other disorders such as postpartum anxiety, postpartum obsessive-compulsive disorder, and postpartum psychosis. The term "baby blues" refers to mild, short-term depressive symptoms many new mothers experience after giving birth, such as feelings of sadness and anxiety, being overwhelmed, experiencing mood swings, having a loss of appetite, having difficulties sleeping, and episodes of crying. The "baby blues" may last for a few days or persist for up to two weeks after giving birth (U.S. Department of Health and Human Services, 2021). Mental health professionals who are aware of the prevalence of the "baby blues" can help mothers navigate these symptoms and be vigilant for any that persist beyond two weeks or are more severe, such as a parent's thoughts about hurting or killing themselves or their baby or lack of interest in their baby, as these are indicative of peripartum depression (U.S. Department of Health and Human Services,

2021). Clinicians need to address any urgent safety needs to protect parents, babies, and families and know the symptoms of psychosis, which we discuss in Chapter 6.

In addition to PPD and the "baby blues," counselors and other mental health professionals should be aware of the prevalence of what is termed "postpartum anxiety" or "peripartum anxiety." While the specifier *"with peripartum onset"* is not included in the DSM-5-TR (2022) for anxiety disorders, pregnant women and new mothers may present with specific anxiety related to the health of their fetus or baby, the progress of their pregnancy, or the fear of childbirth (Thiel et al., 2020). This book addresses anxiety, as well as other presenting problems of the peripartum period, including maternal stress, difficulties with adjustment, and family/relational challenges during the peripartum period.

THE SCOPE OF THE PROBLEM

PPD and other peripartum mood disorders are common, so counselors must be ready to work with women who experience them. For instance, an estimated 1 in 8 women experience depression during pregnancy and after birth in the United States, indicating a significant need for interventions geared toward reducing depressive symptomology (Bauman et al., 2020). As discussed above, the official prevalence rate is likely an underreporting of actual prevalence, which means that more women are experiencing PPD than are accounted for in official tallies (O'Hara & McCabe, 2013). Because of the prevalence rates of PPD, many babies are exposed to maternal depression and accompanying behaviors that may be detrimental to their attachment and developmental trajectory (Bernard et al., 2018). Effectively addressing and treating PPD helps mothers, their babies, and the entire family. Counselors and other mental health professionals can also advocate for policy changes that would help mothers, partners/fathers, infants, and their families.

In addition to the high rates of women experiencing PPD and other related mental health challenges, effective treatment can be hard to access. For example, mothers who need inpatient treatment face challenges, as there are few inpatient facilities that allow a mother and baby to remain together. If the mother and baby are separated so that the mother can obtain needed psychiatric services in an inpatient facility, this can lead to premature or unwanted cessation of breastfeeding. As breastfeeding has been shown to be a protective factor for women, situations in which a mother is forced to choose between her own mental health and continuing to remain with her infant and breastfeed are not beneficial (Mezzacapa, 2004; Haga et al., 2012). Best practice approaches would allow mothers and infants to remain together as a unit (Dembosky, 2021; Bray, 2019). Maternal mental health inpatient programs, which treat mothers and allow their infants to remain with them, are needed. Attempts in the United States to create such facilities have been hampered by cultural and structural challenges (Dembosky, 2021). Such facilities include appropriate childcare while mothers are in treatment as well as therapeutic support for healthy mother–infant interactions.

Access to treatment is a key social justice, and equity issues are pertinent to maternal mental health. Counselors and other mental health professionals should be concerned about these barriers to treatment and the scarcity of inpatient programs tailored for mothers with PPD and other mood disorders. There are serious potential risks for mothers who do not receive needed treatment and who are dealing with severe depression. Key among these risks is suicide, which is one of the leading causes of maternal death in the perinatal period (Gressier et al., 2017). As counselor educators working to train new generations of counselors, the co-authors were motivated to write this book to raise awareness of this important mental health issue. We want to raise awareness around the significance of this topic and increase access to information and resources for clinicians, women and families, and counseling and psychology graduate students.

Another important aspect of accessing treatment is a mother's fear of revealing symptoms or mental health concerns. Many mothers fear stigma and may avoid revealing their mental health concerns, perhaps worrying that their competency as a mother may be questioned. Many also feel shame that they are not experiencing the maternal "bliss" of caring for their infant that is culturally expected of mothers. As mental health professionals, we can advocate for the needs of new mothers, their partners, and families. We can build a culture of acknowledgment and support to counter the message that problems should be silenced, and that women should project an image of happiness even when they are having symptoms of a maternal mood disorder. Effective treatment to address the sources of the mood disturbance should be promoted to help women truly feel and engage with the joys of interacting with their infant.

COMMON STRESSORS DURING THE PERIPARTUM PERIOD

As described in the case study, women frequently experience a range of stressors during the peripartum period, some related directly to pregnancy. Counselors and other mental health professionals who are aware of the common stressors and mood changes during the peripartum period will be more likely to be attuned to emergent symptoms of a possible mood disorder. Although there has been an increased focus on women's postpartum experiences, peripartum depression is underdiagnosed and undertreated for a variety of reasons, including societal expectation for expectant and new mothers to be happy, the common tendency to focus on the baby's health, the stigma associated with mental illness, as well as social isolation that many new moms experience. Becoming a mother is a profound role and identity shift for women, as well as a profound relational change for couples, families, and the extended family (Thompson, 2019). There is frequently a lack of support for this shift, as families and even medical professionals focus on the baby, not the mother. Focusing on the mother's mental health is necessary, especially for women who may be at risk of developing a peripartum mood disorder because "the perinatal period—broadly defined as the interval in which women are planning pregnancy, pregnant, or postpartum— is a high-risk time for major depressive episodes"

(Miklowitz et al., 2015, p. 590). This definition of the perinatal period includes the period of pregnancy itself as well as the time after the birth of the baby. Mothers experience a major life change and the accompanying adjustments and stress, whether they are first-time mothers or expanding their families. The DSM-5 (2013) diagnostic criteria for major depressive disorder with peripartum onset includes pregnancy itself, a shift from the previous postpartum timeframe. This supports the imperative of screening all pregnant women for depressive symptoms.

New mothers, whether they are first-time mothers or already have a child (or children) are navigating a host of changes, including how and/or whether to breastfeed, dealing with sleep disruptions, and finding ways to care for themselves and their families along with meeting the needs of their newborn(s) (Simkin et al. 2010). Mothers without partners are navigating these changes without the support of a spouse, but may offset this with extended family support (Thompson, 2019). For fathers and partners, the baby's birth is the start of a major adjustment process. For first-time fathers/same-sex partners, this process involves the shift to the role of being a parent, which is a profound life role change (Newman & Newman, 2018). For fathers/same-sex partners who are already parents, adjusting to the birth of another baby (or babies) can bring added pressures, including time, resources, and financial concerns. When a baby arrives, the entire family changes (Newman & Newman, 2018).

We recommend that counselors and other mental health professionals take time to inquire about a woman's experiences of conception, pregnancy, birth, and the immediate postpartum, as these experiences (and her subjective perceptions of them) can impact her emotional wellbeing, mental health, and overall adjustment as a mother. If a woman experiences birth trauma during childbirth, this can increase her risk of developing psychopathology, specifically post-traumatic stress disorder (Ayers, 2017). Conversely, if a woman experiences a birth process in which she feels supported, this may buffer her from stress (Newman & Newman, 2018). One source of birth support that is receiving more research attention is that of trained birth doulas, who provide a continuous presence during the process. They can offer physical support such as massage, emotional support such as listening and reframing, as well as information. They also seek to empower their clients (Steel et al., 2015). Mental health professionals who are aware of the options that women and families can choose from, as well as the stressors they face during the perinatal period, will be more prepared to effectively assess and then aid them in treatment.

Career concerns and family life can be stressors for new mothers after the baby's birth. During pregnancy and after the baby's arrival, families face choices about how to manage work roles and financial concerns. Depending on the family's nation of residence, national policy may be supportive of mothers and their partners during the perinatal period or there may be a dearth of social policies to aid families during this critical time. In the United States there are no national laws in place guaranteeing paid maternity and paternity leave, making it the only industrialized nation that does not offer paid maternity leave, although an estimated 70 percent of women have paid employment (Shepherd-Banigan & Bell, 2014; U.S. Bureau of Labor Statistics [BLS],

2014). The *Family Medical Leave Act of 1993* (FMLA) allows for 12 weeks of leave and guarantees that the position will be protected so that they can return, but many working mothers do not qualify for FMLA (Andres et al., 2016). American mothers have limited options for taking time away from paid employment after giving birth and some have six weeks of maternity leave or none at all (Grice et al., 2011).

Due to the challenges described above, families are often left struggling to determine a course of action for the postpartum period that is both financially viable and consistent with their needs and values. Thus, many mothers return to work before they feel ready, and the transition back can be a time of intense stress. Mothers who return to work in the United States often do so while their infants are very young. Various forms of work–family conflict can develop as a result of this early return to work, as families consider how to have their infants cared for and fed while their mothers are working.

In addition to these adjustments outside the home, life at home is markedly different with a newborn in the house. For first-time parents, the arrival of a newborn can change previously established patterns and routines. It is typically the mother who handles more infant care, regardless of whether or not she is breastfeeding (Katz-Wise et al., 2010). For first-time parents who are members of an opposite-sex couple, the arrival of a baby increases the likelihood of the parents falling into stereotypical gendered roles, even if they had previously endorsed egalitarian values in domestic labor (Katz-Wise et al., 2010). This means that it is frequently a new mother who is handling diaper changes and infant feedings, along with other household responsibilities, which can lead to resentment and relationship dissatisfaction. Counselors and other mental health professionals should keep in mind that couples who have recently had a baby may experience conflict around parenting, chores, and household responsibilities that they did not anticipate.

Counselors and other mental health professionals should also be attuned to the needs of same-sex parents and gender-nonbinary parents. Any expectant mother/parent undergoes psychological changes during pregnancy, but mothers/parents who are in same-sex relationships or are gender nonbinary have specific concerns and stressors, including societal discrimination. Partners undergo psychological adjustment as they integrate this identity into their lives and prepare for parenting. Although childbearing is frequently conceptualized from a cisgender perspective, trans men also become pregnant and bear children (Petit et al., 2017). All relationships undergo changes during pregnancy, as the birthing parent, partner, and family prepare to welcome a new baby, so the needs of the partner must be attended to as well.

Life with a newborn is full of changes, and counselors who express empathy and have awareness about what topics to discuss can enhance their therapeutic rapport with clients who are new parents. Self-care can be especially challenging in the immediate postpartum. Another major adjustment that mothers face is short sleep duration, and sleep disruption and deprivation (Demirci et al., 2012). Most women experience sleep disruption and deprivation at least for the first several months of an infant's life as they attend to their needs. Many women experience sleep deprivation for months and years after giving birth, as some babies have more challenges with sleeping for longer periods. Newborn babies have a different sleeping and eating timetable from that of adults, and typically go through several cycles of sleeping, eating, and wakefulness through a 24-hour day. Researchers have found that breastfeeding is not associated with shorter sleep duration, which is good information for mental health professionals who are working with breastfeeding new mothers (Demirci et al., 2012). There are natural variations between infants regarding sleep duration, and when an infant has a short sleep duration it negatively impacts the mother's sleep and contributes to maternal sleep disruption (Demirci et al., 2012). Sleep deprivation and disruption are associated with daytime sleepiness and other negative consequences (Demirci et al., 2012), as well as mood disturbance and the development of mental health disorders. These sleep disruptions can have a more significant impact on mothers who work, particularly those who work full time despite being tired and overworked at home.

IMPACTS OF PERIPARTUM DEPRESSION

PPD and other maternal mood disorders can have profound impacts on mothers, families, and infants. The risks of untreated or undertreated peripartum depression are significant for the mother, baby, family, and mother's work roles outside the home (Stuart-Parrigon & Stuart, 2014; Gjerdingen et al., 2008). PPD can have negative impacts on a child's development during infancy and beyond (Stuart-Parrigon & Stuart, 2014). Developmental issues among babies and children whose mothers experience PPD can include problems with breastfeeding, insecure-anxious attachment patterns, and social problems that can persist into adolescence (Hübner-Liebermann et al., 2012). Maternal depression can impact parenting quality and the development of attachment relationships (Hayes et al., 2013).

Counselors and other mental health professionals should explore a mother's relationship with her infant and support mothers in bonding with their infants. One key aspect of effective parenting with an infant is sensitivity. Sensitivity in parenting involves "attentiveness to an infant's state, accurate interpretation of the infant's signals, well-timed responses that promote mutually rewards interactions" (Mesman et al., 2012, as cited in Newman & Newman 2018, p. 155). Infants want to connect with their caregivers, but caregivers who are not psychologically or emotionally available may provide inconsistent care. Maternal depression can negatively impact mother–infant interactions in a variety of impactful ways; for instance infants of depressed mothers may avert their gaze from their mothers (Boyd et al., 2006). Maternal depression may also interfere with maternal sensitivity, which has been defined as "the ability to detect and respond appropriately to infants' cues" (Bernard et al., 2018, p. 579). So, mothers experiencing PPD may sometimes miss cues or be unresponsive. Even if they see the cues, depressed mothers may lack the energy or emotional fortitude to appropriately respond. These behaviors can disrupt mother–infant synchrony, lead to problems with infant attachment, and reduce the satisfaction that mothers get from their caregiving relationship.

PPD during pregnancy can also have a negative effect on infant attachment style, if the infant experiences parenting that is less than optimal in the three months after birth.

Hayes et al. (2013, p. 1) point out:

> Results revealed that infants classified as disorganized had mothers with higher levels of depressive symptoms during pregnancy compared to infants classified as organized. Maternal parenting quality moderated this association, as exposure to higher levels of maternal depressive symptoms during pregnancy was only associated with higher rates of infant disorganized attachment when maternal parenting at three months was less optimal.

This suggests that early intervention during pregnancy and immediately after birth to help mothers experiencing depression find relief from their symptoms, and support to enhance their parenting to effectively interact with their infants, can have a positive impact.

While many clinicians receive training and coursework in diagnosis and treatment, few receive specialized training in working with women, their partners, and their families in the peripartum period, let alone in working with women experiencing PPD or related mood disorders. Some graduate programs address women's mental health generally and child psychology or child psychopathology, but few emphasize maternal mental health and specific disorders such as PPD. This lack of specific coursework and training on maternal mental health can result in a gap between the competencies that mental health professionals should have to help women and their families in the perinatal period, especially those women experiencing PPD, and their actual readiness to implement best practices in support of maternal mental health. This book is intended to help bridge that gap, providing extensive information about women's needs during the perinatal period, effective ways to screen mothers at risk of developing mood disorders such as PPD, as well as best practices to meet the specific treatment needs of women experiencing PPD.

AN OVERVIEW OF SCREENING AND PREVENTATIVE APPROACHES

What is the current role of counselors and other mental health professionals in help women with PPD and other maternal mood disorders? And perhaps more importantly, what could it be? The current role of mental health professionals could be expanded to provide more support to women and families in this crucial peripartum period. Many women have more contact with their infants' pediatrician in the first months after birth than with their own healthcare providers but may fear judgment about their parenting efficacy or other negative repercussions if they are open about any symptoms of depression (Heneghan et al., 2004). In the United States, many models of peripartum care include a six-week postpartum visit. While screening during this visit is important, it may be belated to help women already experiencing symptoms who could have benefited from earlier intervention. Further, we recommend that women be screened for depression and other mood disorders during pregnancy. Mental health professionals have the training to effectively screen women, but typically are not partnered with obstetrician/gynecologists (OB/GYNs) or midwives who provide prenatal and peripartum care.

Moreover, mental health professionals providing services to pregnant women to address common stressors and to help prepare for the demands of caring for a newborn would be a wonderful way to integrate mental health professionals earlier in the process. Timely treatment would also prevent symptoms from becoming severe and disrupting family functioning. Providing effective screening to all pregnant women and new mothers would be a very positive step in the direction of reducing new incidences and the severity of PPD.

IMPACT OF THE COVID-19 PANDEMIC

In addition to the changes inherent in pregnancy itself and in welcoming a baby, mothers and families also experience stressors associated with broader changes in society. During the writing of this book, the world faced the COVID-19 pandemic. The pandemic changed society and lifestyles, as people adjusted to social distancing recommendations and/or quarantine requirements. The effects of the pandemic have been extensive in the United States, with the high case load and death rate. The pandemic impacted pregnant women, new mothers, their babies, and their partners and families. Reports indicate that pregnant women and their families, as well as new mothers and parents, have faced extra stress due to the pandemic and its consequences. Pregnancy is "a unique immune condition" (Mor & Cardenas, 2010, p. 426) and, as such, pregnant women were advised to be extra cautious during this pandemic (CDC, 2021). Furthermore, many hospitals changed their protocols, limiting how many people could accompany a birthing mother in labor and delivery. While protocols vary, some hospitals only allowed one person, while others did not allow anyone to accompany the birthing mother. This limited the options for birthing women, who faced unwelcome choices between a spouse or another companion, such as a birth doula or their mother or other trusted companion. While these sorts of restrictions have eased during the writing of this book, the ongoing pandemic has continued to create challenges for pregnant people. For instance, becoming infected with the coronavirus during pregnancy, especially during the third trimester, has been associated with higher rates of preterm birth (Neelam et al., 2022).

In addition to impacting pregnancy and birth experiences, the COVID-19 pandemic changed the experiences of new mothers, leading some to feel more isolated due to concerns about their infants' health and more anxious about protecting their children from viral exposure (Walsh et al., 2022). Furthermore, many women and their immediate families live away from extended family and some have struggled with isolation as new mothers even prior to the pandemic. Women whose jobs provided a main source of socialization may also struggle with the isolation of maternity leave or remote work. These factors were compounded by the pandemic and recommendations during the early months/years of the pandemic to avoid close sustained social contact with people outside one's household. Also, many of the in-person settings where mothers meet and talk about their experiences and receive social and practical support, such as breastfeeding support groups, were not available during the early part of the pandemic. Online forums may serve as an alternative, although lacking in the personal touch of in-person interactions. In contrast, the pandemic-related changes to mental health service delivery may have had some positive aspects for new mothers, as the increase in telehealth services may serve new mothers who may struggle to obtain childcare to be able to attend in-person therapy services. Mental health professionals who want to provide services and outreach to pregnant women and new mothers may want to partner with OB/GYNs and/or midwifes to promote their services and make providers aware of telehealth options for services.

THEORETICAL PERSPECTIVES

This book is framed in a strengths-based perspective to help mental health professionals highlight and leverage mothers', fathers', partners' and families' strengths, even in the face of a daunting diagnosis such as peripartum depression. By examining strengths, we can see our clients in a new way and help them recognize their own resilience and courage as they face the grave challenge of PPD. This book is guided by Bronfenbrenner's Bioecological Systems Theory and informed by feminist and multicultural theories as we address the contextual factors that impact women and the biases they face when they become mothers. Further, in Chapter 3 we examine the health disparities that women of color experience during pregnancy, childbirth, and as mothers, and address the need for counselors and other mental health professionals to demonstrate cultural competence in order to practice ethically and work effectively with diverse mothers and families.

This book is intended to provide support, encouragement, and resources for counselors and other mental health professionals working with mothers, partners/fathers, and families after the birth of a baby (or babies), as well as those experiencing PPD or other mood disturbances. In Chapter 2, we present the STRENGTHS model of case conceptualization and treatment, which we apply to case studies throughout the book. We explore a range of factors that can impact a person's experience of the peripartum period and either enhance or decrease their wellbeing. This book also describes evidence-based treatment approaches and ways to apply a post-traumatic growth perspective to the treatment of PPD, which are consistent with the strengths-based framework of the STRENGTHS model presented in Chapter 2.

CONCLUSION

Becoming a mother in the United States of America has become more dangerous in recent years. The United States has one of the highest rates of preventable maternal mortality as compared with ten other high-income countries (Gunja et al., 2022). Black mothers in the United States are at especially high risk of negative maternal health outcomes, including dying during pregnancy, childbirth, or in the first year after giving birth, as the maternal mortality rates are differentially impacting Black women (Gunja et al., 2022; Hoyert, 2022). There is a need to address systemic factors that increase the risk Black mothers face during pregnancy, childbirth, and postpartum. Mental health professionals can play a powerful role in addressing the urgent need to advocate for mothers'/parents' wellbeing, to fight to reduce maternal mortality and morbidity rates, and to reduce the negative impact of PPD and other mental health disorders on mothers/parents and their families.

REFERENCES

Abu-Rish Blakeney, E., Bekemeier, B., & Zierler, B. K. (2020). Relationships between the great recession and widening maternal and child health disparities: Findings from Washington and Florida. *Race and Social Problems, 12*(2), 87–102. doi:10.1007/s12552-019-09272-1

American Psychiatric Association (APA). (2000). *Diagnostic and statistical manual of mental disorders* (4th ed.; text revision).

American Psychiatric Association (APA). (2013). *Diagnostic and statistical manual of mental disorders* (5th ed.).

American Psychiatric Association (APA). (2022). *Diagnostic and statistical manual of mental disorders* (5th ed.; text revision).

Andres, E., Baird, S., Bingenheimer, J. B., & Markus, A. R. (2016). Maternity leave access and health: A systematic narrative review and conceptual framework development. *Maternal and Child Health Journal, 20*, 1178–1192. doi:10.1007/s10995-015-1905-9

Ayers, S. (2017). Birth trauma and post-traumatic stress disorder: The importance of risk and resilience. *Journal of Reproductive and Infant Psychology, 35*(5), 427–430. doi:10.1080/02646838.2017.1386874

Bauman, B. L., Ko, J. Y., Cox, S., D'Angelo, D. V., Warner, L., Folger, S., Tevendale, H. D., Coy, K. C., Harrison, L., & Barfield, W. D. (2020). Vital signs: Postpartum depressive symptoms and provider discussions about perinatal depression—United States, 2018. MMWR *Morbidity and Mortality Weekly Report, 69*, 575–581. doi:10.15585/mmwr.mm6919a2

Bernard, K., Nissim, G., Vaccaro, S., Harris, J. L., & Lindhiem, O. (2018). Association between maternal depression and maternal sensitivity from birth to 12 months: A meta-analysis. *Attachment & Human Development, 20*(6), 578–599. doi:10.1080/14616734.2018.1430839

Blevins, C. A., Weathers, F. W., Davis, M. T., Witte, T. K., & Domino, J. L. (2015). Posttraumatic Stress Disorder Checklist for DSM-5. doi:10.1037/t51564-000

Boyd, R. C., Zayas, L. H., & McKee, M. D. (2006). Mother–infant interaction, life events and prenatal and postpartum depressive symptoms among urban minority women in primary care. *Maternal and Child Health Journal, 10*(2), 139–148. doi:10.1007/s10995-005-0042-2

Bray, B. (2019, April). Bundle of joy? *Counseling Today, 61*(10), 30–35. https://ct.counseling.org/2019/03/bundle-of-joy/

Center for Disease Control and Prevention. (CDC) (updated 2021, August). Pregnant and recently pregnant people at risk of severe illness from Covid-19. https://www.cdc.gov/coronavirus/2019-ncov/need-extra-precautions/pregnant-people.html

Cox, J. L., Holden, J. M., & Sagovsky, R. (1987). Edinburgh Postnatal Depression Scale. doi:10.1037/t01756-000

Dekel, S., Ein-Dor, T., Ruohomäki, A., Lampi, J., Voutilainen, S., Tuomainen, T.-P., Heinonen, S., Kumpulainen, K., Pekkanen, J., Keski-Nisula, L., Pasanen, M., & Lehto, S. M. (2019). The dynamic course of peripartum depression across pregnancy and childbirth. *Journal of Psychiatric Research, 113*, 72–78. doi:10.1016/j.jpsychires.2019.03.016

Dembosky, A. (2021). A humane approach to caring for new mothers in psychiatric crisis. *Health Affairs, 40*(10), 1528–1533. doi:10.1377/hlthaff.2021.01288

Demirci, J. R., Braxter, B. J., & Chasens, E. R. (2012). Breastfeeding and short sleep duration in mothers and 6–11-month-old infants. *Infant Behavior and Development, 35*(4), 884–886. doi:10.1016/j.infbeh.2012.06.005

El-Sayed, A. M., Finkton, D. W., Paczkowski, M., Keyes, K. M., & Galea, S. (2015). Socioeconomic position, health behaviors, and racial disparities in cause-specific infant mortality in Michigan, USA. *Preventive Medicine, 76*, 8–13. doi:10.1016/j.ypmed.2015.03.021

Family and Medical Leave Act of 1993, 29 U.S.C. §§ 2601–2654 (2006).

Figueiredo, F. P., Parada, A. P., de Araujo, L. F., Silva, W. A., Jr., & Del-Ben, C. (2015). The influence of genetic factors on peripartum depression: A systematic review. *Journal of Affective Disorders, 172*, 265–273. doi:10.1016/j.jad.2014.10.016

Gjerdingen, D., Katon, W., & Rich, D. E. (2008). Stepped care treatment of postpartum depression. *Women's Health Issues, 18*(1), 44–52. doi:10.1016/j.whi.2007.09.001

Gressier, F., Guillard, V., Cazas, O., Falissard, B., Glangeaud-Freudenthal, N. M.-C., & Sutter-Dallay, A.-L. (2017). Risk factors for suicide attempt in pregnancy and the post-partum period in women with serious mental illnesses. *Journal of Psychiatric Research, 84*, 284–291. doi:10.1016/j.jpsychires.2016.10.009

Grice, M. M., McGovern, P. M., Alexander, B. H., Ukestad, L., & Hellerstedt, W. (2011). Balancing work and family after childbirth: A longitudinal analysis. *Women's Health Issues, 21*(1), 19–27. doi:10.1016/j.whi.2010.08.003

Gunja, M. Z., Seervai, S., Zephyrin, L., & Williams II, R. D. (2022, April). Health and health care for women of reproductive age: How the United States compares with other high-income countries. *The Commonwealth Fund Issue Briefs*. https://www.commonwealthfund.org/publications/issue-briefs/2022/apr/health-and-health-care-women-reproductive-age

Haga, S. M., Ulleberg, P., Slinning, K., Kraft, P., Steen, T. B., & Staff, A. (2012). A longitudinal study of postpartum depressive symptoms: Multilevel growth curve analyses of emotion regulation strategies, breastfeeding self-efficacy, and social support. *Archive of Women's Mental Health, 15*, 175–184. doi:10.1007/s00737-012-0274-2

Hayes, L. J., Goodman, S. H., & Carlson, E. (2013). Maternal antenatal depression and infant disorganized attachment at 12 months. *Attachment & Human Development, 15*(2), 133–153. doi:10.1080/14616734.2013.743256

Heneghan, A. M., Mercer, M. B., & DeLeone, N. L. (2004). Will mothers discuss parenting stress and depressive symptoms with their child's pediatrician? *Pediatrics, 113*(3), 460467. doi:10.1542/peds.113.3.460

Hoyert, D. L. (2022). Maternal mortality rates in the United States, 2020. NCHS Health E-Stats. 2022. doi:10.15620/cdc:113967

Hübner-Liebermann, B., Hausner, H., & Wittmann, M. (2012). Recognizing and treating peripartum depression. *Deutsches Ärzteblatt International, 109*(24), 419–424. doi:10.3238/arztebl.2012.0419

Katz-Wise, S. L., Priess, H. A., & Hyde, J. S. (2010). Gender-role attitudes and behavior across the transition to parenthood. *Developmental Psychology, 46*(1), 18–28. doi:10.1037/a0017820

Kress, V. E., & Paylo, M. J. (2019). *Treating those with mental disorders: A comprehensive approach to case conceptualization and treatment* (2nd ed.). Pearson. https://www.amazon.com/Treating-Those-Mental-Disorders-Conceptualization/dp/0134814568

Kroenke, K., Spitzer, R. L., & Williams, J. B. W. (1999). Patient Health Questionnaire-9. doi:10.1037/t06165-000

Lindahl, V., Pearson, J. L., & Colpe, L. (2005). Prevalence of suicidality during pregnancy and the postpartum. *Archives of Women's Mental Health, 8*(2), 77–87. doi:10.1007/s00737-005-0080-1

Lougheed, S. C. (2019). Strengths-based creative mindfulness-based group work with youth aging out of the child welfare system. *Social Work with Groups, 42*(4), 334–346. doi:10.1080/01609513.2019.1571762

Mezzacappa, E. S. (2004). Breastfeeding and maternal stress response and health. *Nutrition Reviews, 62*(7), 261–268. doi:10.1111/j.1753-4887.2004.tb00050.x

Miklowitz, D. J., Semple, R. J., Hauser, M., Elkun, D., Weintraub, M. J., & Dimidjian, S. (2015). Mindfulness-Based Cognitive Therapy for perinatal women with depression or bipolar spectrum disorder. *Cognitive Therapy and Research, 39*, 590–600. doi:10.1007/s10608-015-9681-9

Mor, G., & Cardenas, I. (2010). The immune system in pregnancy: A unique complexity. *American Journal of Reproductive Immunology, 63*, 425–433. https://10.1111/j.1600-0897.2010.00836.x

Neelam, V., Reeves, E. L., Woodworth, K. R., O'Malley Olsen, E., Reynolds, M. R., Rende J., Heather Wingate, H., Manning, S. E., Romitti, P., Ojo, K. D., Silcox, K., Barton, J., Mobley, E., Longcore, N. D., Sokale, A., Lush, M., Delgado-Lopez, C., Diedhiou, A., Mbotha, D., Simon, W., Reynolds, B., Hamdan, T. S., ... Gilboa, S. M. (2022). Pregnancy and infant outcomes by trimester of SARS-CoV-2 infection in pregnancy–SET-NET, 22 jurisdictions, January 25, 2020–December 31, 2020. *Birth Defects Research*, 1–15. doi:10.1002/bdr2.2081

Newman, B. M., & Newman, P. R. (2018). *Development through life: A psychosocial approach*. Cengage Learning.

O'Hara, M. W., & McCabe, J. E. (2013). Postpartum depression: Current status and future directions. *Annual Review of Clinical Psychology, 9*(1), 379–407. doi:10.1146/annurev-clinpsy-050212-185612

Petit, M.-P., Julien, D., & Chamberland, L. (2017). Negotiating parental designations among trans parents' families: An ecological model of parental identity. *Psychology of Sexual Orientation and Gender Diversity, 4*(3), 282–295. doi:10.1037/sgd0000231

Roberts, L., Davis, G. K., & Homer, C. S. (2019). Depression, anxiety, and post-traumatic stress disorder following a hypertensive disorder of pregnancy: A narrative literature review. *Frontiers in Cardiovascular Medicine, 6*. doi:10.3389/fcvm.2019.00147

Simkin, P., Whalley J., Keppler, A., Durham, J., & Bolding, A. (2010). *Pregnancy, childbirth, and the newborn: The complete guide* (4th ed.). Meadowbrook Press.

Shepherd-Banigan, M., & Bell, J. F. (2014). Paid leave benefits among a national sample of working mothers with infants in the United States. *Maternal and Child Health Journal, 18*, 286–295. doi:10.1007/s10995-013-1264-3

Steel, A., Frawley, J., Adams, J., & Diezel, H. (2014). Trained or professional doulas in the support and care of pregnant and birthing women: A critical integrative review. *Health & Social Care in the Community, 23*(3), 225–241. doi:10.1111/hsc.12112

Stowe, Z. N., Hostetter, A. L., & Newport, D. J. (2005). The onset of postpartum depression: Implications for clinical screening in obstetrical and primary care. *American Journal of Obstetrics and Gynecology, 192*(2), 522–526. doi:10.1016/j.ajog.2004.07.054

Stuart-Parrigon, K., & Stuart, S. (2014). Perinatal depression: An update and overview. *Current Psychiatry Reports, 16*(9). doi:10.1007/s11920-014-0468-6

Sue, D. W., Sue, D., Neville, H. A., & Smith, L. (2022). *Counseling the culturally diverse: Theory and practice* (9th ed.). John Wiley & Sons.

Tebeka, S., Le Strat, Y., & Dubertret, C. (2016). Developmental trajectories of pregnant and postpartum depression in an epidemiologic survey. *Journal of Affective Disorders, 203*, 62–68. doi:10.1016/j.jad.2016.05.058

Thiel, F., Iffland, L., Drozd, F., Haga, S. M., Martini, J., Weidner, K., Eberhard-Gran, M., & Garthus-Niegel, S. (2020). Specific relations of dimensional anxiety and manifest anxiety disorders during pregnancy with difficult early infant temperament: A longitudinal cohort study. *Archives of Women's Mental* Health, *23*, 535–546. doi:10.1007/s00737-019-01015-w

Thompson, I. A. (2019). Pregnancy and delivery. In J. Ponzetti (Ed.), *Macmillan encyclopedia of families, marriages, and intimate relationships, volume 2* (pp. 689–691). Macmillan.

U.S. Bureau of Labor Statistics (BLS). (n.d.). *2014 home*. U.S. Bureau of Labor Statistics. https://www.bls.gov/opub/mlr/2014/home.htm

U. S. Department of Health and Human Services (2021). Office on Women's Health - Depression during and after pregnancy. https://www.womenshealth.gov/a-z-topics/depression-during-and-after-pregnancy

Walsh, T. B., Reynders, R., & Davis, R. N. (2022). New parent support needs and experiences with pediatric care during the COVID-19 pandemic. *Maternal and Child Health Journal*, *26*, 2060–2069. doi:10.1007/s10995-022-03496-1

Wisner, K. L., Jennings, K. D., & Conley B. (1996). Clinical dilemmas due to the lack of inpatient mother-baby units. *International Journal of Psychiatry in Medicine*, *26*(4), 479–493. doi:10.2190/NFJK-A4V7-CXUU-AM89

2

A Strengths-Based Approach to Case Conceptualization

Vanessa Beatriz Teixeira

This chapter describes a strengths-based approach to treating mothers with peripartum depression (PPD) and other varying mental health symptoms during the peripartum period, such as mania and postpartum anxiety, which will also be highlighted throughout the book. The authors of this book have approached the treatment of PPD considering the role of mothers, their relationship to their infants, and other important contextual factors.

Clinical case conceptualization is an important part of treatment for clients presenting with any DSM-5-TR diagnosis (Kress & Paylo, 2019). This comprehensive process is a way for clinicians to better understand the nature of presenting symptoms from a biopsychosocial perspective (Sperry & Sperry, 2020). This understanding helps clinicians formulate individualized and appropriate treatment goals based on individual needs as seen from a systemic and cultural perspective. A case conceptualization for PPD should include a comprehensive assessment of individual, family, societal, and cultural factors, including specific strengths and resources related to each factor.

Accordingly, a comprehensive strengths-based approach that addresses multiple aspects of a woman's identity has been developed. This book introduces the STRENGTHS model of case conceptualization for helping women and families struggling during the peripartum period (Figure 2.1). Our hope is that counselors can use this case conceptualization and treatment model to feel more confident, knowledgeable, and skilled in the unique treatment of PPD.

SIGNIFICANT INDIVIDUAL, INFANT, FAMILY, SOCIETAL, AND CULTURAL FACTORS

The STRENGTHS approach acknowledges that mothers, along with their families, are directly impacted by their environment. This concept is derived from the Ecological Systems Theory (Bronfenbrenner, 1979), which posits that social environments influence our development. This significant model theorizes that human beings are shaped by various systems. The first part of the STRENGTHS model begins with the mother's microsystem and extends to her macrosystem. It

Figure 2.1
STRENGTHS Model

S	•Significant Individual, Infant, Family, Societal, and Cultural Factors
T	•Treatment Barriers
R	•Risk Factors
E	•Enlisting Support from Family, the Community, and Medical Professionals
N	•Noticeable Symptoms, Severity, & DSM-5-TR Diagnosis OR Needs Identified by Family & Treatment Team
G	•Goals Identified by Family
T	•Treatment Recommendations
H	•Helpful, Protective, and Resilience Factors
S	•Self-Care & Wellness

is important to understand that as an individual person, the mother will have a connection and relationship with all parts of her ecological system, which can be important factors in treating PPD. The microsystem encompasses the mother as an individual with her own strengths, limitations, values, wants, and needs. Factors related to the mother's unique individual circumstances should be considered first. Some examples of significant individual factors can include the mother's pregnancy and postpartum experience, her beliefs about herself as a person and her role as a mother, and her physical and emotional health during and after pregnancy. Subsequently, infant factors can be complex in that, during pregnancy, the baby is physically part of the mother, slowly developing as a fetus and growing to a baby. Important factors related to the baby inside the womb can include the baby's health and growth, movement and response to outside stimuli, and other factors that can impact the mother, such as the pregnancy causing nausea and other physical or emotional ailments. After birth, the mother and newborn detach physically, but have almost non-stop interactions through feeding, changing, and other infant needs. Significant infant factors after birth can include the baby's temperament, physical health, potential physical trauma experienced during labor and delivery, latching challenges, developmental milestones, and sleep patterns.

The mother's microsystem is also impacted by her immediate home environment to include other children, her spouse/significant other, or close family members residing in the home. Immediate family members should be considered in the treatment of PPD, as family interactions and support, or lack thereof, can have a significant impact on both mother and baby (Sampson et al., 2014). Factors related to other children in the home can include a disruption of sibling birth order, a child with special needs, opposing schedules of older children, or behavioral issues/concerns. If the mother is in a romantic relationship, factors associated with the significant other can include lack of paternity leave, difficulty adjusting to the parenting role, relationship problems, partner's mental health issues, or parenting disagreements. Other family members residing in the home such as a mother-in-law can also add a different dynamic to the role of being a new parent. Significant factors related to other family members in the home can include communication difficulties or opposing views on parenting issues such as whether, or how, to breastfeed, co-sleep, or take care of a sick baby. Cultural norms and generational gaps can also impact the parenting role, especially when close family members confront a different style of parenting. Expanding outside of the home environment and immediate family unit, the mother may have numerous interactions with neighbors, co-workers, friends, distant relatives, pediatricians, children's schoolteachers, family doctors, or pastors. Her relationships and connections, or lack thereof, outside of the home environment can have a major impact in the treatment of PPD.

On a more global level, the mother's macrosystem will consist of societal and cultural factors that are oftentimes outside of the individual's control. For example, a health insurance plan that has a high deductible may impact financial planning related to having a new baby, labor and delivery costs, and all the extra spending that comes with a newborn. If the mother has no insurance at all, she may not be able to afford an efficient breast pump or a consultation appointment with a lactation consultant, which could potentially hinder her breastfeeding knowledge, confidence, and ability. Cultural or societal norms may also significantly impact goals and decisions related to breastfeeding or formula feeding. For example, there is a substantial disparity in breastfeeding for Black and White mothers, with White mothers breastfeeding their children at much higher rates than Black mothers (Anstey et al., 2017). Other societal factors can include the mother's community, and the availability of support and resources such as access to high-quality daycare, public transportation, high-income jobs, paid maternity leave, and safe schools and neighborhoods. Similarly, cultural factors are also important to consider, as culture can play an important role throughout the pregnancy and postpartum experience. A mother's culture can determine if she has a hospital or home birth, her beliefs and decision about birth control or abortion, whether she chooses to breastfeed or formula feed, and the decisions of her church or her family about mental health treatment. Counselors can seek to understand and explore the mother's culture and be sensitive to the multidimensional values and beliefs held by the family unit.

In the treatment of PPD, counselors should pay special attention to the various complex individual, infant, family, societal, and cultural factors that are present during the peripartum period. These factors are not isolated and are almost always connected, interrelated, and transactional. Effective treatment of PPD involves a holistic perspective of the mother's inner and outer world, and how each factor can positively or negatively impact her perinatal experience.

Treatment Barriers

Research indicates that nearly 50 percent of women do not seek professional help for symptoms of depression (Nadeem et al., 2009). Nadeem et al. (2009) identified various barriers that women face with accessing treatment, from a woman denying that she has a problem, to being afraid of the stigma that comes with seeking counseling or other forms of professional help. In order for counselors to provide successful treatment for the concerning symptoms of PPD, the first step is that mothers and their families recognize a need for treatment and commit to the counseling process. This section highlights some significant barriers to the treatment of PPD from both individual and societal levels.

When looking back at the mother's microsystem, numerous individual challenges can be identified in seeking treatment for PPD, including limited time for self-care, lack of knowledge and understanding of depressive symptoms, fear of feeling stigmatized for having a mental illness, and perceived racism from professionals (Freed et al., 2012). A mother's deep cultural beliefs may also serve as a treatment barrier for seeking professional help. One study found that African American mothers often feel strong pressure to hide symptoms of PPD due to the belief that new mothers should be strong and independent, and endure the challenges of motherhood without showing weakness. When these mothers did divulge their mental health symptoms to close family members and friends, their depressive symptoms were dismissed or denied. Mothers reported not seeking treatment for the fear of being labeled as "crazy" or having their children taken away (Sampson et al., 2014). Similar results were found with Latina mothers, who reported the need to hide their emotions for the fear of being judged by family members for having PPD (Sampson et al., 2021). Being aware of individual barriers for seeking treatment, especially among women from underrepresented or marginalized backgrounds, is an important consideration for counselors.

Barriers to seeking treatment can also be present among close family members such as a romantic partner, the mother's parents or in-laws, or other close relatives who may help or hinder the mother's openness to treatment. Mothers often report a lack of support from their partner or other close family members, especially when they are experiencing emotional challenges. This lack of support can present itself in many ways, such as not showing the mother appreciation, poor communication skills, not helping with housework or the baby, not being aware of what depressive symptoms look like, not taking the mother's symptoms seriously, or not taking the mother to doctor's appointments (Alfayumi-Zeadna et al., 2019). Recognizing that lack of support from family members presents as a major barrier to seeking professional help for mental health symptoms, counselors can ensure that treatment for PPD actively involves the family unit.

Outside of the mother's microsystem, societal barriers for seeking treatment can be even more challenging, as they are mostly outside of the individual's or family's control. Examples of societal barriers can include lack of healthcare or availability of transportation to see a doctor, having to wait weeks or months to schedule a doctor or psychiatrist appointment, healthcare professionals' lack of understanding and screening for PPD, low socioeconomic status or financial strain to pay for therapy or other treatments, society's negative stigma of PPD, and lack of childcare when the mother can attend doctor's appointments (Alfayumi-Zeadna et al., 2019). For instance, a mother with multiple children residing in a low-income neighborhood might have difficulty attending a doctor's appointment if she does not have childcare or transportation. Her priority might be taking care of her children and ensuring their needs are met before her own. If she does not have health insurance, she might face an additional barrier in seeking treatment or finding a doctor who can help her. If she has limited education, she might not recognize the signs of PPD or believe there is anything wrong with how she is feeling, possibly attributing symptoms of depression to being a tired mother. Counselors should be aware of the many barriers women face when seeking treatment for PPD and help eliminate significant barriers so mothers can get the professional help they need.

With all the individual, family, and systemic barriers many women face during the peripartum period, it is no wonder nearly half of women don't seek treatment when they experience symptoms of PPD. Working with the community and healthcare providers to reduce and remove these barriers would greatly benefit women and their families during the vulnerable time of pregnancy and after birth. Furthermore, counselors must pay special attention to cultural barriers and ensure they are culturally competent when working with diverse women, children, and families during the peripartum period.

RISK FACTORS

Qualitative and quantitative research related to risk factors associated with PPD has been conducted for over 30 years and appears to have been relatively constant during the past three decades (Beck, 2001; Garcia et al., 2021; Hain et al., 2016; O'Hara & Swain, 1996; Robertson et al., 2004). It is vital for counselors to be aware of significant PPD risk factors for the purpose of helping and educating women and their families on what may increase the risk of developing symptoms of PPD and other peripartum mood disorders during the peripartum period.

A strongly correlated risk factor for developing PPD is a history of mental health symptoms, especially depression prior to the woman's pregnancy. For women with a personal or family history of bipolar disorder, the risk for developing a postpartum episode with psychotic features increases. Also, experiencing depression and anxiety during pregnancy, as well as experiencing the "baby blues" shortly after birth, greatly increases a woman's chance of developing PPD (APA, 2013). Counselors can work collaboratively with women who have a history of mental health issues if they are currently pregnant or planning to become pregnant in the future. Being proactive by discussing symptoms of PPD and developing a plan for early treatment options can help women take charge of their mental health and better prepare and cope with a potential PPD diagnosis.

Another strong risk factor for developing PPD is a wide variety of maternal life stressors during the peripartum period (Julian et al., 2021). It should be noted that life stressors can be related or unrelated to motherhood and are connected to other strongly correlated PPD risk factors, such as marital problems, limited social support, obstetric complications, and infant temperament. While these risk factors are generally separated in research literature, we have linked them in this section to generalize maternal life stressors. These life stressors can be acute and temporary or chronic and persistent, depending on the mother's life circumstances. Examples of short-term maternal life stressors can include childcare stress, challenging infant temperament, pregnancy and childbirth complications, and difficulties with breastfeeding. Long-term life stressors can include persistent financial issues or lower socioeconomic status, prolonged marital conflict, and a continual lack of social support. Understanding that certain factors can increase a mother's chances for developing PPD is an important part of treatment. Counselors can help clients recognize, reduce, and even eliminate certain life stressors that are strongly correlated to developing PPD (Figure 2.2). More detailed information on risk factors related to PPD can be found in Chapter 4.

Figure 2.2
Risk Factors for PPD

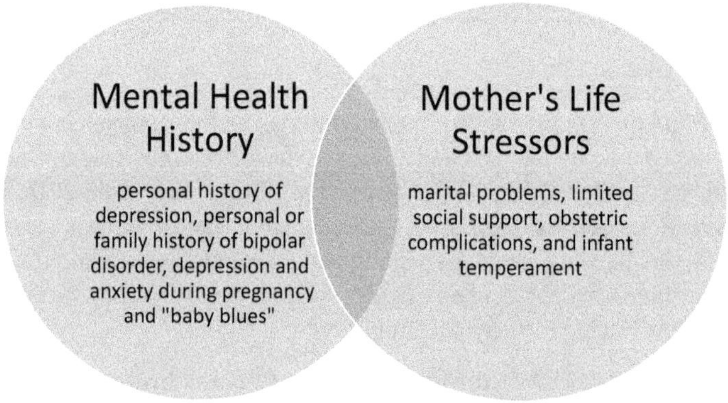

Mental Health History
personal history of depression, personal or family history of bipolar disorder, depression and anxiety during pregnancy and "baby blues"

Mother's Life Stressors
marital problems, limited social support, obstetric complications, and infant temperament

ENLISTING SUPPORT FROM FAMILY, THE COMMUNITY, AND MEDICAL PROFESSIONALS

It is widely recognized that lack of social support is a longstanding risk factor for developing PPD, as well as a treatment barrier for seeking treatment for PPD symptoms. Hence, enlisting social support from the mother's family members, her community, and medical professionals is essential to effective treatment. Since some women may feel hesitant about reaching out to their support network for help, counselors can educate women on the importance of enlisting social support and encourage mothers to identify and successfully communicate their needs during the perinatal period.

Support from family members is key to maternal wellbeing and is broadly known as a protective factor for PPD. Mothers continue to report fewer depressive or anxiety symptoms when they feel more supported at home during the peripartum period (Arnold & Kalibatseva, 2021). Specifically, emotional support from a romantic partner has proved to be vital during pregnancy and after birth, reducing the risk of PPD (Kızılırmak et al., 2020). Support can look different depending on the mother's needs and wishes. It may be helpful for counselors and women to identify what kind of support a mother would like from different family members. From her partner, she might need emotional intimacy such as a soothing massage, or she may need physical support such as help with household chores. From other family members, she may need more practical help with childcare or transportation to doctor's appointments. Since family support is essential for mothers during the peripartum period, counselors should encourage mothers to regularly communicate their specific needs to family members.

Counselors can be open to working with family members to educate them on the importance of social support as a buffer against developing PPD and other maternal mood disorders. Additionally, family members can be useful in assisting mothers with enlisting outside social supports from the community and medical professionals. Community supports can vary widely depending on the mother's pregnancy or postpartum needs. In the past decade, mothers have started seeking community support via online and social media groups. Recent research indicates that mothers find solace, connection, and support through social media platforms. These platforms allow mothers to access helpful information day or night, and even increases their confidence in parenting decisions (Bridges, 2016). Community supports for peripartum women can also be found locally through non-profit organizations, hospitals, birth centers, and community centers. Counselors can work with families to find community supports that are most beneficial for them, whether it's a virtual support group for new mothers that meets weekly on Zoom, a social media platform with discussion posts for parents of twins, or a monthly in-person meet-up at a local library for adoptive mothers. Counselors can work collaboratively with the mother and family to find the right type of support the mother needs. The more community resources counselors are aware of, the more social supports they can recommend to new parents.

While family and community support can be substantially beneficial for mothers, support from medical professionals is often valuable and necessary. New mothers often have access to pediatricians, gynecologists, and/or midwives during the peripartum period. Asking questions and communicating concerns with healthcare professionals can be a helpful way for mothers to feel more confident during pregnancy and postpartum. For example, mothers who are experiencing excessive worry, pain, or bleeding during pregnancy can contact their doctor, talk to a nurse, or schedule a check-up to ease their worries. For mothers who are having difficulties with breastfeeding, a lactation consultant can be particularly helpful with latching concerns, diagnosing tongue or lip ties, and providing tips for successful breastfeeding. Mothers who are concerned about their child not meeting developmental milestones can contact their pediatrician to discuss their concerns and possible specialist referrals. Counselors can encourage mothers to develop a positive, trusting relationship with medical professionals so they can successfully communicate their needs throughout the postpartum period. If the mother provides consent, counselors can look for opportunities to work alongside healthcare professionals to collaborate on the mother's treatment and family goals. Diverse ways to advocate for mothers' needs by collaborating with other healthcare providers in their treatment will be discussed throughout this book.

NOTICEABLE SYMPTOMS, SEVERITY, AND DSM-5-TR DIAGNOSIS OR NEEDS IDENTIFIED BY FAMILY AND TREATMENT TEAM

As mental health counselors, we recognize that while mothers may experience varied symptoms of anxiety, depression, or other mental health issues during the peripartum period, it does not mean they will meet DSM-5-TR criteria and be formally diagnosed with PPD. Hence, this section is divided into two parts; the first part will highlight DSM-5-TR diagnoses with evident symptoms of PPD, while the second part will emphasize specific needs identified by the family and treatment team, regardless of a formal diagnosis.

When reading through the DSM-5-TR, counselors will notice that PPD is not a stand-alone diagnosis. Rather, it is a specifier for major depressive disorder, bipolar I disorder, bipolar II disorder, and brief psychotic disorder (APA, 2022). This specifier, *'with peripartum onset,'* can be utilized with the most recent mood episode during pregnancy and up to four weeks postpartum. The DSM-5-TR refers to peripartum-onset mood episodes as either major depressive or manic episodes that can occur with or without psychotic features. Clearly, these severe DSM-5-TR disorders and accompanying symptoms can be debilitating for a pregnant or postpartum mother. Symptoms of peripartum onset mood episodes can vary widely, both in their presentation and severity. A major depressive episode during pregnancy can look like a mother who is lethargic, apathetic, crying daily, unable to care for her hygiene, and having thoughts of suicide. In contrast, a manic episode can look like a mother with abnormally elevated mood and rapid speech, engaging in risky or dangerous behaviors, staying up all night without feeling tired, and experiencing major distractibility. Both mood episodes can present with psychotic features such as delusions, hallucinations, disorganized speech, and/or disorganized or catatonic behaviors. When experiencing a psychotic episode, mothers can lose touch with reality and potentially become a danger to themselves or others. Thus, counselors should be mindful of suicidal or homicidal thoughts or behaviors when treating

PPD or other peripartum-onset disorders and screen for suicidality and other safety issues. More detailed information about screening, diagnosis, and assessment of PPD can be found in Chapter 6.

For women who may not meet the full criteria for one of the DSM-5-TR diagnoses described above with peripartum onset, counselors can shift the focus to specific needs identified by the family and/or treatment team. Generally, women have identified four main categories of needs during the perinatal period (Slomian et al., 2021). First and foremost, mothers report *needing information*. Pregnant and postpartum women often seek information related to various perinatal issues such as questions about their pregnancy, medical issues, breastfeeding, sleeping patterns, and newborn concerns. Regarding the need for information, counselors can provide pregnant and postpartum mothers with helpful community resources as well as accurate and current psychoeducation about pregnancy and newborn issues. In order to provide such accurate information, mental health professionals working with new mothers must educate themselves and seek training, supervision, or consultation in this area. Endorsing recommendations from the American Pediatric Association can be a helpful resource for counselors.

Moreover, women report a need for *psychological support* (Slomian et al., 2021). Many women feel socially isolated, especially after giving birth. Some mothers report a strong desire for encouragement and reassurance that they are doing a good job in their role as a mother. This social and psychological support is especially important when it comes from their partners (Slomian et al., 2017). Regarding the need for psychological support, counselors can encourage mothers to actively seek social support and communicate their need for encouragement and reassurance. Counselors can also work with the mother's family to provide psychoeducation about the importance of giving this type of social support to new mothers.

Another common need mothers report during the perinatal period is the *sharing of experiences* (Slomian et al., 2017). Many mothers express a desire to communicate with other women about motherhood, with the hopes of gaining insight into their own experience as a mother and to also compare if what they are experiencing is normal or abnormal. These conversations help mothers feel more supported and understood, while feeling less lonely and isolated. Counselors can assist women in finding a healthy support network of mothers with whom they can share their experiences. The final common need mothers have identified is the need for *practical and material support*. Practical needs include managing the household with typical chores such as shopping, cleaning the house, and cooking. New mothers report seeking this type of help so they can spend more time with their newborn and less time doing housework (Slomian et al., 2017). Counselors can help women brainstorm and explore different ways they can ask for and receive support for their practical needs. Once again, involving the mother's close and extended support network appears to be essential to successfully meeting diverse motherhood needs (see Figure 2.3).

Figure 2.3
Four Main Needs Identified by Mothers

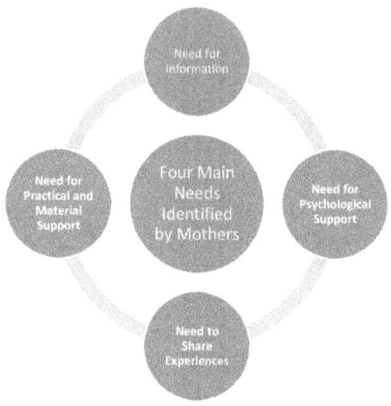

While considering specific needs identified by the mother is important, counselors should also consider needs identified by the family and treatment team. Family members may be useful in identifying concerns the mother may not be able to recognize, such as psychosis. Involving close family members can generate a more comprehensive perspective of the mother's needs. If the mother has a treatment team, such as a psychiatrist, communicating with healthcare professionals can be useful. The treatment team could be used to identify mental health patterns or needs, such as the need for medication for more severe mental health symptoms. Including the family and treatment team throughout the treatment process can be both holistic and advantageous to treating PPD.

GOALS IDENTIFIED BY FAMILY

Working collaboratively to explore *specific, measurable, attainable, relevant, and timely* (SMART; Doran, 1981) treatment goals is an important part of treatment for PPD. When working with mothers, promoting positive perinatal mental health is essential in treatment and goal planning. Since mother and baby often influence each other's physical and emotional health, goals should not only include the mother's, but the infant's needs as well. When thinking about developing treatment goals, counselors should consider the STRENGTHS model and some of the previously discussed sections that may impact goal setting. Counselors are encouraged to reflect on significant individual, infant, family, societal, and cultural factors, as well as treatment barriers, risk factors, availability of support from the family, community, and medical professionals, the mother's DSM-5-TR diagnosis, or specific needs that have been identified by the client, family, and/or treatment team.

Developing SMART goals can be challenging, especially considering the many diverse and complex issues related to the peripartum period. Using a structured and systematic way of creating treatment goals can be helpful. To begin, SMART goals must be *specific*. This means the goal clearly and simply details exactly what is expected of the client during treatment. A specific goal is easily understood by the clinician, client, family, and other treatment team members. Next, goals should be *measurable*. This means the goal can be quantified in some way to assess change and evaluate the client's treatment progress. In addition, goals should be *attainable*. Clients should be able to realistically achieve treatment goals by using their skillsets and having access to available resources. SMART goals should also be *relevant*. Clients should feel that treatment goals are important to them and in alignment with their values and long-term objectives. Lastly, goals must be *timely*. Clients should know there is a certain timeline and deadline for achieving goals during treatment. Counselors can educate clients and their families about SMART goals when creating a plan for treatment.

Knowing that mothers greatly benefit from receiving social support during the peripartum period, counselors should include the mother, infant, supportive family members, and the mother's treatment team when identifying and developing goals for PPD treatment. Creating treatment goals should be a collaborative, creative, and ongoing process. Counselors are encouraged to think outside the box, while emphasizing that both the mother's and infant's needs are central to goal development. Table 2.1 shows some helpful examples of SMART goals for women experiencing different mental health symptoms during the peripartum period.

Table 2.1
SMART Goals

	Larissa is experiencing depression and anxiety during the second trimester	Sasha recently gave birth and is struggling with breastfeeding and feelings of failure	Arleen gave birth two months ago was recently hospitalized for suicidal thoughts
Goal #1	Larissa will practice one mindfulness activity (i.e., deep breathing, yoga, grounding) every night for 30 minutes before going to bed for the next three months.	Sasha will meet with a lactation consultant 3× per week for the next two weeks to assist with breastfeeding challenges.	Arleen will attend psychoeducational groups 4× per week at a partial hospitalization program, as recommended by her treatment team for the next two months.
Goal #2	Larissa will join an online or local support group for pregnant mothers and reach out to this support group at least 2× per week for the next three months to gain support and help reduce feelings of depression and anxiety.	Sasha will join a support group for breastfeeding mothers and reach out to that support group 2× per week for one month.	Arleen will take medications as prescribed by her psychiatrist for the next six months.

(Continued)

Table 2.1 **(Continued)**
SMART Goals

	Larissa is experiencing depression and anxiety during the second trimester	Sasha recently gave birth and is struggling with breastfeeding and feelings of failure	Arleen gave birth two months ago was recently hospitalized for suicidal thoughts
Goal #3	Larissa will meet with a counselor 1× per week for three months to discuss treatment progress and different ways to reduce symptoms of anxiety and depression.	Sasha will practice saying positive affirmations about her role as a mother at least 1× per day for the next two months.	Arleen will attend therapy with her partner 1× per week to discuss safety planning and ways her family can support her treatment goals.

TREATMENT RECOMMENDATIONS

Treatment for depression can be separated into two categories: pharmacological and non-pharmacological treatments. While mothers tend to prefer non-pharmacological treatment interventions during the peripartum period, medications may be necessary for some women who experience more severe symptoms related to PPD (Battle et al., 2013; Guille et al., 2013). This section will briefly outline both categories of treatments. More detailed information on PPD treatment recommendations can be found in Chapter 11.

The first approach to treating PPD should be through non-pharmacological treatment interventions (Dominiak et al., 2021). It is widely recognized that both cognitive behavioral therapy (CBT) and interpersonal psychotherapy (IPT) are evidence-based practices for the treatment of depression in pregnant and postpartum women (Dominiak et al., 2021; Nillni, 2018). CBT interventions for this population vary widely and can include psychoeducation about pregnancy, birth, and newborn care, assertiveness skills to learn how to communicate more effectively, cognitive restructuring to challenge negative thoughts and formulate more positive ones, self-esteem training to boost the mother's self-confidence, and "baby and me" sessions to help mothers form healthier interactions with their baby. In contrast, IPT focuses more on interpersonal issues and clients become more aware of how their thoughts and feelings impact their interactions with others. There is an emphasis on improving interpersonal relationship functioning and increasing social support (Nillni, 2018). Alternative and complementary non-pharmacological treatment interventions have also been recommended for PPD, including exercise, yoga, prenatal massage, acupuncture, mindfulness, and music (Nillni, 2018; Khowaja & Rind, 2021).

Pharmacological treatments for PPD should be used as a second-line treatment for clients who either have not benefited from psychological treatment approaches or present with more severe, and potentially dangerous, mental health symptoms (Dominiak et al., 2021). It should be noted that despite their increased use, there exists limited evidence-based research in the effectiveness of psychopharmacological interventions for PPD (Nillni, 2018). Nevertheless, some mothers may require medication for management of depressive or psychiatric symptoms to maintain positive mental health and the safety of mother and baby. A combination of anti-depressant medications with evidence-based psychotherapy provides the most ideal outcome when treating PPD as compared with medication alone (Hantsoo et al., 2014). Counselors should encourage mothers to continue therapy sessions while also speaking with their psychiatrist or primary-care doctor about different pharmacological treatment options for PPD. Overall, adherence and compliance with medication management can be greatly beneficial for both mother and baby in the perinatal period.

Helpful, Protective, and Resilience Factors

Working with mothers through a strengths-based perspective can be both helpful and refreshing to the therapeutic process. Exploring and identifying helpful, protective, and resilience factors related to the mother's inner and outer world is an important part of effectively preventing and treating PPD. In therapy sessions, counselors can collaborate with women during the perinatal period, or even prior to conception, to discover a variety of factors that can positively contribute to perinatal mental health.

Research indicates numerous helpful, protective, and resilience factors that act as a buffer to PPD. The most widely recognized and evidence-based factor is social support during the perinatal period. While social support has many components, women report that the most meaningful relationships are ones in which they can consistently count on the other person for assistance as well as relationships in which their worth is reassured by the acknowledgment of their skills and abilities. Mothers commonly report that social support not only significantly reduces their parenting stress, but also increases their quality of life (Milgrom et al., 2019). Knowing that lack of social support is a risk factor for PPD, counselors can encourage women to develop, nurture, and rely on their support network during pregnancy and postpartum.

Another protective factor for developing PPD relates to the mother's inner strengths and positive coping skills (Julian et al., 2021). Specifically, mothers who believe they can solve their own problems and have control over what happens in their lives are less likely to struggle with PPD. Similarly, a mother's high level of resilience, or ability to modulate and control her emotions and adjust to life's stressors, appears to act as a buffer to PPD (Hain et al., 2016). Possessing positive affect, such as being friendly, cheerful, trusting, and good-natured has also been found to be a protective factor (Bos et al., 2013). Understanding the importance of cultivating a woman's inner strengths and positive coping skills is essential to preventing PPD. Counselors can help mothers develop resilience, positive affect, self-esteem, and self-confidence in therapy sessions. Lastly, breastfeeding, and close touch immediately after giving birth have been found to reduce PPD symptoms in mothers (Bayri Bingol & Demirigoz Bal, 2020). Hence, counselors can encourage mothers, family members, and health professionals to facilitate breastfeeding or other bonding activities immediately after birth.

SELF-CARE & WELLNESS

A broadly accepted definition of self-care includes "routine positive practices and mindful attention to one's physical, emotional, relational, and spiritual selves in the context of one's personal and professional lives" (Wise & Barnett, 2016, p. 210). Similarly, the term wellness refers to the "process and state of a quest for maximum human functioning that involves the body, mind, and spirit" (Archer et al., 1987, p. 311). Self-care and wellness among mothers is a fundamental necessity to foster and promote positive perinatal mental health (Kim & Dee, 2017). In the early postpartum period, however, a mother's main priority is to care for the needs of her newborn baby. As a result, mothers often ignore important self-care needs like hygiene, sleeping, eating, and healing from childbirth (Lambermon et al., 2020). Counselors can promote positive perinatal mental health by advocating for mothers to establish and maintain a self-care and wellness routine during the peripartum period.

The Self-Care Wheel promotes life balance and wellness in six essential life areas: *physical, psychological, emotional, spiritual, personal,* and *professional* (Phoenix, 2013). These six categories of self-care are pertinent for establishing and maintaining positive perinatal mental health. *Physical* self-care includes basic human needs such as safe housing, medical care, healthy eating and exercise, quality "me" time, hygiene, sexuality, and getting enough sleep. Since newborns create their own schedule for eating and sleeping, it is important for mothers to find time in between their baby's schedule to take care of their own basic needs. This becomes more difficult if the mother is breastfeeding and is the only one who can feed the baby throughout the night. Counselors can encourage mothers to elicit help from their partner or other family members to care for the baby while the mother showers, eats, naps, and takes care of other physical self-care needs.

Psychological self-care focuses on the mother's mental health needs such as attending individual therapy or a support group, taking time for self-reflection and self-awareness, journaling, and asking for help (Phoenix, 2013). Mothers may neglect this type of self-care due to the many demands of motherhood. However, psychological self-care can often be done while the mother is taking care of other needs such as changing or breastfeeding the baby, taking a shower, walking the dog, or cleaning up the house. For example, a mother can talk on the phone with a friend while taking her baby for a walk in the stroller or playing in the park. Reflecting on her own psychological wellbeing does not need to take up time from a mother's busy schedule and can be done on a regular basis during other daily activities. Similarly, *emotional* self-care can also be done routinely and without taking up much time. This type of wellness emphasizes self-love and self-compassion by practicing positive affirmations, engaging in a fun hobby, laughing, cathartic crying, and taking care of other emotional needs (Phoenix, 2013). Both psychological and emotional self-care focus on the mother's inner world and her core mental health needs. Counselors can help mothers identify what is important to them and how they can foster positive mental health without taking up time from their busy life.

Spiritual self-care involves getting in touch with one's spirituality in a variety of ways, including being in nature, meditating, singing, dancing, playing, doing yoga, praying, and practicing self-forgiveness (Phoenix, 2013). While spirituality can include religious beliefs, it certainly does not require them. Spiritual values can help individuals explore the meaning of the universe and what purpose they have for being alive (Corey, 2006). Mothers can explore and focus on their spirituality while taking care of their babies or by requesting support from others for a brief period of time to engage in practices like meditation that require more concentration. Counselors can encourage mothers to share and introduce their newborn to important spiritual values, beliefs, and traditions. *Personal* self-care focuses on the mother's desires and plans for her life. This type of self-care includes fostering friendships, going on dates, relaxing, spending time with family, making a vision board and indulging in hobbies (Phoenix, 2013). Mothers often struggle with feelings of guilt and believe they must spend all their free time with their children (Prikhidko & Swank, 2018). Counselors can assist mothers with the personal process of discovering and nurturing who they are as a person, outside of being a mother.

Finally, *professional* self-care is the last category identified in the Self-Care Wheel, and includes setting firm boundaries at work, taking mental health, vacation, and sick days, planning a next career move, or taking a class (Phoenix, 2013). This is an important type of self-care, as working mothers often report feelings of guilt and intense pressure related to balancing work and family life (Forbes et al., 2021). While many mothers go back to work after childbirth, counselors must be sensitive to the needs of both working mothers and mothers who stay at home. Not every mother wants to work or is able to work when taking care of children. While professional self-care may not fully apply to every mother, counselors can explore a mother's future career plans or educational goals. In Chapter 10, we will explore more aspects related to motherhood, career, and identity.

Balancing self-care and family care is a source of stress and guilt for many mothers (Prikhidko & Swank, 2018). The task of caring for our needs while also caring for a child can leave many mothers feeling burned out, tired, and at risk for developing PPD. Thus, self-care and wellness are essential in the effective prevention and treatment of PPD. The Self-Care Wheel can be a helpful tool for promoting positive perinatal mental health and wellness. Counselors can become familiar with different types of self-care and help mothers establish and maintain a healthy life balance during the perinatal period.

Another helpful resource mental health professionals can use to address wellness is the Indivisible Self Model of Wellness (Myers & Sweeney, 2005), which is a way to conceptualize and address a client's overall wellness in counseling as well as focus on specific factors, including self-care, that either positively or negatively impacting their wellness. This model structures various factors of wellness within five selves: *Creative, Coping, Physical, Essential,* and *Social Selves. Thinking, emotions, work, control,* and *positive humor* are the factors that make up the *Creative Self.* The *Coping Self* comprises *leisure, stress management, self-worth,* and *realistic beliefs.* Exercise and *nutrition* are the two factors that make up the *Physical Self.* The *Essential Self* comprises *spirituality, gender identity, self-care,* and *cultural identity. Friendship* and *love* comprise the *Social Self.* Counselors and other mental health professionals can assess clients' wellness using the Five Factor Wellness Inventory (5F-WeL; Myers & Sweeney, 2005). Using this model, counselors can also work with clients to develop tailored self-care and wellness plans to help them meet their self-care and wellness needs and support their overall progress in treatment.

This chapter introduced various significant factors incorporated in a strengths-based approach to treating women with PPD. The STRENGTHS model is a comprehensive and multicultural treatment approach that addresses a variety of factors related to the peripartum period. While this model is focused on PPD, it can be applied to a variety of peripartum presenting problems, including peripartum anxiety, which has not yet been defined by the DSM-5-TR, but may be a primary presenting concern for many mothers. This model is highlighted in every book chapter to assist counselors in better understanding women, their peripartum experiences, and the complexities of treating PPD and other related peripartum mood disorders and presenting problems. Counselors are strongly encouraged to apply this model with any client who is experiencing varying mental health symptoms during the pregnancy and postpartum period.

Case Study: Leila

Leila, a 23-year-old Hispanic female, gave birth to a healthy baby girl two weeks ago at a birth center. Throughout her pregnancy, Leila regularly met with her midwife for prenatal care and concerning pregnancy symptoms. Leila admitted that during her first, second, and third trimesters, she regularly felt exhausted, had very low energy, and trouble sleeping. She also had trouble concentrating when doing her college schoolwork and felt sad and hopeless most days. Leila reported that, after finding out she was pregnant, her boyfriend was unfaithful and did not show much interest in being part of the pregnancy or the baby's life. Leila spent many of her days crying and felt a great deal of anxiety about raising the baby alone. While she currently resides with her mother, father, and younger sister, she often feels guilty about having a child without the emotional and financial support of a romantic partner. At her two-week postpartum check-up with her midwife, Leila appeared disheveled and tired. She reported having a great deal of difficulty with breastfeeding but feels a lot of pressure from her family to continue trying to breastfeed her baby and not use formula. When asked about feelings of anxiety and depression,

Leila began crying and told her midwife that she feels hopeless and wishes she could "disappear." She continues to struggle with sleep, feels tired and lacks energy during the day, and has difficulty focusing on tasks. When she looks at social media, she often feels lonely and isolated, especially when she sees pictures of her ex-boyfriend with his new girlfriend. Leila often finds herself crying after checking her social media accounts and sometimes wishes she had never got pregnant. Leila reported that she is also feeling guilty because she does not feel like she's a good mother and is not bonding with the baby like she thought she would. Leila denied thoughts of hurting herself or others, but stated, "somedays, I wonder if she would be better off without me and my mother can just take care of her." Leila's midwife recommended that Leila see a therapist right away regarding her symptoms of anxiety and depression. Leila stated that she does not have any insurance and is unsure if she can afford a therapist with all the birth center bills. Leila left her midwife's office feeling defeated and hopeless.

Reflection Questions for Clinicians

- What steps could the midwife take to help Leila connect with a mental health clinician?
- How could you help Leila gain access to care?
- What cultural considerations can serve as strengths or barriers to treatment?

APPLYING THE STRENGTHS MODEL—THE CASE OF LEILA

Significant Individual, Infant, Family, Societal, and Cultural Factors

Leila is a Hispanic woman currently residing with her family of origin and her new baby. The baby's father does not reside with Leila, and they are not currently romantically involved. As a new mother, she has various stressors that impact and influence her mental health. To start, Leila's culture is an important factor that counselors should attend to. In Hispanic culture, family influence and collectivistic values are a crucial part of life and are a source of strength for Leila. Leila's parents are a big part of her life, and she currently resides in their home, along with her younger sister. While Leila is having difficulty breastfeeding, her family would like for her to continue breastfeeding without the use of formula, which is also an important part of her culture's expectations of new mothers.

Treatment Barriers

Treatment barriers related to Leila's family and culture should be considered. Leila is a first-time mother and appears to be having difficulties bonding with her baby. Lack of knowledge related to being a parent and understanding her own mental health can be a barrier to treatment. She is also experiencing significant life stressors, including a recent break-up. Her culture can also serve as a barrier, as Hispanic families may be less supportive about seeking counseling and understanding or identifying symptoms of PPD in new mothers (Sampson et al., 2021). Also, giving the baby formula instead of breastfeeding can be viewed by others as "lazy" or not wanting what is best for her child. The value placed on breastfeeding by Leila's family and society can become a major stressor for Leila if she has difficulties with initiating or sustaining breastfeeding, and she may not see formula as an equally viable option. Leila's parents will also be financially supporting Leila and her baby, which can become a stressor for Leila to be able to make her own decisions regarding the baby and her role and authority as a mother. Additionally, Leila does not currently have health insurance and worries about affording mental health counseling services.

Risk Factors

Leila is a new single mother who recently went through a break-up with the baby's father. This is a significant stressor for Leila, who has become increasingly upset about being a single mother and raising a child without a partner. This stressor is further exacerbated by seeing pictures of the baby's father on social media. A lack of sexual or romantic intimacy may also be a factor contributing to her loneliness and isolation. Leila does not mention any friendships or social supports outside of her home, which can further increase loneliness and isolation from the outside world. She had social and peer interactions while working on college classes during her pregnancy, but she has not mentioned attending any classes since giving birth. Additionally, Leila is not currently working, does not have health insurance, and is struggling to pay her birth center bills. Since she does not have any financial help from the baby's father, she may have additional financial worries that contribute to her PPD. Regarding her mental health, Leila experienced symptoms of depression during her pregnancy, which increases the risk of PPD after birth. All these stressors could be contributing to, and exacerbating, her lack of bond with her baby and symptoms of PPD.

Enlisting Support from Family, the Community, and Medical Professionals

Hispanic families tend to be close to extended family members like aunts and cousins, providing Leila with outside support to aid in her feelings of loneliness and isolation. Further, her family's spirituality can also be a significant strength, as Hispanic families often use religion as a focal point to feel deeply connected to one another through spiritual traditions. If Leila's family is part of a church, that can also be a great benefit, as church resources can offer Leila assistance with finances, returning to college, seeking financial help from the baby's father, and searching for free or reduced-pay mental health counseling. Enlisting support from Leila's midwife can be valuable. Leila's mental status exam (MSE) could be completed by her midwife to assess some important factors about Leila such as her appearance, mood, cognitions, perceptions, thoughts, behaviors, insight, and judgment. While midwives generally lack training and confidence in conducting an MSE, it is becoming an increasingly important skill for maternity medical professionals (McCauley et al., 2021). Since Leila gave birth at a birth center, she may not have had access to lactation consultants, who are available at hospitals. Enlisting support from a lactation consultant could be helpful due to her breastfeeding difficulties.

Noticeable Symptoms, Severity, & DSM-5-TR Diagnosis/Needs Identified by Family & Treatment Team

During pregnancy, Leila reported low energy, difficulty sleeping and trouble concentrating. After giving birth, Leila mentioned feelings of hopelessness and sadness related to being a new mother due to a lack of self-efficacy in her role as a new mother and not having a strong bond with her baby like she expected. She often feels guilty about not being a good mother and has expressed thoughts of "disappearing." During her two-week postpartum appointment, Leila appeared tearful and disheveled when talking to her midwife. She presented for the appointment with a great deal of anxiety about her experiences as a new mother. She continues to struggle with sleep, feeling tired, lack of energy, and has difficulty focusing. While she reported feelings of depression, she did not indicate any suicidal ideation, homicidal ideation, hallucinations, or orientation impairments. She is currently feeling both defeated and hopeless. Based on Leila's presenting symptoms, a possible DSM-5-TR diagnosis is *major depressive disorder, recurrent episode, moderate, with peripartum onset* (APA, 2022).

Goals Identified by Family

While Leila didn't mention specific treatment goals, her midwife recommended that Leila attend therapy due to her symptoms of anxiety and depression. Decreasing negative emotions and increasing positive feelings associated with being a mother can be a helpful goal. Since Leila is a first-time mother, she may not be aware of useful goals related to being a new mother, such as needing information, practical and material support, psychological support, and sharing experiences with others (Slomian et al, 2021). These can be added to her treatment plan. Considering Leila's family and their importance in her life, she mentioned her family wanting her to continue breastfeeding rather than formula feed her baby.

> **Examples of SMART treatment goals for Leila**
>
> - Leila will attend therapy with a counselor 1× per week for the next two months to decrease depressive symptoms.
>
> - Leila will join and attend a local support group for new mothers 1× per week to increase support and decrease isolation.
>
> - Leila will attend virtual "mommy and me" groups 1× per week to learn new skills focused on increasing feelings of bonding with her baby.
>
> - Leila will meet with a lactation consultant at least 1× per week to address current breastfeeding issues.

Treatment Recommendations

Based on Leila's presenting symptoms, recommendation for treatment should start with non-pharmacological treatment interventions, such as Cognitive Behavioral Therapy (CBT). Specific interventions can include psychoeducation about being a new mother, assertiveness skills to learn how to communicate more effectively with her family about her breastfeeding concerns, self-esteem training to boost her confidence as a new mother, and "baby and me" sessions to help increase feelings of bonding. Since Leila reported feelings of guilt about not bonding with her baby, she may benefit from therapy focused on maternal and infant mental health.

Helpful, Protective, and Resilience Factors

While Leila is currently facing numerous systemic, cultural, and societal stressors related to her pregnancy and birth, there are also many strengths that clinicians should emphasize. Leila has a strong and supportive family system, providing her with basic survival needs such as safe shelter, nutritious food, financial help, and strong emotional family support. Although Leila is currently not working and does have financial stressors associated with healthcare costs, she is not in immediate crisis related to finances and providing for her child. Her family currently provides her with a positive and nurturing home environment, allowing her plenty of time and space to bond with her child without the burden of excessive worry about working or finances. Leila has numerous individual strengths that allowed her to graduate from high school and be accepted into college.

Self-Care & Wellness

As a new mother, Leila is learning about how to approach her own self-care and wellness and care for her infant. Since her parents and sister can help with taking care of the baby, Leila will be able to rest and spend time away from childcare responsibilities to focus on self-care. This self-care time can be spent on personal hobbies, attending mental health counseling, going outside of the house for a mental health day, and reaching out to friends. Attending college classes when she feels ready could be an important part of getting in touch with her individual needs outside of being a mother.

REFERENCES

Alfayumi-Zeadna, S., Froimovici, M., Azbarga, Z., Grotto, I., & Daoud, N. (2019). Barriers to postpartum depression treatment among Indigenous Bedouin women in Israel: A focus group study. *Health & Social Care in the Community, 3*, 757–776. doi:10.1111/hsc.12693

American Psychiatric Association. (APA). (2013). *Diagnostic and statistical manual of mental disorders* (5th ed.). doi:10.1176/appi.books.9780890425596

American Psychiatric Association. (APA). (2022). *Diagnostic and statistical manual of mental disorders* (5th ed., text rev.). doi:10.1176/appi.books.9780890425787

Anstey, E. H., Shoemaker, M. L., Barrera, C. M., O'Neil, M. E., Verma, A. B., & Holman, D. M. (2017). Breastfeeding and breast cancer risk reduction: Implications for black mothers. *American Journal of Preventive Medicine, 53*(3S1), S40–S46. doi:10.1016/j.amepre.2017.04.024

Archer, J., Probert, B. S., & Gage, L. (1987). College students' attitudes toward wellness. *Journal of College Student Personnel, 28*(4), 311–317.

Arnold, M., & Kalibatseva, Z. (2021). Are "Superwomen" without social support at risk for postpartum depression and anxiety? *Women & Health, 2*, 148–159. doi:10.1080/03630242.2020.1844360

Battle, C. L., Salisbury, A. L., Schofield, C. A., & Ortiz-Hernandez, S. (2013). Perinatal antidepressant use: Understanding women's preferences and concerns. *Journal of Psychiatric Practice, 19*(6), 443–453. doi:10.1097/01.pra.0000438183.74359.46

Bayri Bingol, F., & Demirgoz Bal, M. (2020). The risk factors for postpartum posttraumatic stress disorder and depression. *Perspectives in Psychiatric Care, 56*(4), 851–857. https://doi.org/10.1111/ppc.12501

Beck, C. T. (2001). Predictors of postpartum depression: An update. *Nursing Research, 50*, 275–285. doi:10.1097/00006199-200109000-00004

Bos, S. C., Macedo, A., Marques, M., Pereira, A. T., Maia, B. R., Soares, M. J., Valente, J., Gomes, A. A., & Azevedo, M. H. (2013). Is positive affect in pregnancy protective of postpartum depression? *Brazilian Journal of Psychiatry, 35*(1), 5–12. doi:10.1016/j.rbp.2011.11.002

Bridges, N. (2016). The faces of breastfeeding support: Experiences of mothers seeking breastfeeding support online. *Breastfeeding Review, 24*(1), 11–20.

Bronfenbrenner, U. (1979). *The ecology of human development: Experiments by nature and design*. Harvard University Press.

Corey, G. (2006). Integrating spirituality in counseling practice. *Vistas Online*. Retrieved from https://www.counseling.org/docs/default-source/vistas/integrating-spirituality-in-counseling-practice.pdf?sfvrsn=7ddd7e2c_10

Dominiak, M., Antosik-Wojcinska, A. Z., Baron, M., Mierzejewski, P., & Swiecicki, L. (2021). Recommendations for the prevention and treatment of postpartum depression. *Ginekologia Polska, 92*(2), 153–164. doi:10.5603/GP.a2020.0141

Doran, G. T. (1981). There's a S.M.A.R.T. way to write management's goals and objectives. *Management Review, 70*(11), 35–36. http://www.ctwomen.org/blog/?offset=1525436874947

Forbes, L. K., Lamar, M. R., & Bornstein, R. S. (2021). Working mothers' experiences in an intensive mothering culture: A phenomenological qualitative study. *Journal of Feminist Family Therapy*, *33*(3), 270–294. doi:10.1080/08952833.2020.1798200

Freed, R. D., Chan, P. T., Boger, K. D., & Tompson, M. C. (2012). Enhancing maternal depression recognition in health care settings: A review of strategies to improve detection, reduce barriers, and reach mothers in need. *Families, Systems, & Health*, *30*(1), 1–8. doi:10.1037/a0027602

Garcia, V., Meyer, E., & Witkop, C. (2021). Risk factors for postpartum depression in active duty women. *Military Medicine*, *187*(5-6), e562–e566. doi:10.1093/milmed/usab161

Guille, C., Newman, R., Fryml, L. D., Lifton, C. K., & Epperson, C. N. (2013). Management of postpartum depression. *Journal of Midwifery & Women's Health*, *58*(6), 643–653. doi:10.1111/jmwh.12104

Hain, S., Oddo-Sommerfeld, S., Bahlmann, F., Louwen, F., & Schermelleh-Engel, K. (2016). Risk and protective factors for antepartum and postpartum depression: A prospective study. *Journal of Psychosomatic Obstetrics & Gynecology*, *37*(4), 119–129. doi:10.1080/0167482X.2016.1197904

Hantsoo, L., Ward-O'Brien, D., Czarkowski, K., Gueorguieva, R., Price, L., & Epperson, C. (2014). A randomized, placebo-controlled, double-blind trial of sertraline for postpartum depression. *Psychopharmacology*, *231*(5), 939–948. doi:10.1007/s00213-013-3316-1

Julian, M., Le, H.-N., Coussons-Read, M., Hobel, C. J., & Dunkel Schetter, C. (2021). The moderating role of resilience resources in the association between stressful life events and symptoms of postpartum depression. *Journal of Affective Disorders*, *293*, 261–267. doi:10.1016/j.jad.2021.05.082

Khowaja, B., & Rind, K. (2021). Efficacy of complementary and alternative medicine in treatment of postpartum depression: A situation analysis. *Global Journal of Public Health Medicine*, *3*(2), 386–395. doi:10.37557/gjphm.v3i2.85

Kim, Y., & Dee, V. (2017). Self-Care for health in rural Hispanic women at risk for postpartum depression. *Maternal & Child Health Journal*, *21*(1), 77–84. doi:10.1007/s10995-016-2096-8

Kızılırmak, A., Calpbinici, P., Tabakan, G., & Kartal, B. (2020). Correlation between postpartum depression and spousal support and factors affecting postpartum depression. *Health Care for Women International*, *42*(12), 1325–1339. doi:10.1080/07399332.2020.1764562

Kress, V. E., & Paylo, M. J. (2019). *Treating those with mental disorders: A comprehensive approach to case conceptualization and treatment* (2nd ed.). Pearson.

Lambermon, F., Vandenbussche, F., Dedding, C., & van Duijnhoven, N. (2020). Maternal self-care in the early postpartum period: An integrative review. *Midwifery*, *90*, 102799. doi:10.1016/j.midw.2020.102799

McCauley, K., Elsom, S., Muir-Cochrane, E., & Lyneham, J. (2011). Midwives and assessment of perinatal mental health. *Journal of Psychiatric and Mental Health Nursing*, *18*(9), 786–795. doi:10.1111/j.1365-2850.2011.01727.x

Milgrom, J., Hirshler, Y., Reece, J., Holt, C., & Gemmill, A. W. (2019). Social support—A protective factor for depressed perinatal women? *International Journal of Environmental Research and Public Health*, *16*(8), 1426. doi:10.3390/ijerph16081426

Myers, J. E., & Sweeney, T. J. (2005). The Indivisible Self: An evidence-based model of Wellness (reprint). *The Journal of Individual Psychology*, *61* (1), 269–279.

Nadeem, E., Lange, J. M., & Miranda, J. (2009). Perceived need for care among low-income immigrant and US-born black and Latina women with depression. *Journal of Women's Health*, *18*, 369–375. doi:10.1089/jwh.2008.0898

Nillni, Y. I., Mehralizade, A., Mayer, L., & Milanovic, S. (2018). Treatment of depression, anxiety, and trauma-related disorders during the perinatal period: A systematic review. *Clinical Psychology Review*, *66*, 136–148. doi:10.1016/j.cpr.2018.06.004

O'Hara, M., & Swain, A. (1996). Rates and risk of postpartum depression—A meta-analysis. *International Review of Psychiatry*, *8*(1), 37–54.

Phoenix, O. (2013). The Self-Care Wheel. www.OlgaPhoenix.com. https://olgaphoenix.com/self-care-wheel/

Prikhidko, A., & Swank, J. M. (2018). Motherhood experiences and expectations: A qualitative exploration of mothers of toddlers. *The Family Journal*, *26*(3), 278–284. doi:10.1177/1066480718795116

Robertson, E., Grace, S., Wallington, T., & Stewart, D. E. (2004). Antenatal risk factors for postpartum depression: A synthesis of recent literature. *General Hospital Psychiatry*, *26*, 289–295. doi:10.1016/j.genhosppsych.2004.02.006

Sampson, M., Duron, J. F., Maldonado Torres, M. I., & Davidson, M. R. (2014). A disease you just caught: Low-income African American mothers' cultural beliefs about postpartum depression. *Women's Healthcare: A Clinical Journal for NPs*, *2*(4), 44–50. http://npwomenshealthcare.com/wp-content/uploads/2014/10/PostPart_N14.pdf

Sampson, M., Yu, M., Mauldin, R., Mayorga, A., & Gonzalez, L. G. (2021). "You withhold what you are feeling so you can have a family": Latinas' perceptions on community values and postpartum depression. *Family Medicine & Community Health*, *9*(3), 1–9. doi:10.1136/fmch-2020-000504

Slomian, J., Reginster, J. Y., Emonts, P., & Bruyère, O. (2021). Identifying maternal needs following childbirth: Comparison between pregnant women and recent mothers. *BMC Pregnancy and Childbirth*, *21*(1), 1–15. doi:10.1186/s12884-021-03858-7

Slomian, J., Emonts, P., Vigneron, L., Acconcia, A., Glowacz, F., Reginster, J. Y., … & Bruyère, O. (2017). Identifying maternal needs following childbirth: A qualitative study among mothers, fathers and professionals. *BMC Pregnancy and Childbirth*, *17*(1), 1–13. doi:10.1186/s12884-017-1398-1

Sperry, J., & Sperry, L. (2020, December 7). Case conceptualization: Key to highly effective counseling. *Counseling Today*. https://ct.counseling.org/2020/12/case-conceptualization-key-to-highly-effective-counseling/

Wise, E. H., & Barnett, J. E. (2016). Self-care for psychologists. In J. C. Norcross, G. R. VandenBos, D. K. Freedheim, & L. F. Campbell (Eds.), *APA handbook of clinical psychology: Education and profession* (pp. 209–222). American Psychological Association. doi:10.1037/14774-014

3

Social and Cultural Factors Associated with Peripartum Depression and Maternal Stress

Isabel A. Thompson

Personal Narrative

As a first generation Mexican American, my husband and I were over the moon about having our first child, and I felt that since I am Mexican, I had all the answers about motherhood as well as my mother's help with being a first-time mom. When the time came to ask for help, however, my mother would tell me, "I don't know I had you and your sisters 20 years ago." I should have considered that from the beginning and just realized that I should have taught myself more than what was expected. I had imagined that things would start off great, but it was a nightmare that I could not escape. I was breastfeeding as much as I could, but my mother's doubts kept creeping in and saying that I should consider formula. "Why would my mom say this to me? Weren't we created to nurture our own blood?" Eager to prove her wrong, I kept insisting I could breastfeed my child. When my son was around two months old, I noticed a change in me. I cared less about my appearance and personal hygiene, ordered take-out food all the time, and laid in the same position all day and night; to the point I made a marking on my bed. Because of my husband's demanding work schedule, I was alone physically and mentally. No one in my family noticed at all. I'm pretty good at putting up a fake smile when needed. I never sought help because I didn't want to feel labeled as depressed. I didn't want to take any medication for it because it just wasn't for me even though it was necessary. My postpartum won the battle and it seemed like even if I tried I just didn't care to pull myself out.

—*Anonymous*

In the personal narrative above, expectations about motherhood related to this mother's cultural background impacted her perception of herself as a mother and her competency. Moreover, the lack of expected familial support seemed to further exacerbate this mother's symptoms. In this text we acknowledge that peripartum depression (PPD) does not arise in a vacuum; in fact, social and cultural factors may contribute to maternal stress and to the development of PPD and other related peripartum mood disorders. Therefore, we use a multicultural/feminist lens to frame the issues related to the development, screening, diagnosis, and treatment of PPD

DOI: 10.4324/9780429440892-3

within the broader socio-cultural context. This chapter also explores social and cultural factors relevant to working with military families and veterans, persons with disabilities (PWDs), same-sex parents, transgender parents, and those who have expansive gender identities.

SOCIAL AND CULTURAL FACTORS

Social and cultural factors shape a person's upbringing, worldview, identity, sense of themselves, and impact how a person is perceived by others, what we perceive as the appropriate role for a mother or parent, how someone sees themselves as a mother, and whether they view themselves as succeeding in this role. These factors impact mothers' and families' experiences during pregnancy and after birth and how any mood changes are perceived and understood during the peripartum period.

Social and cultural factors also influence a mother's help-seeking behaviors, the accessibility of treatment, and the efficacy of treatment interventions. People from marginalized groups may have more barriers accessing needed and wanted healthcare (Zittel-Palamara et al., 2008) or avoid seeking care due to fear of or previous experiences with medical racism, heterosexism, or other biases imposed by healthcare providers. Maternal health disparities, including maternal mental health and maternal mortality rates (Glazer & Howell, 2021) as well as infant health disparities, including racial and ethnic differences in infant mortality rates (Abdulrahman et al., 2015; CDC, n.d.-b), are significant and negatively impact members of marginalized and disadvantaged groups. The United States is experiencing a current crisis of maternal mortality, with the highest rate of any industrialized country (Glazer & Howell, 2021). Counselors and other mental health professionals need to be aware of the current crisis with maternal mortality rates, especially related to racial and ethnic health disparities. Counselors and other mental health professionals must also be aware of the negative impact of societal racism and other forms of prejudice including but not limited to classism, sexism, ageism, xenophobia, heterosexism, homophobia, and transphobia, when working clients during the sensitive peripartum period.

UNDERSTANDING THE ROLE EXPECTATIONS RELATED TO MOTHERHOOD

Motherhood is idealized in many cultures, and may be viewed unrealistically, which can be detrimental to mothers themselves, their infants, and their families. There are frequently unwritten rules about what it means to be a "good" mother, including myths such as "A mother should always be happy caring for their children." These gendered cultural expectations include that mothers are fulfilled by motherhood and caring for their infant (Hogan, 2017). Compounding the stigma associated with mental illness in general, the stigma seeking help for PPD may in part be due to the cultural expectation about motherhood. Mothers sometimes fear disclosing PPD or other postpartum mood symptoms, or minimize their symptoms (Ugarriza, 2004). Depressive symptoms impact a mother's mood and day-to-day functioning (Haga et al., 2012) and mothers may fear that this reflects on how well they are doing as mothers.

Gender-based assumptions around motherhood and parenthood are pervasive and reflect societal expectations about the roles that parents should have based on their gender (Forbes et al., 2020, 2021). Navigating gender-based stereotypes is often an unwelcome aspect of becoming a mother, as mothers deal with expectations around their role as a caregiver, and issues around career and childcare (Forbes et al., 2020). Motherhood implies female gender in its very definition, and this can be especially problematic for parents who identify as transgender, gender non-binary, or have other expansive gender identities. Even for those who identify as cisgender women, the role of "mother" brings a cascade of expectations that tend to reinforce traditional gender roles and can be uncomfortable. Furthermore, one of the most common questions people tend to ask pregnant individuals is, "What are you having? A boy or a girl?" For families who do not want to reinforce traditional gender roles, this question can be uncomfortable and reveals the pervasiveness of binary gendered societal expectations.

SOCIO-CULTURAL VALUES AND LACK OF MATERNITY, PATERNITY, AND PARENTAL LEAVE

Despite the rhetoric surrounding the importance of motherhood and family life in the United States, there is a lack of funding and other forms of support that would significantly aid mothers and families. Key among these absences is the lack of laws guaranteeing paid parental leave after the birth or adoption of a child. Although over 70 percent of women in the United States have paid employment, the United States of America is the only industrialized nation that does not offer paid maternity leave (Shepherd-Banigan & Bell, 2014). This is a noteworthy deviance from a broader global norm of paid maternity leave (Addati et al., 2014). Mothers who have recently given birth often return to work before they feel ready or have recovered from childbirth. Partners are also negatively impacted by the lack of paid parental leave and cannot spend as much time supporting their partner and bonding with their baby. The pressure on families can be enormous. While the US government does allow for up to 12 weeks of unpaid leave without risk of job loss through the Family and Medical Leave Act of 1993 (FMLA; 2006), this law only applies workers at companies with over 50 people who have been employed for at least 12 months (Andres et al., 2016; Slopen, 2020). Unfortunately, many working parents do not qualify for FMLA (Slopen, 2020).

Employees taking FMLA may be able to create a composite of paid and unpaid leave, depending on company benefits. In a study examining New York City mothers' FMLA leave, Slopen found that Black mothers were more likely to take unpaid leave than White mothers, while mothers with college degrees were more likely to have access to paid leave (2020). Jou et al. (2018) reported that paid leave was associated with positive health outcomes for mothers and their babies and higher chances of participation in behaviors like exercise.

Some mothers take a shorter leave than the maximum 12 weeks allowed due to the financial strain involved but then struggle with the costs of childcare (Slopen, 2020). Moreover, even if they take the full 12 weeks of leave, this is still shorter than the leave time for mothers in many other countries. The United States deviates from norms of high-income countries in the short timeframe of the allowed leave period along with the lack of guaranteed paid leave (Addati et al., 2014; Khan, 2020; Slopen, 2020). Many other nations have more generous laws, with duration of leave and the guarantee of payment. Paid leave of sufficient duration has benefits for mothers and babies, including improved health outcomes for mothers and children and increased financial stability (Addati et al., 2014). Paid leave also increases the likelihood that women will participate in the paid workforce after becoming mothers (Khan, 2020). Longitudinal research conducted in Europe indicates that generous maternity leave policies have long-term benefits for mothers by providing stress reduction after childbirth (Avendano et al., 2015). The positive effects among women who had longer maternity leave include decreased depression scores, even decades after giving birth (Avendano et al., 2015). Countries that adopt guaranteed paid maternity leave policies show decreased rates of infant, neonatal, and under-five mortality, with benefits demonstrable two years after policy adoption (Khan, 2020). The benefits of paid maternity leave to babies, children, and mothers are clear and there is an urgent need to advocate for guaranteed paid maternity leave in the United States (Schindler-Ruwisch & Eaves, 2022).

The lack of guaranteed federal paid parental leave translates into lots of stress for many families, juggling the needs of their newborn, while trying to stay financially afloat, manage childcare, and navigate career decisions (Slopen, 2020). Mothers may quit paid employment even when they want to return. Childcare is a huge cost to most families, and many families face challenging decisions about whether and when a birthing parent should return to work, often considering if a parent's paycheck is substantial enough to cover childcare costs. It is often the mother who gives up paid employment: "Cultural norms of intensive mothering and resulting unequal caregiving responsibilities create expectations that mothers need to earn enough to cover the cost of care to remain employed" (Ruppanner et al., 2021, p. 4). Further, expensive childcare differentially impacts the employment of mothers with lower levels of education (Ruppanner et al., 2021).

Cultural Norms of Support after Childbirth

The lack of parental leave in the United States may also be reflective of broader sociocultural values that prioritize individualism over the collective good. In addition to the lack of parental leave, many mothers in the United States do not receive systemic support to reduce their workload at home after birth. Many women struggle in the immediate postpartum, as their partners return to work quickly. Depending on cultural and family norms, new mothers may be largely alone, trying to take care of their newborns while also trying to care for themselves.

However, if a new mother perceives help as intrusive or the help is provided by someone she is not comfortable with, this can increase depressive symptoms. In the Chinese tradition, it is usually the new mother's mother or mother-in-law who provides the in-home support (Bina, 2008). In a literature review comparing studies of cultural factors and PPD, Bina (2008) reported that in a study of Taiwanese mothers, receiving support from their own parents was associated with fewer depression symptoms as compared with receiving unwanted emotional support from their in-laws, which was associated with depressive symptoms. These results suggest that a mother's needs, their comfort level with the support person, and their preferences should be honored in the postpartum.

RACIAL AND ETHNIC MATERNAL HEALTH DISPARITIES

Maternal health disparities between White women and women of color are pronounced and have persisted through time (Wang et al., 2021). These racial and ethnic disparities impact both maternal physical and mental health, as well as rates of severe maternal morbidity and maternal mortality (Wang et al., 2021). According to the US Centers for Disease Control and Prevention, "Severe maternal morbidity (SMM) includes unexpected outcomes of labor and delivery that result in significant short- or long-term consequences to a woman's health" (CDC, n.d.-a). SMM has been increasing for all birthing parents from 1993 to 2014 in the United States, with 2014 being the most current year for which national data is available (CDC, n.d.-a). In a qualitative study that included 20 mothers from different racial and ethnic backgrounds almost all the mothers "reported distressing childbirth experiences related to their maternal morbidity" (Wang et al., 2021, p. 77), but especially the Black and Latina women. Clinicians should be attentive to their clients' experiences of childbirth and any related trauma associated with childbirth and be aware of the need to address this with Black and Latina mothers (Wang et al., 2021). Counselors can help women to identify and process distressing birth experiences such as obstetrical complications and birth trauma by inviting them to share about their childbirth experiences and explore their feelings about what transpired during the birth (Gamble & Creedy, 2004).

Maternal mortality rates show clear disparities between women of color and White women (Hoyert, 2022). Maternal mortality "refers to the death of a woman from complications of pregnancy or childbirth that occur during the pregnancy or within 6 weeks after the pregnancy ends" (Eunice Kennedy Shriver National Institute of Child Health and Human Development, n.d.). The concerning upward trend in maternal mortality in the United States is accounted for by an increase in deaths among non-Hispanic Black women and Hispanic Women (Hoyert, 2022). The National Center for Health reported that the "maternal mortality rate for 2020 was 23.8 deaths per 100,000 live births compared with a rate of 20.1 in 2019" with significant increases in maternal mortality rates for non-Hispanic Black women and Hispanic women, but not for White mothers (Hoyert, 2022, p. 1). The risks of childbirth and the postpartum period are high for Black mothers in the United States, as the "maternal mortality rate for non-Hispanic Black women was 55.3 deaths per 100,000 live births, 2.9 times the rate for non-Hispanic White women" (Hoyert, 2022, p. 1). This concerning statistic reveals the risks that Black mothers in the United States face while pregnant, giving birth, and in the first year postpartum. It is not only mothers who are impacted by disparities in mortality rates; infant mortality rates are higher among Black, Native Hawaiian or other Pacific Islander, Native American/Alaska Native and Hispanic babies (CDC, n.d.-b.), so advocating for the needs of mothers and babies is acutely needed. From an intersectional framework, counselors who advocate for the needs of Black and Hispanic mothers who are disproportionately represented in the disturbing national maternal mortality statistics would be acting consistent with the Multicultural and Social Justice Counseling Competencies discussed later in the chapter.

MATERNAL MENTAL HEALTH DISPARITIES

Maternal mental health is an important consideration during the peripartum period, as peripartum depression and other maternal mood disorders can affect mothers of any cultural background or socioeconomic status. However, certain risk factors for the development of PPD, such as poverty or the stressors associated with marginalization, may be more prevalent in certain groups. It is important to recognize and address these risk factors to ensure that all mothers have access to the support and resources they need to maintain their mental health during this critical time. For example, researchers reported a higher rate of postpartum depression among a Native American sample than the general population (Baker et al., 2005). Moreover, mothers of color n may have a harder time accessing desired or needed treatment than White women (Zittel-Palamara et al., 2008). Furthermore, mothers from marginalized and minoritized backgrounds may be less likely to pursue treatment for PPD or other perinatal mood symptoms due to mistrust in the existing systems of care available (Conteh et al., 2022). In addition to factors of race and ethnicity, pregnant women from low-income backgrounds who have increased stress levels may also have increased risk of developing PPD (Scheyer & Urizar, 2016).

WORKING WITH MOTHERS FROM MARGINALIZED RACIAL AND ETHNIC BACKGROUNDS

Since racial and ethnic maternal health disparities are a significant risk to women of color (and their babies) during the peripartum time, there is an urgent need for culturally competent counselors who effectively work with clients directly, provide support to broader communities, and advocate for systemic change in maternal healthcare delivery and mental healthcare access. To be effective, counselors need to address their own potential implicit biases in working with peripartum clients from marginalized backgrounds.

It is recommended in the counseling literature that counselors broach the topic of racial, ethnic, and cultural difference with their clients through the practices of cultural broaching (Day-Vines et al., 2007; King, 2021). Cultural broaching is not a one-time event, but rather a multidimensional process in which counselors broach topics of race, ethnicity, and culture, and validate experiences of discrimination and build the therapeutic alliance (Day-Vines et al., 2020).

Demonstrating cultural humility is also recommended. Cultural humility has been described as "an approach and process" (Mosher et al., 2017, p. 221). It includes both intrapersonal and interpersonal aspects such as openness to the lived experiences of others (Mosher et al., 2017) and understanding cultural aspects of clients' identity from a place of humility (Choe et al., 2022). In the peripartum context, this would include an openness to understanding the intersections of clients' racial and ethnic identities with their parental identity.

Multicultural and Social Justice Counseling Competencies

The Association for Multicultural Counseling and Development (a national division of the American Counseling Association) and the American Counseling Association endorsed the *Multicultural and Social Justice Counseling Competencies* (MSJCC) to provide a framework for counselors to effectively address various forms of oppression, experiences of marginalization, intersectional identities, and privilege in all aspects of the counseling field, including counseling practice (Ratts et al., 2015). Bell (2023) defines oppression as "the interlocking forces that create and sustain injustice" (p. 5). Oppression occurs in various forms including racism, sexism, ableism, heterosexism, ageism, classism, and other forms of discrimination based on group identity (Bell, 2023). Furthermore, people are not just oppressed based on one dimension of their identity but on their various intersectional identities (Bell, 2023).

Intersectionality refers to how aspects of identity are socially constructed and interrelate in complex ways with various forms of oppression (Ratts et al., 2016). In foundational writings, Crenshaw stated that: "because the intersectional experience is greater than the sum of racism and sexism, any analysis that does not take intersectionality into account cannot sufficiently address the particular manner in which Black women are subordinated" (1989, p. 140). The intersectional nature of oppression is catalyzing and, concomitantly, failure to recognize intersectionality is exclusionary. Maternal/parental group level identities are intersectional aspects of identity that impact a person's life and experiences of privilege and marginalization.

The MSJCC is structured to examine the various ways in which privileged identities interact with marginalized identities and addresses the following professional relationship dyads: privileged counselor–marginalized client; privileged counselor–privileged client; marginalized counselor–privileged client; marginalized counselor–marginalized client (Ratts et al., 2016).

One example of this dynamic (when a counselor is not demonstrating cultural competence) would be a counselor from a privileged background recommending that a new mother from a less privileged background take additional leave from work to reduce her stress level and bond with her new baby. Instead of imposing a solution from a privileged perspective, this counselor could approach the client from a stance of cultural humility and use cultural broaching skills to develop the therapeutic alliance.

Figure 3.1
Multicultural and Social Justice Counseling Competencies

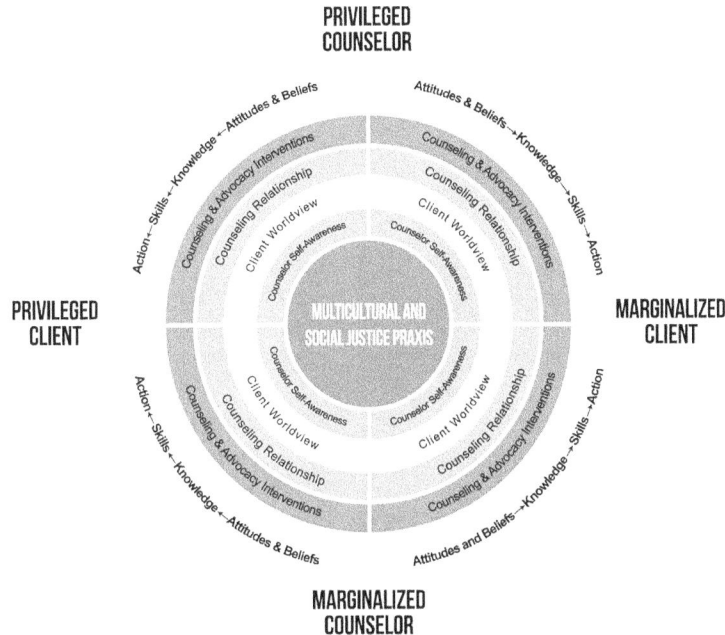

Source: *Multicultural and Social Justice Counseling Competencies.* Copyright 2015 by M. J. Ratts, A. A. Singh, S. Nassar-McMillan, S. K. Butler, & J. R. McCullough. Reprinted with permission.

This MSJCC addresses four domains of cultural and social justice competency: Counselor Self-Awareness, Client Worldview, Counseling Relationship, and Counseling and Advocacy Interventions (Ratts et al., 2015). Table 3.1 examines some specific competencies with applications for counseling clients with peripartum-related issues. For the full document with all the competencies, please see: www.multiculturalcounselingdevelopment.org/competencies

Table 3.1
Applying the Multicultural and Social Justice Counseling Competencies

Specific Themes/Competencies	Application to Counseling in the Peripartum Period
Counselor Self-Awareness 1. "Attitudes and Beliefs: Privileged and marginalized counselors are aware of their social identities, social group statuses, power, privilege, oppression, strengths, limitations, assumptions, attitudes, values, beliefs, and biases."	Counselors engage in self-reflection to examine their own identities as well as their attitudes and beliefs, specifically as they relate to cultural values, attitudes, biases, and beliefs about pregnant people, childbirth, mothers, parenting, and related topics.

(Continued)

Table 3.1 **(Continued)**
Applying the Multicultural and Social Justice Counseling Competencies

Specific Themes/Competencies	Application to Counseling in the Peripartum Period
Client Worldview 3. "Skills: Privileged and marginalized counselors possess skills that enrich their understanding of clients' worldview, assumptions, attitudes, values, beliefs, biases, social identities, social group statuses, and experiences with power, privilege, and oppression."	Counselors demonstrate skills with understanding diverse worldviews, regarding differing "assumptions, attitudes, values, beliefs, biases" about pregnancy, birth, parenting, and caring for an infant. Counselors demonstrate skill in addressing "social identities, social group statuses, and experience with power, privilege and oppression," specifically with regards to experiences of conception, pregnancy, birth, and the postpartum period.
Counseling Relationship 2. "Knowledge: Privileged and marginalized counselors possess knowledge of how client and counselor worldviews, assumptions, attitudes, values, beliefs, biases, social identities, social group statuses, and experiences with power, privilege, and oppression influence the counseling relationship." IV. *Counseling and Advocacy Interventions* "Privileged and marginalized counselors intervene with, and on behalf, of clients at the intrapersonal, interpersonal, institutional, community, public policy, and international/global levels."	Counselors need to possess a knowledge base of the various social identities and worldview factors that shape expectations, cultural beliefs, values, and practices associated with pursuing parenthood, pregnancy, childbirth, and parenting. They also understand how social group identities and statuses impact clients' experiences of parenting and the counseling relationship. Counselors take action and intervene at various levels, including within the person, (e.g., address distressing thoughts or feelings a pregnant person is experiencing), interpersonal level (e.g. address family dynamics that may be unhealthy), institutional, (e.g., identifying stressors such as an unsupportive supervisor who is inflexible regarding childcare disruptions), community levels (e.g., providing low-cost or free support groups for new parents in community settings), public policy, (e.g., advocating for paid parental leave in the United States; advocate for systemic and policy change to address racial disparities in the maternal mortality and infant mortality rates), and international/global levels (e.g., address the need for a focus on maternal mental health internationally).

Note: The themes/competencies on the lefthand side of the table are quoted from the *Multicultural and Social Justice Counseling Competencies* (Ratts et al., 2015, pp. 5–11).

PREGNANCY AND DISABILITY

Disability has been defined by the Americans with Disabilities Act as "a physical or mental impairment that substantially limits a major life activity" and the US Supreme Court furthers that this disability is permanent or long term and interferes with activities of daily living (Gladding & Newsome, 2018, p. 81). Approximately 1 in 5 people in the United States has a disability, with rates rising due to the aging demographic, socioeconomic barriers to accessing healthcare, emerging conditions (such as chronic fatigue syndrome), and advances in medical interventions that help people survive injuries (Newsome & Gladding, 2018). Experiencing pregnancy and childbirth as a person with a disability adds additional layers of consideration and challenges to the complex peripartum time (Mitra et al., 2016). Counselors can help people with disabilities consider what resources and supports they already have or want to have in place to reduce stress in the peripartum period.

Some maternal mental health disorders could constitute a disability, depending on the severity, duration, and impact on functioning. Pregnancy or childbirth can lead to a temporary disability or permanent acquired disability if someone experiences severe medical or mental health complications during pregnancy or after birth. Pregnant individuals may qualify for temporary disability status, needing documentation from their doctors to qualify for different duties during pregnancy (such as no heavy lifting or reduced standing while at work) or take leave using FMLA (U.S. Department of Labor, n.d.).

The American Rehabilitation Counseling Association (ARCA) is a national division of the American Counseling Association focused on individuals with disabilities. The ARCA Task Force on Competencies for Counseling Persons with Disabilities developed the *Disability-Related Counseling Competencies* to guide counselors to work effectively with clients who have disabilities, addressing how disability status cuts across all other forms of diversity and impacts all segments of the population (Chapin et al., 2018). Ableism is defined as:

> A worldview in which being able-bodied is assumed and acted on as the unquestioned norm for the way things are and should be. Because the ableist viewpoint is so systemically dominant and ingrained in the culture, people are typically unaware of its influence on how they perceive and act (e.g., designing buildings and homes with steps for entering instead of ramps, which everyone can use and which some persons or situations require).
>
> (Chapin et al., 2018, p. 10)

Table 3.2

Clinical Considerations Related to Disabilities in the Peripartum Periodz

Categories of Disabilities	Examples	Clinical Considerations during the Peripartum Period
Physical	Sensory loss (such as blindness or deafness), orthopedic impairments, congenital conditions (such as spina bifida), chronic illnesses (such as multiple sclerosis (MS) and diabetes.	Pregnant people who have existing physical disabilities may experience bias in medical settings, may face challenges navigating the medical system (Mitra et al., 2016) and/or have additional medical complications due to pregnancy.
Cognitive	Alzheimer's disease, developmental disabilities, learning disabilities.	Pregnant people with existing cognitive disabilities may face discrimination in healthcare settings.
Psychiatric	Mood disorders, disorders that cause psychosis, substance use disorders.	Pregnancy and childbirth increase the risk of a birthing parent developing a mood disorder (APA, 2022).

Note: Information about types of disabilities and examples of disabilities drawn from Gladding and Newsome (2018, p. 81).

Table 3.2 includes information about some disabilities that are readily observable by others, and other disabilities that can be "hidden." Individuals with these types of disabilities may have decisions about whether to disclose their disability status. Mood disorders or other physical chronic illnesses can sometimes be "hidden" by the person or are not observable upon initial contact, but still impair functioning. An acquired disability is: "A condition that occurs suddenly or develops gradually during the lifespan; thus, the person has had prior experiences, expectations, and identity as a non-disabled person" (Chapin et al., 2018, p. 10). An ARCA committee developed the *Disability-Related Counseling Competencies*, which uses the term persons with disabilities (PWDs) (Chapin et al., 2018). PWDs who are seeking to become pregnant, who are pregnant, or are new parents may experience discrimination in healthcare settings (Mitra et al., 2016). For example, pregnant people with mobility disabilities have reported experiencing barriers to receiving supportive care, including healthcare providers who lack knowledge about their disability or have negative viewpoints and challenges with physically accessing healthcare buildings (Mitra et al., 2016). Counselors can support clients with disabilities and encourage self-advocacy in navigating these complex systems (that are often ableist in their structure and norms). Table 3.3 highlights specific competencies and how they can be applied in counseling, especially for clients in the peripartum period.

Table 3.3

Applying the Disability-Related Counseling Competencies

Specific Competencies	Application to Counseling Clients with Peripartum Concerns
"A.1 Understand that PWDs, like all people, can live full and productive lives, and they deserve to have encouragement and opportunities to develop and express themselves as they progress through every stage of the lifespan."	Counselors must be sensitive to the needs of PWDs who may be seeking to conceive, are pregnant, or are new parents. Awareness that pregnancy itself can result in temporary disability.
"B.1. Advocate for equality of opportunity to achieve full inclusion and participation in all aspects of society."	Be affirmative and supportive in advocating for the needs of PWDs during the peripartum period, including conception, pregnancy, birth, and postpartum.
"C.2. Make efforts to ensure the accessibility of technology used for distance counseling, websites, social media sites, software, and computer applications."	Ensure websites are accessible, provide resources in advance of appointments that can be accessed in different formats and provide telehealth services with adaptive technology such as closed captioning (U.S. Department of Health and Human Services [HHS], 2022). Seek training and consultation if they need support to make their communication and digital platforms more accessible to PWDs.
"E.2. Understand the systems of discrimination that PWDs may experience in their education, job search, and employment, and how their high rate of unemployment and under-employment may affect their ability to function effectively in other spheres of life (e.g., housing, physical and emotional health, ability to support a family)."	Counselors working with pregnant PWDs, and their families should be aware of the intersections of identity and how ableist employment discrimination can impact a person's experience of pregnancy, birth, and the postpartum. Counselors should also be aware of the protections afforded by the *Pregnancy Discrimination Act of 1978* for expectant mothers (see Chapter 10 for more details).

Note: The competencies on the lefthand side of this table are quoted from the *Disability-Related Counseling Competencies* (Chapin et al., 2018).

SPIRITUALITY AND RELIGIOUS DIVERSITY

In addition to differences related to culture, ethnicity, sexuality, gender identity, and class, women and families also come from different worldviews and spiritual and/or religious backgrounds. While it is challenging to define spirituality, the Association for Spiritual, Ethical, and Religious Values in Counseling (ASERVIC), a national division of the American Counseling Association, has developed a document to illuminate what is meant by the term spirituality and help counselors understand it.

> Spirit may be defined as the animating life force, represented by such images as breath, wind, vigor, and courage. Spirituality is the drawing out and infusion of spirit in one's life. It is experienced as an active and passive process. […] Spirituality is also defined as a capacity and tendency that is innate and unique to all persons. This spiritual tendency moves the individual toward knowledge, love, meaning, peace, hope, transcendence, connectedness, compassion, wellness, and wholeness. Spirituality includes one's capacity for creativity, growth, and the development of a value system. Spirituality encompasses a variety of phenomena, including experiences, beliefs, and practices.
>
> (ASERVIC, n.d.-b, p. 1)

This definition of spirituality provides insight into what clients may be referring to when they discuss their spirituality. As counselors, it is recommended to remain open to how the client is defining spirituality and what it means in their lives. It further elaborates that spirituality may be experienced or approached in a variety of ways, including through religion (ASERVIC, n.d.-b). For some clients, their religion and spirituality may be closely aligned. Other clients may not identify with a particular religion but may identify as spiritual and non-religious.

Religion, in contrast to spirituality, is usually more clearly defined and associated with a particular set of beliefs and practices in an organized or group setting (Hyman & Handal, 2006). While there is some overlap between religion and spirituality, religion was viewed by religious professionals "as objective, external, and ritual or organizational practices that one performs in a group setting and that guide one's behavior; while spirituality was defined as internal, subjective, and divine experience or direct relationship with God" (Hyman & Handal, 2006, p. 264). While this quotation includes a reference to God, the ASERVIC definition of spiritualty does not reference God or a higher power and is applicable to clients who identify as spiritual, agnostic, non-theistic, or atheistic.

When assessing the impact of a client's spirituality and/or religion, counselors can consider spiritual and religious beliefs on a life-affirming to life-constricting continuum (Gladding & Newsome, 2018). For instance, positive religious coping can be a source of support for parents who are navigating life with a new baby (Van Tongeren et al., 2018). In another study of diverse mothers from marginalized backgrounds, spiritual and religious beliefs and practices were a resource to help them cope with depressive symptoms and reconnect with meaningful motivations and sources of inner strength and succor (Curtis et al., 2018). In other situations, specific spiritual or religious beliefs are life-constraining and at odds with other dimensions of a person's identity. Furthermore, people can experience crisis of faith or spiritual conflicts that negatively impact their functioning and wellbeing overall, such as some parents with babies in the Neonatal Intensive Care Unit (NICU) experiencing spiritual struggles such as questioning ultimate meaning in life (Brelsford & Doheny, 2022). Counselors can support new mothers by learning more about their worldview, sense of meaning and purpose, and their spiritual or religious beliefs and the impact of those beliefs on their experience of motherhood.

Modern Western society does not fully embrace rituals to mark a woman's passage to motherhood, which can hinder mothers in their successful transition to motherhood. In the United States it is common to have a baby shower celebrating a baby's imminent arrival. Baby showers include gifts for the baby (and often gifts for the mother as well) and offer a space for a mother's community of family and friends to mark the upcoming arrival of the new baby. Baby showers can function as an "ordinary" ritual that is meaningful to expectant mothers, especially first-time mothers (Han, 2013, as cited in Williams et al., 2022). When "ordinary" pregnancy rituals are lacking or missing, such as during the early days of the COVID-19 pandemic, with in-person baby showers canceled, new mothers reported feeling isolated, without the same sense of community support and acknowledgment (Williams et al., 2022).

Clinicians should be prepared to explore the spiritual and/or religious dimensions of motherhood, the rituals or practices that are meaningful to her, as well as a mother's experience of PPD or other mood symptoms (if applicable). For example, if a woman experiencing PPD believes in fate or karma, this may impact her understanding of how and why the PPD developed as well as her views about how she can recover. For some mothers, connecting with a higher power or with God could be a helping factor in treatment, while for mothers who do not believe in God or a higher power, the approach described above would be counterproductive. Therefore, assessing clients' worldview and spiritual beliefs is essential for providing counseling services in ethically and culturally competent ways. Further, exploring the meaning that each woman ascribes to her PPD, if any, would be an important aspect of treatment.

Applying the *Competencies for Addressing Spiritual and Religious Issue in Counseling*

ASERVIC has developed a helpful resource entitled the *Competencies for Addressing Spiritual and Religious Issue in Counseling* (https://aservic.org/spiritual-and-religious-competencies/). The competencies are grouped into six sections: Culture and Worldview, Counselor Self-Awareness, Human and Spiritual Development, Communication, Assessment, and Diagnosis and Treatment. The first section situates these competencies in the domain of multicultural competencies that counselors have a responsibility to master and practice consistently with the underlying ethical principles of avoiding causing harm, being of benefit, and respecting clients' autonomy (American Counseling Association, 2014). Table 3.4 includes specific applications of these competencies for peripartum clients.

Table 3.4

Applying the *Competencies for Addressing Spiritual and Religious Issue in Counseling*

Specific Competencies	Application to Counseling in the Peripartum
"1. The professional counselor can describe the similarities and differences between spirituality and religion, including the basic beliefs of various spiritual systems, major world religions, agnosticism, and atheism."	Counselors have general knowledge about faith traditions and belief systems and are prepared to discuss issues of beliefs, worldview, spirituality, and religion with their clients. For example, if a new mother seeking treatment shares that she is Sikh, the counselor should already have general knowledge about Sikhism and not expect the client to educate them about it.
"2. The professional counselor recognizes that the client's beliefs (or absence of beliefs) about spirituality and/or religion are central to his or her worldview and can influence psychosocial functioning."	Understand that a person's beliefs or absence of beliefs impact how they view and relate to developmental changes, including conception, pregnancy, and birth.
"4. The professional counselor continuously evaluates the influence of his or her own spiritual and/or religious beliefs and values on the client and the counseling process."	Examining their own spiritual and/or religious beliefs to avoid imposing beliefs or values is especially important so that the counselor can genuinely connect with and create a non-judgmental space for their clients. Many issues in the peripartum period connect to religious beliefs and values, so this is especially pertinent.
"11. When making a diagnosis, the professional counselor recognizes that the client's spiritual and/or religious perspectives can a) enhance well-being; b) contribute to client problems; and/or c) exacerbate symptoms."	In some cases, for some mothers diagnosed with PPD, spiritual beliefs could be a major source of strength as a positive coping strategy as she faces PPD and caring for a new baby. For another mother, spiritual or religious struggles could contribute to her stress. In other cases, spiritual or religious beliefs can exacerbate symptoms.
"13. The professional counselor is able to a) modify therapeutic techniques to include a client's spiritual and/or religious perspectives, and b) utilize spiritual and/or religious practices as techniques when appropriate and acceptable to a client's viewpoint."	Modifying treatment techniques as well as incorporating spirituality and/or religious practices as therapeutically appropriate and if it is considered appropriate from the client's perspective. For example, if a mother shares that prayer has helped her cope with stressful experiences in the past, the counselor could discuss with the mother intentionally integrating prayer into her daily routine as she goes through treatment for PPD and cares for her baby.

Note: The competencies on the lefthand side of the table are quoted from the *Competencies for Addressing Spiritual and Religious Issue in Counseling* (ASERVIC, n.d.-a, pp. 1–2).

The *Competencies for Addressing Spiritual and Religious Issue in Counseling* provide guidance about how clinicians effectively address spirituality and religion in counseling. We recommend that counselors implement these competencies in their work with clients.

WORKING WITH LGBTGEQIAP+ COMMUNITIES

Counselors and mental health professionals working with mothers and families need to be aware and knowledgeable about the needs of parents who identify as LGBTGEQIAP+. Birthing parents who identify as LGBTGEQIAP+ frequently encounter specific challenges and biases when it comes to public perception of their role as parents. LGBTGEQIAP+ is an inclusive initialism that refers to "Lesbian, Gay, Bisexual, Trans, Transgender, & Two Spirit (2S, Native Identity); Gender Expansive, Queer & Questioning, Intersex; Agender, Asexual & Aromantic; Pansexual, Pan/Polygender, & Poly Relationships Systems; and is inclusive of other related identities" (Ausloos, 2020). The process of conception and pregnancy is often conceptualized with a cisgender heteronormative frame (Garbes, 2018). Upon the birth of the baby, LGBTGEQIAP+ mothers/birthing parents may encounter biases and prejudice based on their identity (or how others perceive them) due to heterosexist, homophobic, and transphobic discrimination.

While there has been increased awareness of non-traditional families such as lesbian mothers who choose to adopt or bear children (Hadley & Stuart, 2009), there continue to be unique challenges faced by this population and other sexual and affectional minority populations who seek to become, or are, parents. Furthermore, they may experience a lack of awareness around the process of becoming pregnant and face prejudice, including from healthcare professionals (Markus et al., 2010).

The Society for Sexual, Affectional, Intersex, and Gender Expansive Identities (SAIGE) (formerly the Association for Lesbian, Gay, Bisexual, and Transgender Issues in Counseling; ALGBTIC) has published competencies that can assist counselors in working effectively with members of this population. *Competencies for Counseling with Lesbian, Gay, Bisexual, Queer, Questioning, Intersex, and Ally Individuals* (ALGBTIC LGBQQIA Task Force, Harper et al., 2013) are specific competencies that counselors need to demonstrate to work effectively with clients who are members of these communities. The American Counseling Association's *Competencies for Counseling with Transgender Clients* (ALGBTIC, 2010) is intended to help professional counselors effectively work with transgender clients from a strengths-based and wellness perspective and addresses the need to use gender-affirmative language with transgender clients.

We recommend that counselors familiarize themselves with these competencies and seek support and further education in the form of training, supervision, and consultation if they identify areas in which that they need to develop competence, especially when applying these competencies in the peripartum context, with individuals or couples trying to conceive, those who are pregnant, and new mothers, birthing parents, and their partners/spouses and families.

Applying the *Competencies for Counseling with Lesbian, Gay, Bisexual, Queer, Questioning, Intersex, and Ally Individuals*

The *Competencies for Counseling with Lesbian, Gay, Bisexual, Queer, Questioning, Intersex, and Ally Individuals* were developed by the Lesbian, Gay, Bisexual, Queer, Questioning, Intersex, and Ally (LGBQQIA) Competencies Task Force of the Association for Lesbian, Gay, Bisexual and Transgender Issues in Counseling (ALGBTIC), which is currently called the Society for Sexual, Affectional, Intersex, and Gender Expansive Identities (SAIGE), an organization for counselors and related professionals focused on serving these communities (https://saigecounseling.org/). Table 3.5 highlights specific competencies and applications in the peripartum context.

Table 3.5

Applying the *Competencies for Counseling with Lesbian, Gay, Bisexual, Queer, Questioning, Intersex, and Ally Individuals*

Specific Competencies	Applying Competencies in Counseling in the Peripartum Period
Competent counselors will: A. Human Growth and Development "A.1 Understand that biological, familial, cultural, socioeconomic, and psychosocial factors influence the course of development of affectional orientations and gender identity/expressions."	Understand and effectively address the intersectionality of clients' identities and how these intersect with affectional orientation and gender identity/expressions over the course of the lifespan, including the peripartum period—trying to conceive, pregnancy, birth, and the postpartum.
C. Helping Relationships "C.1. Acknowledge that affectional orientations are unique to individuals and they can vary greatly among and across different populations of LGBQQ people. Further, acknowledge an LGBQQ individual's affectional orientation may evolve across their life span."	Counselors recognize the significance of understanding of the uniqueness of affectional orientation and how it can change over the lifespan (and during the peripartum time) and avoid making assumptions about someone's sexual or affection orientation or gender identity or expression based on pregnancy or family roles.
D. Group Work "D.2. Recognize the power the group process has for LGBQQ members in affirming identity, community development, and connection during all group modalities (e.g., psychoeducation, group tasks, counseling, psychotherapy)."	Develop ways for prospective and expectant and new LGBQQ parents to connect to others who may have similar experiences and can support one another, either through offering counseling groups or providing psychoeducation about the benefits of groups and connections to community resources.

Table 3.5 (Continued)
Applying the *Competencies for Counseling with Lesbian, Gay, Bisexual, Queer, Questioning, Intersex, and Ally Individuals*

Specific Competencies	Applying Competencies in Counseling in the Peripartum Period
E. Professional Orientation and Ethical Practice "E.3. Consult with supervisors/colleagues when their personal values conflict with counselors' professional obligations related to LGBQQ individuals about creating a course of action that promotes the dignity and welfare of LGBQQ individuals."	Counselors have an ethical responsibility to seek supervision/consultation if their own personal values are impeding their ability to provide quality care to LGBQQ clients, including those who are pursuing parenting, pregnancy, surrogacy, adoption, or are new parents.
H. Research and Program Evaluation "H.1. Be aware that the counseling field has a history of pathologizing LGBQQ individuals and communities (e.g., studies of homosexuality as a "disorder" and research agendas that seek to "prove" that affectional orientation and/or gender identity/expression can be "changed"). Understand that these approaches to research and program evaluation have been deemed harmful and unethical in their research goals by professional organizations in the field."	Counselors should acknowledge that the history of pathologizing LGBQQ individuals and communities has an impact on help-seeking behavior. Counselors must strive to communicate affirmatively, challenge heteronormative narratives of pregnancy and new parenthood, and normalize and affirm expectant parenting and new parenting experiences for LGBQQ individuals who are also parents.

Note: The competencies on the lefthand side of the table are quoted from the *Competencies for Counseling with Lesbian, Gay, Bisexual, Queer, Questioning, Intersex, and Ally Individuals* (ALGBTIC LGBQQIA Task Force, Harper et al., 2013, pp. 9–21).

APPLYING THE *COMPETENCIES FOR COUNSELING WITH TRANSGENDER CLIENTS*

The American Counseling Association's *Competencies for Counseling with Transgender Clients* addresses the need for counselors to work effectively with transgender clients. The authors discuss the need for counselors to use transgender-affirmative language, stating "it is important to honor the set of pronouns that clients may identify with and/or select—and to use these pronouns throughout the counseling process" (ALGBTIC, 2010, p. 137). They frame their approach from strengths-based and wellness-oriented theoretical perspectives (ALGBTIC, 2010). In addition, the World Professional Association of Transgender Health (WPATH) *Standards of Care* is a resource for medical and mental health professionals seeking to enhance their understanding of transgender clients' needs and to discuss reproductive health and fertility with clients who are transsexual, transgender, and gender non-conforming, as hormonal therapies impact fertility (WPATH, 2012).

Heteronormative views of pregnancy and new motherhood are dominant, and negatively impact expectant and new mothers/parents who are transgender or gender non-binary or have other expansive gender identities (Garbes, 2018). There is a need for affirming counseling services for transgender and gender-nonconforming parents. It is also recommended that counselors self-reflect on how they define family and invite clients to share their own definition of family and who they consider family, rather than making assumptions based on biology or legal status (ALGBTIC, 2010).

WORKING WITH MILITARY SERVICE MEMBERS, VETERANS, AND THEIR FAMILIES

Military families are those in which a least one individual in the family is currently a member of a branch of the U.S. Armed Forces (Gladding & Newsome, 2018). Military culture is different from civilian culture in terms of ethics, values, and role expectations and those within it face unique stressors (Weiss et al., 2010; Prosek et al., 2018). A taskforce of the Military and Government Counseling Association (a division of the American Counseling Association), developed the *Competencies for Counseling Military Populations*, to help counselors to effectively serve military service members and veterans (Prosek et al., 2018). This document addresses how military and civilian culture differ, the importance of understanding each military branch's subculture, and the unique experiences of reserve members of the military (Prosek et al., 2018).

Pregnancy and parenting as an active-duty service member, or the spouse of an active-duty service member, include a variety of stressors. Sustaining breastfeeding can also be a challenge, although all branches defer deployment in the first six months postpartum (Martin et al., 2015). Counselors providing clinical services to military mothers can invite their clients to share about how their military service has impacted their experience of pregnancy, childbirth, breastfeeding, and caring for their baby.

When someone retires or separates from military service, they are considered a veteran (Prosek et al., 2018) and there is a growing need for clinicians with expertise in working with military veterans (Gladding & Newsome, 2018). Although the veteran suicide rate decreased in both 2019 and 2020, veterans continue to have a higher risk of suicide than the general civilian population (U.S. Department of Veterans' Affairs, 2022). Female veterans have a higher rate of psychiatric disorders and sexual trauma than the general population; researchers have found a significant association between sexual harassment during military service and mothers' peripartum emotional challenges (Miller & Ghadiali, 2018). Therefore, we recommend that clinicians assess military and veteran mothers for sexual harassment and other forms of sexual violence as well as symptoms of PPD. We also recommend that counselors familiarize themselves with the clinical services offered by the Veterans' Administration system.

MULTIPLE PERSPECTIVES: FATHER/PARTNER

Social and cultural expectations of fathers and fatherhood are also shaped by gendered assumptions about what it means to be a father. Another factor that impacts fathers and families is the demand to return quickly to paid employment after their partner gives birth, which can have a negative impact. For instance, a lack of paternal involvement in infant care has been associated with the development of maternal PPD (Séjourné at al., 2012). Supporting fathers can in turn support mothers with postpartum adjustment.

ETHICAL AND LEGAL CONSIDERATIONS

Counselors and other mental health professionals must demonstrate cultural competence with all clients and be prepared to serve diverse clients, as an ethical mandate of the profession (ACA, 2014). It is imperative that counselors demonstrate competence with diverse clients and have knowledge of relevant laws. For instance, the *Competencies for Counseling with Lesbian, Gay, Bisexual, Queer, Questioning, Intersex, and Ally Individuals* specify that counselors should demonstrate understanding and awareness of the key social and historical events, including new legislation, and the meaning of these events for individuals and their mental health (ALGBTIC LGBQQIA Task Force, Harper et al., 2013). Being cognizant of the Americans with Disabilities Act of 1990 and the legal protections for persons with disabilities is imperative to provide ethical care. Further, counselors need to be aware of how legal protections apply in the peripartum context and impact individuals, couples, or families seeking to conceive, birth, adopt, and/or parent a child (or children).

IMPACT OF THE COVID-19 PANDEMIC

COVID-19 made existing gender-based inequalities in workload at home worse (Forbes et al., 2021). Mothers, and especially mothers of color, experienced stress and anxiety during the COVID-19 pandemic (Garland McKinney & Meinersmann, 2022). The COVID-19 pandemic exacerbated existing inequities and disproportionately impacted the Black community (Hassoun Ayoub et al., 2022). In a qualitative study of 35 mothers who were pregnant during the COVID-19 pandemic, all participants reported stress due to public health and conflicting information (Williams et al., 2022). Pregnant Black women reported additional sources of stress compared with White pregnant women due to "heightened awareness of racialized violence" (Williams et al., 2022, p. 1). Being aware of the differential impact of COVID-19 can help counselors to effectively address experiences related to COVID-19 in clinical settings.

CONCLUSION

To provide competent and ethical counseling services, counselors and other mental health professionals working with pregnant individuals and new parents must consider the various dimensions of diversity. Moreover, realizing the intersectionality of identity, counselors, and other mental health professionals should be attuned to ways in which various dimensions of identity intersect and how this relates to a person's experience of privilege and marginality. Furthermore, counselors are ethically mandated to create a safe, inclusive space for all clients, including those who are seeking to start a family, who are pregnant, expectant parents, or who are parents.

> ### Case Study: Cristina—*written by contributor Alexandra Perez*
>
> Cristina begins to struggle emotionally days after giving birth to her daughter. She recently moved from Mexico to the United States, leaving most of her family and friends behind. Due to this recent change and loss of her support system, she is feeling isolated. Cristina lives with her husband and mother-in-law, who since becoming aware of her pregnancy has tried to provide support and advice. Given the good care she received throughout her pregnancy, Cristina was excited to start her family. However, days after giving birth to her first child, Cristina presented to an emergency room given her husband's concern for her wellbeing. When she presented to the emergency room, Cristina's husband reported that she was often tearful, appeared sad, and disengaged. Cristina also appeared tearful, seemed fearful, and did not speak or report on her symptoms to her medical providers or her family members. Cristina only spoke Spanish; however, her husband was bilingual and able to communicate his concerns. A Spanish-speaking crisis worker was able to build rapport and engage Cristina in conversation. The crisis worker validated her feelings of distress and provided information regarding peripartum mood symptoms. Upon further evaluation by crisis workers at the Emergency Room—Psychiatry Department, it became evident that Cristina was presenting with symptoms consistent with peripartum depression, which included: feelings of sadness, feelings of worthlessness, crying easily, difficulty bonding with her newborn, and feelings of failure as a mother. Once suicidal/homicidal ideation was ruled out, the crisis worker was able to walk Cristina over to the hospital's mental health community clinic to complete a thorough evaluation and connect her with appropriate treatment and resources. Through this process Cristina reported feeling helpless due to her inability to properly care for her daughter as expected by others. She identified her inability to breastfeed as a trigger as well. She stated that she had difficulty verbalizing her fears to her husband and mother-in-law due to their expectations of her as a mother. She also reported having difficulty managing the differences in parenting that she and her mother-in-law had. These symptoms were further exacerbated by her feelings of isolation. Cristina informed the crisis worker that she had not been provided with information or education regarding breastfeeding or other childcare needs such as support groups that might be educational and help expand her social support. After this initial evaluation, it was determined that Cristina was experiencing symptoms consistent with peripartum depression. It was evident that cultural and social factors were impacting her emotional wellbeing.

> **Reflection Questions for Clinicians**
>
> - What aspects of Cristina's history/current concerns would you want to follow-up with if you were a counselor/mental health provider?
> - What aspects of Cristina's story may connect with the DSM-5-TR criteria for PPD, or mood symptoms, or the potential development of such symptoms?
> - Are there any aspects of Cristina's story that are personally triggering for you? Are there any aspects of her story that you connect with strongly or feel disconnected from?
> - What social/cultural factors do you believe may be impacting Cristina's level of distress?
> - What intervention/treatment plan/goals would be appropriate in this case?

APPLYING THE STRENGTHS MODEL—THE CASE OF CRISTINA

Significant Individual, Infant, Family, Societal, and Cultural Factors

- Cristina moved from Mexico to the United States.
- Cristina feels isolated due to the loss of a broader support system since her move.
- Cristina started struggling emotionally shortly after giving birth.

Treatment Barriers

- Cristina speaks Spanish and needs treatment providers who speak Spanish fluently.
- Cristina needs access to ongoing services that are affordable.

Risk Factors

- Recent major life transition moving from Mexico to the United States.
- Feeling isolated from broader support system.
- Sadness about inability to breastfeed.

Enlisting Support from Family, the Community, and Medical Professionals

- Family therapy to address family dynamics and help educate her family about her needs for support.
- Include husband in some joint sessions to enhance couple bond.
- Ensure that Cristina has access to ongoing services with a Spanish-speaking provider.

Noticeable Symptoms, Severity, & DSM-5-TR Diagnosis OR Needs Identified by Family & Treatment Team

- Feelings of sadness and worthlessness.
- Crying easily, difficulty bonding with her newborn.
- Feelings of failure as a mother.

Goals Identified by Family

- Her husband is hoping treatment helps Cristina relieve her feelings of sadness and being a failure as a mother.
- Help Cristina function day to day and bond with her daughter.
- Enhance Cristina's wellbeing by building a broader support system in the United States.

Treatment Recommendations

- Address cultural adjustment related to recent move to the United States.
- Interpersonal Therapy to address Cristina's important personal relationships and how she sees herself as a mother.
- Cognitive Behavioral Therapy to address symptoms of depression and distorted cognitions about herself as a mother.

Helpful, Protective, and Resilience Factors

- Cristina has her husband's support.
- Cristina was willing to seek treatment and go the ER due to her husband's concern.
- Cristina has insight into her own symptoms and family dynamics with her mother-in-law that are stressful for her.

Self-Care & Wellness

- Increase Cristina's social support network in the United States.
- Find daily activities that Cristina can do with her baby that are also positive for her, such as taking a daily walk together.

REFERENCES

Abdulrahman M. E., Finkton, D. W., Jr., Paczkowskia, M., Keyesa, K. M., & Galeaa, S. (2015). Socioeconomic position, health behaviors, and racial disparities in cause-specific infant mortality in Michigan, USA. *Preventative Medicine, 76*, 8–13. doi:10.1016/j.ypmed.2015.03.021

Addati, L., Cassirer, N., & Gilchrist, K. (2014). *Maternity and paternity at work: Law and practice across the world*. International Labour Office.

ALGBTIC LGBQQIA Competencies Taskforce: Harper, A., Finerty, P., Martinez, M., Brace, A., Crethar, H. C., Loos, B., Harper, B., Graham, S., Singh, A., Kocet, M., Travis, L., Lambert, S., Burnes, T., Dickey, L. M., & Hammer, T. (2013). Association for Lesbian, Gay, Bisexual, and Transgender Issues in Counseling Competencies for Counseling with Lesbian, Gay, Bisexual, Queer, Questioning, Intersex, and Ally Individuals. *Journal of LGBT Issues in Counseling, 7*(1), 2–43. doi:10.1080/15538605.2013.755444

American Counseling Association. (2014). *2014 Code of Ethics*. https://counseling.org/knowledgecenter/ethics/code-of-ethics-resources

Association for Lesbian, Gay, Bisexual, and Transgender Issues in Counseling. (ALGBTIC). (2010). American Counseling Association Competencies for Counseling with Transgender Clients. *Journal of LGBT Issues in Counseling, 4*(3), 135–159. doi:10.1080/15538605.2010.524839

Andres, E., Baird, S., Bingenheimer, J. B., & Markus, A. R. (2016). Maternity leave access and health: A systematic narrative review and conceptual framework development. *Maternal and Child Health Journal, 20*, 1178–1192. doi:10.1007/s10995-015-1905-9

Association for Spiritual, Ethical, and Religious Values in Counseling (ASERVIC). (n.d.-a). *Competencies for addressing spiritual and religious issues in counseling*. https://aservic.org/spiritual-and-religious-competencies/

Association for Spiritual, Ethical, and Religious Values in Counseling (ASERVIC). (n.d.-b). *A white paper of the Association for Spiritual, Ethical, and Religious Values in Counseling*. https://aservic.org/aservic-white-paper/

Ausloos, C. D. (2020). LGBTGEQIAP+ initialism. SAIGE Counseling, https://saigecounseling.org/

Avendano, M., Berkman, L. F., Brugiavini, A., & Pasini, G. (2015). The long-run effect of maternity leave benefits on mental health: Evidence from European countries. *Social Science & Medicine, 132*, 45–53. doi:10.1016/j.soscimed.2015.02.037

Baker, L., Cross, S., Greaver, L., Wei, G., & Lewis, R. (2005). Prevalence of postpartum depression in a Native American population. *Maternal and Child Health Journal, 9*(1), 21–25. doi:10.1007/s10995-005-2448-2

Bell, L. A. (2023). Theoretical foundations for social justice education. In Adams, M., Bell, L. A., Goodman, D. J., Shlasko, D., Briggs, R. R., & Pacheco, R. (Eds.), *Teaching for diversity and social justice* (4th ed., pp. 3–26). Routledge.

Bina, R. (2008). The impact of cultural factors upon postpartum depression: A literature review. *Health Care for Women International, 29*, 568–592. doi:10.1080/07399330802089149

Brelsford, G. M., & Doheny, K. K. (2022). Parents' spiritual struggles and stress: Associations with mental health and cognitive well-being following a Neonatal Intensive Care Unit Experience. *Psychology of Religion and Spirituality, 14*(1), 119–127. doi:10.1037/rel0000381

Centers for Disease Control and Prevention (CDC). (n.d.-a). Severe maternal morbidity in the United States. https://www.cdc.gov/reproductivehealth/maternalinfanthealth/severematernalmorbidity.html

Centers for Disease Control and Prevention (CDC). (n.d.-b). Infant mortality. https://www.cdc.gov/reproductivehealth/maternalinfanthealth/infantmortality.htm

Chapin, M., McCarthy, H., Shaw, L., Bradham-Cousar, M., Chapman, R., Nosek, M., Peterson, S., Yilmaz, Z., & Ysasi, N. (2018). *Disability-related counseling competencies*. American Rehabilitation Counseling Association, a division of ACA. http://www.arcaweb.org/key-note-speaker/

Choe, E. J. Y., Jankowski, P. J., Sandage, S. J., Crabtree, S. A., & Captari, L. E. (2022). A practice-based study of cultural humility and well-being among psychotherapy clients. *Counselling & Psychotherapy Research*, doi:10.1002/capr.12599

Conteh, N., Gagliardi, J., McGahee, S., Molina, R., Clark, C. T., & Clare, C. A. (2022). Medical mistrust in perinatal mental health. *Harvard Review of Psychiatry, 30*(4), 238–247. doi:10.1097/HRP.0000000000000345

Crenshaw, K. E. (1989). Demarginalizing the intersection of race and sex: A Black feminist critique of antidiscrimination doctrine, feminist theory and antiracist politics. *University of Chicago Legal Forum, 1989*(1), 139–167.

Curtis, C., Morgan, J., & Laird, L. (2018). Mothers' gardens in arid soil: A study of religious and spiritual coping among marginalized U.S. Mothers with depression. *Journal of Spirituality in Mental Health, 20*(4), 293–320. doi:10.1080/19349637.2018.1428139

Day-Vines, N., Wood, S. M., Grothaus, T., Craigen, L., Holman, A., Dotson-Blake, K., & Douglass, M. J. (2007). Broaching the Subjects of Race, Ethnicity, and Culture During the Counseling Process. *Journal of Counseling and Development, 85*(4), 401–409. doi:10.1002/j.1556-6678.2007.tb00608.x

Day-Vines, N. L., Cluxton-Keller, F., Agorsor, C., Gubara, S., & Otabil, N. A. A. (2020). The multidimensional model of broaching behavior. *Journal of Counseling & Development, 98*(1), 107–118. doi:10.1002/jcad.12304

Eunice Kennedy Shriver National Institute of Child Health and Human Development. (n.d.). Maternal morbidity and mortality. https://www.nichd.nih.gov/health/topics/factsheets/maternal-morbidity-mortality, National Institutes of Health, US Department of Health and Human Services.

Family and Medical Leave Act of 1993, 29 U.S.C. §§2601–2654 (2006).

Forbes, L. K., Donovan, C., & Lamar, M. R. (2020). Differences in intensive parenting attitudes and gender norms among U.S. mothers. *The Family Journal: Counseling and Therapy for Couples and Families, 28*(1), 63–71. doi:10.1177/1066480719893964

Forbes, L. K., Lamar, M. R., Speciale, M., & Donovan, C. (2021). Mothers' and fathers' parenting attitudes during COVID-19. *Current Psychology, 41*(1), 470–479. doi: 10.1007/s12144-021-01605-x

Gamble, J., & Creedy, D. (2004). Content and processes of postpartum counseling after a distressing birth experience: A review. *Birth, 31*(3), 213–218. doi:10.1111/j.0730-7659.2004.00307.x

Garbes, A. (2018). *Like a mother: A feminist journey through the science and culture of pregnancy*. Harper Wave.

Garland McKinney, J. L., & Meinersmann, L. M. (2022). The cost of intersectionality: Motherhood, mental health, and the state of the country. *Journal of Social Issues*, 1–21. doi:10.1111/josi.12539

Gladding, S. T., & Newsome, D. W. (2018). *Clinical mental health counseling in community and agency settings* (5th ed.). The Merrill Counseling Series. Pearson.

Glazer, K. B, & Howell, E. A. (2021). A way forward in the maternal mortality crisis: Addressing maternal health disparities and mental health. *Archives of Women's Mental Health, 24*(5), 823–830. doi:10.1007/s00737-021-01161-0

Hadley, E., & Stuart, J. (2009). The expression of parental identifications in lesbian mothers' work and family arrangements. *Psychoanalytic Psychology, 26*(1), 42–68. doi:10.1037/a0014676

Haga, S. M., Ulleberg, P., Slinning, K., Kraft, P., Steen, T. B., & Staff, A. (2012). A longitudinal study of postpartum depressive symptoms: Multilevel growth curve analyses of emotion regulation strategies, breastfeeding self-efficacy, and social support. *Archives of Women's Mental Health, 15*(3), 175–184. doi:10.1007/s00737-012-0274-2

Hassoun Ayoub, L., Partridge, T., & Gómez, J. M. (2022). Two sides of the same coin: A mixed methods study of black mothers' experiences with violence, stressors, parenting, and coping during the COVID-19 pandemic. *Journal of Social Issues*, 1–27. doi:10.1111/josi.12526

Hogan, S. (2017). The tyranny of expectations of postnatal delight: Gendered happiness. *Journal of Gender Studies, 26*(1), 45–55. doi:10.1080/09589236.2016.1223617

Hoyert, D. L. (2022). Maternal mortality rates in the United States, 2020. NCHS Health E-Stats. 2022. doi:10.15620/cdc:113967

Hyman, C., & Handal, P. J. (2006). Definitions and evaluation of religion and spirituality items by religious professionals: A pilot study. *Journal of Religion and Health, 45*(2), 264–282. doi:10.1007/s10943-006-9015-z

Jou, J., Kozhimannil, K. B., Abraham, J. M., Blewett, L. A., & McGovern, P. M. (2018). Paid maternity leave in the United States: Associations with maternal and infant health. *Maternal and Child Health Journal, 22*(2), 216–225. doi:10.1007/s10995-017-2393-x

Khan, M. S. (2020). Paid family leave and children health outcomes in OECD countries. *Children and Youth Services Review, 116*, 11. doi:10.1016/j.childyouth.2020.105259

King, K. M. (2021). "I want to, but how?" Defining counselor broaching in core tenets and debated components. *Journal of Multicultural Counseling and Development, 49*(2), 87–100. doi:10.1002/jmcd.12208

Markus, E., Weingarten, A., Duplessi, Y., & Jones, J. (2010). Lesbian couples seeking pregnancy with donor insemination. *Journal of Midwifery & Women's Health, 55*(2), 124–132. doi:10.1016/j.jmwh.2009.09.014

Martin, S. E., Emily Drake, E., Yoder, L., Gibson, M., & Litke, C. A. (2015). Active duty women's perceptions of breast-feeding support in the military setting. *Military Medicine, 180*(11), 1154–1160. doi:10.7205/MILMED-D-14-00498

Miller, L. J., & Ghadiali, N. Y. (2018). Mental health across the reproductive cycle in women veterans. *Military Medicine, 183*(5/6), e140–e146. doi:10.1093/milmed/usx094

Mitra, M., Long-Bellil, L. M., Iezzoni, L. I., Smeltzer, S. C., & Smith, L. D. (2016). Pregnancy among women with physical disabilities: Unmet needs and recommendations on navigating pregnancy. *Disability and Health Journal, 9*(3), 457–463. doi:10.1016/j.dhjo.2015.12.007

Mosher, D. K., Hook, J. N., Captari, L. E., Davis, D. E., DeBlaere, C., & Owen, J. (2017). Cultural humility: A therapeutic framework for engaging diverse clients. *Practice Innovations, 2*(4), 221–233. doi:10.1037/pri0000055

Prosek, E. A., Burgin, E. E., Atkins, K. M., Wehrman, J. D., Fenell, D. L., Carter, C., & Green, L. (2018). Competencies for counseling military populations. *Journal of Military and Government Counseling, 6*(2), 87–99. https://veteranmentalhealth.com/wp-content/uploads/2019/11/Counseling-Competencies.pdf

Ratts, M. J., Singh, A. A., Nassar-McMillan, S., Butler, S. K., & McCullough, J. R. (2015). Multicultural and social justice counseling competencies. https://www.multiculturalcounselingdevelopment.org/competencies

Ratts, M. J., Singh, A. A., Nassar-McMillan, S., Butler, S. K. and McCullough, J. R. (2016). Multicultural and social justice counseling competencies: Guidelines for the counseling profession. *Journal of Multicultural Counseling and Development, 44*(1), 28–48. doi:10.1002/jmcd.12035

Ruppanner, L., Collins, C., Landivar, L. C., & Scarborough, W. J. (2021). Norms, childcare costs, and maternal employment. *Gender & Society, 35*(6), 910–939. doi:10.1177/08912432211046988

Scheyer, K., & Urizar, Jr., G. G. (2016). Altered stress patterns and increased risk for postpartum depression among low-income pregnant women. *Archive of Women's Mental Health, 19*, 317–328. doi:10.1007/s00737-015-0563-7

Schindler-Ruwisch, J., & Eaves, T. (2022). Maternity leave in America during a pandemic: The impact of leave on family wellbeing. *Families, Systems & Health, 40*(1), 132–135. doi:10.1037/fsh0000629

Séjourné, N., Vaslot, V., Beaumé, M., Goutaudier, N., & Chabrol, H. (2012). The impact of paternity leave and paternal involvement in child care on maternal postpartum depression, *Journal of Reproductive and Infant Psychology, 30*(2), 135–144. doi:10.1080/02646838.2012.693155

Shepherd-Banigan, M., & Bell, J. F. (2014). Paid leave benefits among a national sample of working mothers with infants in the United States. *Maternal and Child Health Journal, 18*, 286–295. doi:10.1007/s10995-013-1264-3

Slopen, M. (2020). Type and lengths of family leave among New York City women: Exploring the composition of paid and unpaid leave. *Maternal and Child Health Journal, 24*(4), 514–523. doi:10.1007/s10995-020-02884-9

Ugarriza, D. N. (2004). Group therapy and its barriers for women suffering from postpartum depression. *Archives of Psychiatric Nursing, 18*(2), 39–48. doi:10.1053/j.apnu.2004.01.002

U.S. Department of Health and Human Services (2022, July 27). Improving access to telehealth. https://telehealth.hhs.gov/providers/health-equity-in-telehealth/improving-access-to-telehealth/

U.S. Department of Labor (n.d.). What to expect from your employer when you are expecting. https://www.dol.gov/agencies/whd/maternal-health

U.S. Department of Veterans' Affairs (2022). 2022 National veteran suicide prevention annual report. https://news.va.gov/108984/2022-national-veteran-suicide-prevention-annual-report/

Van Tongeren, D. R., Worthington, E. L., Jr., Davis, D. E., Hook, J. N., Reid, C. A., & Garthe, R. C. (2018). Positive religious coping in relationships predicts spiritual growth through communication with the sacred. *Psychology of Religion and Spirituality, 10*(1), 55–62. doi:10.1037/rel0000120

Wang, E., Glazer, K. B., Sofaer, S., Balbierz, A., & Howell, E. A., (2021). Racial and ethnic disparities in severe maternal morbidity: A qualitative study of women's experiences of peripartum care. *Women's Health Issues, 30*(1), 75–81. doi:10.1016/j.whi.2020.09.002

Weiss, E. L., Coll, J. E., Gerbauer, J., Smiley, K., & Carillo, E. (2010). The military genogram: A solution-focused approach to resiliency building in service members and their families. *The Family Journal, 18*(4), 395–406. doi:10.1177/1066480710378

Williams, C. E., Berkowitz, D., & Rackin, H. M. (2022). Exploring the experiences of pregnant women in the U.S. during the first year of the Covid-19 pandemic. *Journal of Social Issues*, 1–29. doi:10.1111/josi.12567

World Professional Association of Transgender Health (WPATH). (2012). Standards of care for the health of transsexual, transgender, and gender-nonconforming people. 7th version.

International Journal of Transgenderism, 13(4), 165–232. doi:10.1080/15532739.2011.700873

Zittel-Palamara, K., Rockmaker, J., Schwabel, K. M., Weinstein, W. L., & Thompson, S. J. (2008). Desired assistance versus care received for postpartum depression: Differences by race. *Archive of Women's Mental Health, 11*(2), 81–92. doi:10.1007/s00737-008-0001-1

4

Assessing Risk Factors for Peripartum Depression and Enhancing Protective Factors to Support Wellbeing

Isabel A. Thompson
with contributor Jamie Hildebrandt Jerome

Personal Narrative

One woman, two pregnancies, and two very different pregnancies at that. My first pregnancy (although medically I had some challenges), mentally it was flawless. I could not wait to be a mom, to be her mom. I delivered my daughter at 38 weeks and 4 days due to IUGR (intrauterine growth restriction). She stopped growing at 32 weeks, so the doctors monitored me heavily. Labor was easy but after birth she was whisked away by the NICU team, as she was considered a preemie based on her weight. When they finally handed her to me, I could breathe again. My little girl was here. For the next 18 months we stayed by other's side, she was my "mini-me," my "partner in crime." Our close bond is why, even though our second pregnancy was planned, and we wanted our children close in age, I believe I began to have perinatal anxiety during my pregnancy with our second child.

During the pregnancy with our second, I had days where I would stay in bed and sit in a dark room because I felt that anyone was better suited to be a mother to my children than myself. I had both panic and anxiety attacks. I could not breathe; my heart would be racing a mile a minute. My fear was all consuming. I also have a personal history of depression as a teenager after my cousin's death, who was a close friend.

When I found out I was pregnant with our second child; my immediate feeling was excitement and joy. That quickly changed to "Is my daughter going to hate me?" and "Am I ruining her life?" Questions like these ran rampant throughout my pregnancy and did not subside. Medically, this pregnancy was fine, although I had morning sickness up until I delivered my son. Mentally this pregnancy took its toll.

When I went into labor with our second, I had just dropped my daughter off at school and made the 30-minute trek to Trader Joe's grocery store. I called my

DOI: 10.4324/9780429440892-4

best friend who is an OB/GYN [obstetrician/gynecologist], and she suggested I go to the hospital immediately. I was not mentally prepared to have the baby that day, I was scheduled to be induced the following week. I was not ready for someone else to pick up my daughter from school, especially since I did not prepare her for that and picked her up. Later we went to the hospital and although I was having contractions, they were not close enough and I went home. The next day my doctor recommended I go back to the hospital. I was sent to Labor and Delivery and immediately my emotions went from guilt and fear to excitement.

My son's delivery was even quicker than my daughter's. Immediately I felt as I did when she was born, and I could not stop smiling or stop smothering him in kisses. The next morning my parents brought our daughter to meet her baby brother. The first few weeks as a family of four were flawless.

I am not able to breastfeed, something we discovered after my daughter's birth, so we made the decision to have a nurse help us so I could sleep and be my best for both kids. This was the same nurse who took care of my daughter, so we had what we thought was a great relationship. We knew her routine, and she knew ours. After a few weeks of her being in our home, something shifted, and I was pushed to the back burner. She acted as if our son was hers, as if she knew him better. She brushed aside things I said because she had more experience with babies.

I can pinpoint the exact moment that an internal switch flipped, and I went from "fine" to "not fine." My daughter was at school, our baby nurse was caring for my son, and I decided to do something for myself by getting a haircut. My mother called me while I was parking to tell me that the stylist was canceling my appointment. I felt defeated. It seems so silly, over a haircut, but the symbolism was deeper. It was the first time, in probably two years, I had any time for myself, and experiencing a cancellation made me feel as though I, as a mom, would never matter again. I came home and got into bed—defeated—over something that normally I would not care about. I told my husband something was wrong and asked him to call my best friend (who is an OB/GYN). I wished that someone, anyone had asked me questions during my pregnancy about how I was feeling, because maybe it would not have been so severe.

After feeling this way for a few days, I decided to call a therapist who specialized in postpartum. Immediately after my first session, everything improved, and a weight was lifted. I gained more confidence in my mothering after each session. I went to therapy for about six months when I felt better and took a step back from therapy but began having panic attacks. I went back to therapy quickly and began weekly sessions again. Six months after going back I made the decision to seek a psychiatrist to discuss medications to help in my healing.

> I continued therapy weekly and then saw my therapist monthly. This support was the biggest factor in me coming through the other side of postpartum depression and anxiety. I vividly remember my first session of therapy and my therapist said to me "Postpartum is not normal, it's common." The feelings and emotions women feel in the postpartum are unique to any other feeling and there is no way to prepare for how we will feel after birth. Remembering we are not alone, and it is so important that we speak up on behalf of all mothers to help everyone get the help and support new mothers, and not-so-new mothers need.
>
> —*Jamie Hildebrandt Jerome*

In this chapter, we examine various risk factors associated with the development of peripartum depression (PPD) as well as protective factors that buffer mothers against developing PPD and other maternal mood disorders. We discuss how counselors can assess significant personal risk factors associated with the development of PPD and explore how to assess these risk factors to enhance preventative efforts as well as implement effective early intervention. We also focus on ways to enhance protective factors to build on mothers' and families' strengths. We discuss ways to improve prenatal screening, and to effectively take action to connect mothers with needed treatment. Further, we discuss risk and protective factors associated with the development of peripartum suicidality and the need for screening, early intervention, and treatment to protect mothers and babies.

RISK FACTORS FOR THE DEVELOPMENT OF PPD

> Every year more than 400,000 infants are born to mothers who are depressed, making PPD the most under-diagnosed obstetric complication in America. Most women typically only have 1–2 postpartum visits with their obstetricians, where depression screening may not always occur. For low-income women, particularly minorities, the risk of undiagnosed and untreated depression is especially high because of below-average rates of postpartum follow-up visits with obstetricians.
> (Postpartum Support International (PSI), n.d.-a)

There are numerous risk factors associated with the development of peripartum depression including lack of support from one's partner, the experience of judgment, lack of familial support, a personal history of depression or anxiety, familial history of depression or bipolar disorder, low maternal age, psychosocial risk factors such as stressful life events, and many more (Dagher et al., 2021; Davey et al., 2011; Silverman et al., 2017). Often, these risk factors are intertwined; counselors working with new mothers should consider various risk and protective factors in their case conceptualization and treatment process. It is essential for counselors to listen closely to a woman's narrative, her pregnancy, birth, and postpartum experience, as well as screen for PPD and other mood disorders.

The quote above from Postpartum Support International reveals the staggering numbers of women, babies, and families impacted by PPD and the dearth of care women often receive after childbirth. No matter the type of birth, vaginal or cesarean, a woman's body experiences stress and sometimes trauma during birth, and that stress and trauma, both mental and physical, deserves the necessary time, support, and treatment to allow for healing. It is hard for a mother to be healthy and confident when she herself is healing, often with limited support from healthcare providers. In addition, lack of partner support and increased conflict is associated with PPD symptoms (Hassert & Kurpius, 2011). Counselors can provide support for the mother and father/same-sex partner, while assessing for risk factors, bolstering protective factors, and advocating for the support mothers need. We begin by examining the importance of partner support for new mothers.

THE SIGNIFICANCE OF PARTNER SUPPORT

Partner support is crucial for new mothers' wellbeing whereas a lack of partner/spousal support has been associated with developing PPD (Kettunen & Hintikka, 2017; Hassert & Kurpius, 2011). Partner support can buffer women from the risk associated with a personal history of depression. In a study of over 1,500 mothers who had recently given birth, researchers found that "supportive couples' relationships protected women from PPD symptoms even when the women were at risk for PPD because of the biological risk factor of a history of depression" (Banker & LaCoursiere, 2014, p. 507). Despite the benefits of partner social support, sometimes new mothers do not get the partner support they want and need. First-time partners/fathers may experience a lack of support for their role transition into parenthood and this, in turn, may impede their ability to support the new mother. Fathers/partners who are welcoming another child into the family experience pressures to parent their older child (or children), while simultaneously supporting the partner who gave birth and bonding with the new baby. Further, fathers and same-sex partners who did not give birth are expected to return to work quickly and may not integrate the birth experience and their parental roles.

The quality of the partner relationship can impact both partners. For instance, poor quality of romantic relationship has been associated with paternal depression in a study of Mexican American fathers (Roubinov et al., 2014). Mothers who feel a lack of support from their partners may be at a greater risk of developing PPD (Kettunen & Hintikka, 2017). In another study, women who reported less marital conflict and increased perceived support reported significantly fewer PPD symptoms than women who reported increased conflict and decreased support (Hassert & Kurpius, 2011).

LACK OF SOCIETAL SUPPORT

A major stressor for many new mothers and fathers/partners is the lack of paid leave from employment, which constitutes a lack of societal support. Paid parental leave is critically important, but as of this writing there is no federally guaranteed paid family leave (United States Department of Labor, n.d.). FMLA (Family and Medical Leave Act) can be used by families to cobble together leave time to be with their baby (or babies), but it is unpaid (unless a worker can use paid leave, or an employer voluntarily pays), and only applies to certain workers in specific employment settings (Andres et al., 2016). Although awareness of the need for paid parental leave is growing and more companies are offering paid leave; this depends on the nature and quality of employment.

SOCIETAL JUDGMENT

Society places a great deal of pressure on mothers which impacts how mothers are judged and evaluated by members of their family and the public, as well as how they judge themselves. Every choice a mother makes is seemingly up for judgment, which can have a negative impact on mothers. As Meeussen and Van Laar (2018) mention, "women's feelings of being pressured to be a perfect mother are related to increased maternal guilt, lower self-efficacy beliefs, and higher stress levels" (p. 2). A mother's self-worth and efficacy are negatively impacted when family, friends, or even strangers judge and evaluate their parenting choices.

Mothers need and deserve support, and instead of receiving support (during what is most likely the most vulnerable time in their lives), they often experience judgment. While this judgment may be well-meaning, the impact is negative as it undermines a mother's confidence. As counselors, is it essential to avoid judging a client's mothering, as this can damage the therapeutic relationship and replicate the experiences of judgement mothers face in broader society.

Judgment Related to Breastfeeding Decisions

Women who choose not to breastfeed or are unable to breastfeed often feel judged. Whether a woman chooses not to breastfeed (for any reason) or is simply unable to is a decision for that woman and family, but unfortunately mothers often face judgment instead of support as they navigate how to feed their baby. Challenges with breastfeeding are common, such as perceived insufficient milk supply, which can be a source of distress in the early postpartum and a contributor to early cessation of breastfeeding (Peacock-Chambers et al., 2017). Some women experience pain and discomfort with breastfeeding, which is a factor in stopping breastfeeding (Hauck et al., 2011). Breastfeeding challenges can have a negative mental health effect. Kristen Thompson, a contributor for *Today Parenting*, shared her midwife's response to her decision not to breastfeed: "whatever was best for my mental health was best for my baby and gave me a hug. It was one of the most liberating moments of my life, and I learned to simply enjoy feeding my baby" (2020, para. 12).

Some women feel the pressure to breastfeed at the expense of their own physical or mental health or their baby's health. For a mother trying to breastfeed but experiencing challenges, it is crucial that the baby be nourished whether with breastmilk or formula (Mohrbacher & Kendall-Tackett, 2010). While overall breastfeeding has been associated with a reduction in depressive symptoms, experiencing problems with initiating or sustaining breastfeeding can increase depressive symptoms (PSI, n.d.-a; Hahn-Holbrook et al., 2013; Figueiredo et al. 2014).

PERSONAL HISTORY OF DEPRESSION

A mother's personal history of mental illness, specifically depression, is a risk factor for the development of PPD (Meltzer-Brody et al., 2013; Baker et al., 2005). Researchers examining a range of risk factors in a nationally representative epidemiological study in the United States reported that personal history of a mental disorder was a strong predictor of a woman experiencing peripartum depression; specifically "depression," "substance use disorder," "bipolar disorder," "and history of suicide attempt" (Tebeka et al., 2016, p. 62). Clinicians are advised to comprehensively screen for the mother's personal history of mental illness, as well as her family history of mental illness. Researchers have also identified history of premenstrual dysphoric disorder (PMDD) (Bloch et al., 2005) and premenstrual syndrome (Gastaldon et al., 2022) as risk factors for PPD. Obtaining an accurate medical history and accurate assessment of current symptoms is key to prevention and effective early intervention with PPD.

When a pregnant woman enters her obstetrician's or midwife's office for the first time, she is asked about her medical history, her partner's medical history, and any known conditions within either family. She is also given options for screening tests. For a healthy pregnancy, a woman will go to the OB/GYN's or midwife's office approximately 15 times. For a pregnancy that carries more risk—such as a twin pregnancy, someone with an advanced maternal age (pregnant age 35 or older), diabetes, or other conditions—the woman may be seen more frequently and may also be seen by additional specialists. Despite this, rarely does a provider ask any questions pertaining to her mental health. However, it is crucial that clinicians obtain a comprehensive medical history, including mental health history, as the risk of developing PPD is at least 20 times greater among women with a prior history of depression according to analysis of a population-based study in Sweden (Silverman et al., 2017).

PERIPARTUM SUICIDALITY

Suicidality is a broad term that refers to suicidal ideation (SI), self-harming behaviors with or without the intent to die by suicide, intentional suicide attempts, and death by suicide (Martini et al., 2019). Maternal suicide is one of the leading causes of maternal death in the peripartum period (Gressier et al., 2017). A comprehensive psychosocial history which includes questions about previous SI and suicide attempts, along with information about a mother's sources of social support, is key to assessing both risk and protective factors.

Risk Factors Associated with Maternal Suicide Attempts

Maternal suicide attempts (SA) during pregnancy are associated with maternal alcohol use, smoking while pregnant, and a personal history of miscarriage (Gressier et al., 2017, p. 284). During the postpartum period, SA has been associated with experiencing a major depressive episode or recurrent depression, as well as the younger age of the mother (Gressier et al., 2017). Therefore, clinicians need to gather comprehensive information about a mother's mental health history, symptoms of depression, substance use, and perinatal loss history.

RISK FACTORS FOR POSTPARTUM PSYCHOSIS

Postpartum psychosis (PPP) is rare, with 1–2 in 1,000 of the population experiencing it (PSI, n.d.-b). The DSM-5-TR does not include PPP as a separate diagnosis, but rather uses the term "postpartum psychotic mood episode" or "postpartum mood episode with psychotic features" (APA, 2022, p. 174). Mothers who have had a previous postpartum mood episode with psychotic features, or who have a personal or family history of depression or bipolar I, have a higher risk of developing another episode following delivery (APA, 2022). After a mother has had a postpartum psychotic episode, the risk of episodes for any future birth is 30 percent to 50 percent (APA, 2022). Among women with PPP, there is a 5 percent maternal suicide rate and a 4 percent rate of infanticide (PSI, n.d.-b).

A challenge associated with accurate diagnosis and treatment of mothers in distress who are experiencing psychosis (and preventing maternal infanticide associated with postpartum psychosis) is that postpartum psychosis has not been a diagnosis in the DSM (Spinelli, 2018). The DSM-5-TR specifier "with peripartum onset" can be applied for Brief Psychotic Disorder (APA, 2022) but it does not provide specific diagnoses for peripartum disorders, which is at odds with the hormonal changes associated with childbirth and hinders efforts to advocate for mothers with mental illness in the judicial system (Spinelli, 2018).

MATERNAL AGE

Women who give birth at an early age are at an especially elevated risk of developing PPD, with the greatest risk for the youngest group of women (20 years old or younger) (Meltzer-Brody et al., 2017). Younger age has also been associated with suicide attempts in the postpartum period (Gressier et al., 2017). Women who are over 35 at the start of their pregnancy are at higher risk of developing depressive symptoms. This is significant, given that many women delay childbearing in industrialized societies and, thus, the number of mothers who fall into this category is increasing (García-Blanco et al., 2017). Given the risks associated with PPD at both younger and older maternal ages, there is a u-shaped relationship between maternal age and PPD, with both younger mothers and older mothers at higher risk of developing PPD, albeit for varying reasons, as compared with adult mothers who become pregnant between the ages of 20 and 35.

Teenage Mothers

Mothers who are teenagers are at a higher risk of developing PPD compared with adult mothers between the ages of 20 and 35 (Kim et al. 2014). Social support may play a role in buffering the stress associated with childbirth, but mothers in their teens have less social support compared with adult mothers (ages 20 to 35) and advanced maternal age mothers (over age 35) (Kim et al., 2014). Teenage mothers often face other challenges, such as barriers to completing their education (as in the case study of Juliette at the end of this chapter). They may not be in a stable relationship, they may not have a supportive microsystem at home, and they may have financial stress. It is also important to consider intersectionality, as researchers have found that the "youngest mothers, mothers with short education, and low income had the greatest risk of experiencing PPD" (Meltzer-Brody et al., 2017, p. 1431).

Mothers Who Are Pregnant Over Age 35

Mothers who become pregnant and give birth later in life are also at higher risk of developing PPD (García-Blanco et al., 2017). "Advanced maternal age" is the term applied to primiparous (first-time mothers) at age 35 or above and multiparous (second-time or more mothers) who are 40 or above at the time of delivery (Kim et al., 2017). Women may fear negative outcomes or medical complications, as pregnancy at an advanced maternal age is associated with a higher risk of fetal abnormality (Murakami et al., 2016). Some pregnant people may not be aware of age-specific risks, and it is recommended that they be made aware of prenatal testing options (Murakami et al., 2016).

Women who give birth over age 35 are more likely to have increased cortisol levels and depressive symptoms than mothers who are younger than 35; however, they are also more likely to have social support, which may counterbalance the increased stress they experience (García-Blanco et al., 2017). Counselors can focus on their clients' strengths and resilience, while screening and assessing for mental health risks associated with pregnancy prior to age 20 and pregnancy over age 35 in a non-judgmental way.

PSYCHOSOCIAL RISK FACTORS

In addition to the risk factors detailed above, counselors need to consider the psychosocial risk factors a woman and her family are experiencing, as these can increase her risk of developing PPD or other mood disorders. Past-year predictors of major depressive episodes among peripartum women include experiencing a recent stressful life event such as being dismissed from work or a change in residence, as measured by 12 questions from the Holmes and Rahe Social Readjustment Rating Scale (Tebeka et al., 2016). Bereavement is also associated with the development of a major depressive episode in the peripartum period (Tebeka et al., 2016). Women who are divorced or widowed are at higher risk of developing PPD (Meltzer-Brody et al., 2017). Psychosocial stressors such as experiencing intimate partner violence can increase the risk of developing PPD (Tebeka et al., 2016). Unintended pregnancy has also been identified as a risk factor for development of PPD (Gastaldon et al., 2022). Mental health professionals should screen for psychosocial stressors and risk factors in the peripartum period and provide psychoeducation to partners/families about the importance of supporting new mothers and buffering them from psychosocial risk factors. Mothers often experience more than one life stressor, and the compounded impact of these stressors should be addressed. In addition to addressing stressors, we recommend clinicians focus on enhancing protective factors in treatment, which is a strengths-based approach.

ENHANCING PROTECTIVE FACTORS

Preventative and early intervention efforts to enhance protective factors among all pregnant women, especially those at risk for developing PPD, are recommended. Prenatal screening for depression and anxiety-related disorders is needed during prenatal medical appointments as 50 percent of peripartum depression cases begin during the pregnancy stage (APA, 2022). Prenatal educational classes and psychoeducation about PPD should be more readily available and affordable.

Protective factors buffer mothers from stress in the peripartum period and the potential of developing PPD or another maternal mood disorder. For instance, bonding between mother and baby, especially through close touch and breastfeeding immediately after birth, is a protective factor against the development of PPD symptoms (Bingol & Bal, 2020). Social support is a protective factor that has been shown to alleviate stress and enhance quality of life (Milgrom et al., 2019). Therefore, enhancing mother–baby bonding is essential. Enhancing social support, whether it be familial, social, or professional, is also crucial. Another protective factor is a mother's own level of wellbeing, which can be enhanced through social support and helping the mother establish a self-care routine that is feasible in the postpartum period (Milgrom et al., 2019).

BONDING BETWEEN MOTHER AND BABY

Breastfeeding and close touch immediately after giving birth have been found to reduce PPD symptoms (Bingol & Bal, 2020). However, not all mothers breastfeed, and other ways to promote bonding should be explored. Doctors, nurses, and hospitals need to be better equipped to support a woman with bonding and caring for her baby, regardless of how she chooses to feed her child. For instance, skin-to-skin contact should be encouraged whether a mother breastfeeds or not. Skin-to-skin contact can also support the bonding process between the father (or another parent/caregiver) and the baby.

Breastfeeding and Bonding

While breastfeeding has benefits for both mother and baby, healthcare providers should know "the importance of providing breastfeeding support to women who want to breastfeed; but also providing compassionate support for women who had intended to breastfeed, but who find themselves unable to" (Borra et al. 2015, p. 897). Counselors can be a part of this compassionate care for mothers by helping them to bond with their babies and finding support for their breastfeeding goals, while also normalizing breastfeeding challenges and that some mothers cannot, or choose not to, breastfeed.

Postpartum Support International (PSI) is one of the leading providers for women worldwide. "Depressed mothers are less likely to breastfeed, nurse for shorter durations, and have more negative emotions and experiences toward breastfeeding. New mothers experiencing breastfeeding difficulty may be more likely to be suffering from PPD, highlighting the importance of screening" (PSI, n.d.-a). There is a need for non-judgmental support around breastfeeding goals with an awareness that breastfeeding struggles can increase emotional distress and the risk of PPD. If the benefits of breastfeeding are outweighed by the stress, other options for bonding and close skin-to-skin contact can be explored. Resources such as lactation consultants who have specialized knowledge can help mothers with their breastfeeding goals. Finding social support amongst other mothers, such as with La Leche League, a non-profit organization that provides useful information and support for women who want to breastfeed, can also be beneficial (La Leche League [LLL], n.d.).

ESTABLISHING A SELF-CARE ROUTINE

While establishing a self-care routine as a new mother or parent can be challenging, as previously effective means of self-care (e.g., going to the gym, time alone to meditate) may not be feasible, helping a new parent establish a self-care routine and finding support can be very beneficial. Self-care has been defined as replenishing the sources that sustain you (Skovholt, 2001; Skovholt & Trotter-Mathison, 2011). Despite its importance, new mothers need support for self-care. For example, if a new mother practiced prenatal yoga as a form of self-care, adapting to post-natal yoga with a baby may be challenging. Furthermore, in the immediate postpartum of the first six weeks, most mothers are not yet medically cleared to participate in exercise, but new mothers in the immediate postpartum can alleviate stress in other ways.

Mothers are adapting to major physical, social, emotional, psychological, hormonal, and role changes after the birth of their baby that impacts their self-care activities profoundly. Having time alone may be a form of replenishing self-care for a mother, but that may be the exact thing she cannot get. In many modern Western homes, mothers give birth, and after the hubbub of the birth subsides they are frequently left alone to fend for themselves and their new baby for many hours of the day, many days of the week. This can be due to a lack of paternal/partner leave and other family living in different places, so other family members such as the new mother's mother and father or her in-laws are not available to support her.

Moreover, sometimes out-of-town family want to help and stay as houseguests, which can create a situation in which an already stressed mother, adapting to her new baby, is also hosting a house guest with their own needs (even if it is a well-intentioned family member). This scenario may increase a mother's stress levels and reduce her energy for self-care. If she does schedule a visit, she may miss out on crucial rest time if her baby is sleeping and she is caught talking to guests. Depending on the visitor's sensitivity, and how they relate with the new mother and baby, the mother may feel ignored or devalued as visitors frequently focus on the baby without paying as much attention to the new mother. So, what would be the ideal form of support for a new mother and baby? We recommend that any visits are fully supportive of the mother, and that the household schedule should revolve around the mother's needs for at least the first six weeks after birth. If the mother normally determines what the family will eat, makes dinner, and does the dishes after dinner, these tasks should be delegated to someone else.

In some families, a paid postpartum doula is a good option to help support the mother and infant and provide relief so that the mother can attend to her own needs and know that her infant is in capable hands. Fathers/partners/extended family can also play this role but may not have as much time and/or expertise in tailoring their approach to serve the mother and infant (e.g., well-meaning family members who visit, expect a new mother to handle all meal planning and preparation, and do not give the mother rest).

Incorporating a self-care and wellness focus is consistent with a strengths-based framework. Enhancing a new mother's self-care routine and addressing various aspects of wellness are powerful therapeutic lifestyle changes that complement treatment interventions for PPD or other mood disorders or symptoms.

THE POWER OF SOCIAL SUPPORT

Social support can be defined as "support which is considered functional, and which leads the receiver of the support to feel cared for, valued and with a sense of belonging to a larger network" (De Sousa Machado et al., 2020, p. 3). Mothers, both new and seasoned, can benefit from a larger support network. "Instrumental support plays a significant role in meeting women's basic needs during the postpartum period" (Negron et al., 2014, p. 1). Social support is a protective factor against the development of anxiety and depression (Negron et al., 2014). Women need support. They deserve support; even more so once they become mothers. Immediately after childbirth, women are expected to "bounce-back," to seemingly act as if they did not just go through huge physiological and hormonal changes and often birth trauma, all while experiencing a miracle simultaneously. A woman's body and mind need time to heal after nine (often ten) months of pregnancy and they need a support network that extends beyond a partner.

Mothers and new parents need supportive friendships, especially during the postpartum period. Ideally, someone coming to visit would bring coffee, a prepared meal, or something to lighten the load and dote on the mother as well as the baby. All the simple self-care activities that people take for granted prior to having a newborn (such as taking a shower) become increasingly harder, so new mothers need help with the simplest of tasks. New mothers adjusting to the increased demands of the early postpartum have an increased need for social support (Negron et al., 2014).

A mother's need for support extends beyond the immediate postpartum. Although technically PPD would only be diagnosed within the first four weeks after delivery according to the DSM-5-TR (APA, 2022), many researchers and clinicians consider PPD to be within the first year after delivery (Dekel et al., 2019). Furthermore, a person who becomes a mother never goes back to a pre-parent identity. Even in the case of an infant's/child's death, a person's identity has changed permanently to being a mother. Mothers need support throughout the journey of motherhood and their needs will vary depending on the season of motherhood they are experiencing.

MULTIPLE PERSPECTIVES: FATHER/PARTNER, FAMILY, RELATIONSHIPS

During pregnancy, expectant fathers experience a process of connecting with the developing fetus (called paternal–fetal attachment) (Lagarto & Duaso, 2021). In a qualitative study, themes emerged including fathers feeling lost in their role and needing support, as well as of "a trigger moment" when the reality of their baby became salient (Lagarto & Duaso, 2021). Fathers also reported struggling with a lack of support for their own mental health (Lagarto & Duaso, 2021). The postpartum period is intense for fathers and partners, as well as siblings and extended family. When a new baby joins a family, it impacts everyone, especially family members and loved ones in the baby's household. Fathers (or partners) having leave from work is imperative for their own wellbeing, for bonding with their baby, and to a new mother's health and healing. While over 70 countries have paid paternity leave, the United States is not one of them (Harrington, 2014) and thus U.S. fathers often have difficulty balancing time with their new family versus the desire or financial need to return to work quickly. Some increase their workload to pursue promotion/advancement and for financial security. With paid leave, fathers can help mothers heal by caring for the baby, changing diapers, caring for other children, cleaning, and doing laundry (Harrington, 2014). Same-sex partners also face challenges in providing support to the birthing parent (or primary caregiving parent). Furthermore, the protection provided to same-sex parents is even more tenuous than that of fathers in heterosexual relationships, and they also face societal discrimination and lack of awareness. For example, gay male parents continue to face stigma and barriers to becoming parents (Perrin et al., 2019).

MULTICULTURAL CONSIDERATIONS

The society, culture, and subculture(s) in which a person gives birth make a significant difference in their experience in the peripartum. For instance, in traditional collectivistic cultures there are more rituals and routines to support a mother in her self-care as she adapts to her life with her baby as compared with modern Western culture with its individualistic values. For instance, in the Chinese tradition, an older female relative, typically the new mother's mother or mother-in-law, takes care of work within the home, such as childcare and cleaning and cooking, to allow the new mother time to recuperate (Bina, 2008). In this case, the role of this person is clearly defined and culturally understood as a primary helper to the mother to prioritize the mother's needs.

Partner and extended family support can provide a space for a birthing mother to begin the journey of physical recovery from childbirth and begin to establish effective self-care routines. However, it is important to consider the mother's preferences and comfort in the immediate postpartum; counselors can help mothers explore cultural expectations around birth and the postpartum as well as their preferences and boundaries. They can explore the support mothers want in the postpartum period (e.g., help with childcare for an older child, someone to take care of all laundry, cleaning, and household chores), and identify who they trust and feel comfortable with to provide that support (e.g., mother, paid postpartum doula, mother-in-law etc.).

Socioeconomic status (SES) is an important sociocultural factor, as it is often related to other stressors and risk factors, as well as the forms of paid support that are feasible (such as postpartum doulas or childcare). Low-income pregnant women "whose cortisol and perceived stress levels stay at an abnormally high level after childbirth are at greater risk for PPD" (Sheyer & Urizar, 2016, p. 327). Therefore, assessing socioeconomic stressors, and the resulting overall stress level for the mother and family, is important.

APPLICATIONS TO COUNSELING

Counselors can direct support through counseling services for mothers, fathers, partners, and families and advocate for them. Assessing risk and protective factors as described in this chapter through a clinical interview process and with assessment instruments is also recommended. Counselors should assess an expectant mother's level of perceived stress and the psychosocial stressors she experiences both before and after childbirth to help mitigate the risk of developing PPD or another maternal mood disorder (Tebeka et al., 2016). Pregnancy itself is listed as a stressful life event on one of the first developed stress rating scales, the *Holmes and Rahe Social Readjustment Rating Scale* (Holmes & Rahe, 1967).

In an interview with *Counseling Today*, I (Isabel Thompson) recommended viewing the mother and infant as a unit, at least for the first few months after birth (Bray, 2019). Supporting mother–infant bonding while helping to meet the mother's treatment needs will help the mother meet her baby's needs. Stepped care models of treatment recommend screening for PPD and working collaboratively with healthcare providers to meet the mother's needs (Gjerdingen et al., 2008). If the severity of a mother's mood symptoms makes it difficult for her to respond to her infant's cues, and she is struggling with SI, inpatient hospitalization may be needed. Unfortunately, inpatient settings with mother–baby psychiatric units that allow the infant to stay with the mother overnight are unavailable in the United States, but existing European models of care indicate that these could assist with mother–infant bonding while mothers receive needed treatment (Dembosky, 2021).

ADDRESSING SELF-CARE AND WELLNESS IN TREATMENT

One key area that can help mothers is enhancing self-care and wellness. As mentioned above, peripartum depression begins in pregnancy in up to 50 percent of cases (APA, 2022). Helping pregnant women care for themselves and to seek treatment early when needed can be a major aspect of preventative care. In conceptualizing self-care, counselors and other mental health professionals may benefit from considering the Indivisible Self Model of Wellness (Myers & Sweeney, 2005). This model is evidence-based and conceptualizes wellness as consisting of Five Selves: Creative, Coping, Physical, Essential, and Social. Counselors and other mental health professionals working with new mothers can assess their wellness levels using the Five Factor Wellness Inventory (5F-WEL; Myers & Sweeney, 2005). This can give clinicians an understanding of the areas in which a mother may be struggling and areas in which she is already demonstrating strong levels of wellness.

ENHANCING PARTNER AND SOCIAL SUPPORT IN TREATMENT

Assessing and supporting mothers in enhancing their social support is recommended, as it is a powerful protective factor (Negron et al., 2014). Supporting and enhancing the partner relationship during the transition to parenthood for first-time parents (or with the addition of a child for parents who already have a child or children) is essential. Social support outside of a marriage or partnership is also very important, especially with people who are experiencing similar life changes, so helping a mother connect with other mothers can be a powerful source of social support.

Counselors can support new mothers by helping them to enhance their existing social support networks and/or build strong social support. There are several types of social support described by Sherbourne and Stewart (1991) that new mothers need:

> 1) *emotional support* through understanding and the encouragement to express feelings, warmth nurturance, and reassurance; 2) *informational support* through providing advice and guidance, helping another understand, sourcing resources and/or coping strategies, information, advice and management strategies; 3) *instrumental support* through material, monetary and behavioral tangible assistance, services, specific aid or goods; 4) *appraisal or comparison support* refers to encouragement and advice by those who have been in similar situations and 5) *social companionship* by spending leisure time with others.
> (Ni and Lin, 2011, as cited in De Sousa Machado et al., 2020, pp. 2–3)

When a woman feels supported and encouraged on the journey of motherhood, this is empowering. Supporting a mother's needs and wants during this period is imperative to her mental wellbeing and helps her feel less isolated. Women need to be reminded not to compare their journey into motherhood and their child's developmental journey with those of others as this can become all-consuming. No two moms are alike, just like no two babies are alike; there are many unique ways to be a loving, caring mother. Every individual has their own needs that must be met for their health and safety, and this is no different for a woman's postpartum needs.

SUPPORT RELATED TO FEEDING/BREASTFEEDING

Counselors and other mental health professionals working with new mothers should be aware of how common challenges of breastfeeding are and the availability of lactation consultants and other forms of support, including groups such as La Leche League (n.d.), an international breastfeeding support organization. There are known health benefits of breastfeeding for the baby (Mohrbacher & Kendall-Tackett, 2010) and benefits for the breastfeeding mothers. It stimulates the release of the hormone oxytocin, which reduces postpartum bleeding (Gartner et al., 2005), and it may reduce stress levels in new mothers (Mezzacappa, 2004).

A woman's breastfeeding goals and intentions are important, as intention to breastfeed may mediate the relationship between breastfeeding and positive mental health, such as reduced depressive symptoms (Borra et al., 2014). While supporting a mother who chooses to breastfeed, counselors can normalize how sometimes breastfeeding does not work out, and that feeding the baby formula is a viable and healthy option. Women need to feel empowered and to have support to let go of worry or shame if they do not (or cannot) breastfeed. Maternal mental health matters; and counselors can support mothers with breastfeeding and with the risks and benefits specific to the unique needs of the mother and baby.

BIOPSYCHOSOCIAL THEORETICAL MODEL

Experiencing social isolation, and a lack of family and social support may exacerbate symptoms of PPD (Hassert & Kurpius, 2011). In modern American society, many women return to an empty home after giving birth, and for many women their spouse/partner returns to work only days, maybe a week, after the baby's arrival. In some cases, family may flood in immediately after the birth, but then leave at the six-week mark, which is a critical timeframe in the development of PPD, as the hormones associated with pregnancy decrease. The combination of hormonal changes, role changes, and lack of family support can be extremely detrimental to a woman's mental health. Caring for a newborn in isolation while feeling lonely, coupled with the sleep deprivation typically associated with having a newborn can erode a woman's own wellbeing. Conversely, in cultural subgroups that are more likely to have extended family in the local area who can provide support, women may be buffered from some of these stressors.

ETHICAL CONSIDERATIONS

Counselors and other mental health professionals have an ethical obligation to effectively screen for depression, other maternal mood disorders, and SI during pregnancy and the postpartum. PPD is relatively common, with research-based estimates that 1 in 8 women experience it (CDC, n.d.). Having depression is associated with SI, which is a risk factor for dying by suicide (Bodnar-Deren et al., 2016). Furthermore, SI is relatively common among postpartum mothers. Therefore, in addition to screening for depression, clinicians should screen mothers for SI. The Edinburgh Postnatal Depression Scale (EPDS; Cox et al., 1987) is commonly used to screen for depression among pregnant and postpartum women and has an item that addresses thoughts of self-harm. The Patient Health Questionnaire (PHQ-9) assessment has nine items responding to the question: "Over the last 2 weeks, how often have you been bothered by any of the following problems?" (Kroenke et al., 1999). It has an item that directly addresses SI: "9. Thoughts that you would be better off dead or of hurting yourself in some way" with response options: "not at all," "Several days," "more than half the days," or "nearly every day" (Kroenke et al., 1999). Any positive SI screening result should be addressed immediately, and the person should be assessed to determine what level of care is needed to keep them safe (Bodnar-Deren et al., 2016).

BARRIERS TO TREATMENT

Due to the stigma associated with maternal mental illness, women who are experiencing symptoms of depressive, anxiety, or other mental health symptoms may be fearful to reveal these symptoms to their healthcare provider, for fear of being judged Kleiman & Raskin, 2013. Furthermore, cultural or familial norms may not include seeking services from mental health professionals.

Another major barrier to effective screening and treatment is the insufficient aftercare that many birthing mothers receive. Standard midwifery care includes a home visit within a few days after the birth of the baby, but this is still not sufficient to meet many postpartum mothers' needs, especially mental or emotional health concerns. Women who give birth at a hospital are discharged a few days after giving birth and are not seen again until their six-week checkup at their OB/GYN's office. "Women expressed that insufficient attention was paid to both their own physical health and emotional needs during the postpartum stay in hospital. After the baby was born, they felt neglected because all focus shifted to the baby" (Rudman & Waldenström, 2007, p. 13). Women who have a birth center or home birth are typically seen by a midwife within the first week after birth and at six weeks; this is still less frequent than the prenatal care they received.

In contrast, a new baby sees their doctor just a few days after birth, and most babies see their pediatrician at least five times before their mother has a follow-up appointment with her provider. With the advancement of telemedicine, mothers could check in with their healthcare provider leading up to their six-week postpartum checkup.

Ideally, the pediatricians and OB/GYNs/midwifes would work together to provide a safety net of care for postpartum mothers. Currently, these care systems are separate, and pediatricians do not communicate with the mother's healthcare provider. If counselors were integrated into the prenatal and postpartum care that women receive at all stages of the process, including conception, prenatal appointments, and the postpartum care, screening and treatment could be more proactive.

COVID-19 AND ONLINE SUPPORT

The COVID-19 pandemic increased the sense of responsibility mothers felt for their babies' welfare, while simultaneously disrupting their connection to family and friends, especially during periods of governmental "lockdowns" implementing behavioral controls and closing many non-essential businesses (Gray & Barnett, 2021). New mothers' groups, which were harder to access during the COVID-19 pandemic, can be a wonderful source of meeting other mothers in the same life stage.

While a partner or spouse can be a very strong source of support, at times they simply cannot understand what a mother has been through, both mentally and physically. "Partners were identified as the primary resource for emotional support, but some women also sought out girlfriends, cousins, godmothers, and other mothers from mother support groups to talk about their feelings" (Negron et al., 2014, p. 5). Connecting with other mothers can reduce a mother's loneliness and isolation and encourage her to advocate for her needs, as well as those of her baby. During the pandemic these groups became virtual, using videoconferencing platforms. Online resources such as *Union Square Play* (https://unionsquareplay.com/), *Our Mama Village* (https://ourmamavillage.com/), and *PedsDocTalk* (https://pedsdoctalk.com/) are just a few examples of where mothers can find an online community of other mothers. Sites like *Union Square Play* and *Nine Months to Mom* (https://ninemonthstomom.com/) offer virtual groups for mothers in similar postpartum stages to support one another virtually.

LOOKING FORWARD: ENHANCED SCREENING DURING PRENATAL AND PEDIATRICIAN VISITS

By routinely including mental health history questions during prenatal visits, providers can be a part of screening, prevention, and effective early intervention for PPD, because "minimizing risk factors and fostering protective factors even during pregnancy are the most important starting points for the prevention of peripartum depression" (Hain et al., 2016, p. 125). The health of the expectant mother and the health of her baby are holistically entwined, and the expectant mother's mental well-being or lack thereof matters. Asking about prior depression is essential: "In the largest population-based study to date, the risk of PPD was more than 20 times higher for women with a depression history, compared to women without" (Silverman et al., 2017, p. 2).

As clinicians we need to use all the tools in our arsenal to help women combat depression, hopefully sometimes before it even starts. It is essential for counselors and other mental health professionals to advocate for women during their pregnancy and in what has been called the "fourth trimester" (the three months immediately following birth) (Johnson, 2017). New mothers need more effective and comprehensive screening. Counselors can be advocates, as there needs to be more training for OB/GYNs and other prenatal providers (midwives, doulas) to screen for depression and other maternal mood disorders. Pediatricians' offices can also provide more proactive screening.

Moms need to feel safe to discuss their own wellbeing without fear of judgment or punishment for doing so, as peripartum depression and other maternal mood disorders are treatable and should not be ignored. Doctors are taking steps in the right direction to help support mothers when they need it most. For instance, across the state of Rhode Island, and within the participating practices with the Blue Cross and Blue Shield program, "screening and referral rates improved from 28% to 77%" (BCBS, n.d.). This is an example of the positive benefits of systemic changes. Creating a safety net for new mothers, fathers/partners, families, and their babies can go a long way to addressing maternal mental health needs and implementing prevention and early intervention to reduce the likelihood of developing PPD or severe negative effects from PPD. Counselors who focus on maternal mental health can advocate for the implementation of such systems and also develop relationships with local OB/GYNs and midwives to collaborate in screening, prevention, and early intervention efforts to better serve mothers, their infants, and their families.

CONCLUSION

Counselors and other mental health professionals working with couples and pregnant women as well as mothers/parents who have recently had a baby should be aware of the risk and protective factors associated with PPD. Screening and case conceptualization that examines current life stressors and social support, medical history, and family history of depression and other mood disorders is essential. Furthermore, enhancing strength and protective factors and supporting a mother's efforts to implement self-care, and building a supportive environment for recovery are also essential.

Case Study: Juliette

Juliette is a 17-year-old White American cisgender woman. She currently lives with her mother and two younger brothers in a small apartment. Her socioeconomic status is low income, and she qualifies for free and reduced lunch at school. Juliette's mother does not have health insurance for herself or her children due to the cost. The family's approach to mental health issues is typically that these sorts of problems will resolve on their own. Juliette is currently seven months' pregnant and is struggling with intense anxiety that interferes with her being able to fall asleep and awakens her during the night. Juliette has Hyperemesis Gravidarum and has struggled with severe nausea and vomiting during pregnancy and has lost weight during pregnancy. She is fearful for the health of her developing baby and that she will not be able to handle being a mother and that her life goals will be thwarted. She became pregnant unintentionally. Her boyfriend Nate, who is the baby's father, is also 17 years old. They are both juniors in high school. Early in the pregnancy, they decided to keep the baby, but they feel overwhelmed and scared about how they will manage to finish high school and move forward with their lives while taking care of and supporting a baby. Juliette's mother is very supportive emotionally. She works two jobs to keep up with rent payments and other bills, so is not at home very much to provide instrumental support. Nate's parents are supportive and want to help their future grandchild any way they can. Juliette's high school has worked with her to develop a plan for her to finish up needed credits. Juliette always dreamed of going away to college, and she feels distressed anticipating that her dreams of going away to college may be unachievable or that she may need to complete college closer to home to have the support of her family to care for her baby while she attends classes.

Recently, she was hospitalized for four days to stabilize her medical condition and she also was then put on subsequent bedrest. Her mother visited her as often as she could while she was hospitalized. Currently, she is not able to attend school in person, but her teachers have worked with her to allow to her to complete work at home and submit it so that she can keep up with her academic requirements. Nate is very supportive and visits her daily after school.

Lately Juliette has had difficulty concentrating on her schoolwork and has started missing deadlines. She is worried about wrapping up her junior year prior to the birth of her baby and fears that if she can't complete it, she will fall further behind. Juliette used to enjoy meeting up with friends, but since she has been put on bedrest, fewer friends have come to visit her and she no longer communicates with them as much on social media as she feels that they can't understand what she is going through. She states that she feels hopeless about her future, even though she longs to hold her new baby after the birth.

Case Study: Jaelyn

Jaelyn is 37-year-old African American cisgender woman. She is currently six months' pregnant. She has a history of miscarriage, having experienced two miscarriages prior to this pregnancy. The first miscarriage occurred when she was 33 and the second when she was 36. Jaelyn and her husband David have been wanting to become parents for many years and grieved tremendously after each miscarriage. The two miscarriages have haunted Jaelyn during this pregnancy, and she is constantly worried that something will happen during this pregnancy. She is concerned as she is over 35 and is aware that some risk factors can increase with pregnancy after age 35.

Jaelyn has a personal history of major depressive disorder, having experienced depression during her second year of college after her grandmother's death and experiencing a sexual assault on campus. Jaelyn attempted suicide after the sexual assault and was hospitalized briefly. She had to leave college for a semester while she sought treatment. She transferred to a college new her hometown and completed her degree, and then went to law school.

She met David while she was in law school, and he was studying for his master's degree. They got married when she was 30. She had another major depressive episode after the loss of her second baby to miscarriage, but her strong relationship with her husband and him helping her find treatment helped her. She had been taking antidepressant medication for the past year but came off the medication when she found out she was pregnant again out of fear of potential harm to the developing fetus. She is having intrusive thoughts of something going wrong with this pregnancy and is very cautious about any potential toxin exposures (hence she wanted to stop taking the antidepressant medication). Since coming off the medication, she has felt a lack of energy and spends any time when she is not working lying in bed. She used to meet up with friends usually once a week, but lately has stopped doing so. She has been feeling down and cries frequently. David is worried about her and wants her to get treatment now. She has stopped going to her customary Zumba classes and no longer keeps up with her other main pastimes, which previously included gardening and baking.

Jaelyn is a successful attorney, and her husband David works in human resources at a large cooperation. Jaelyn plans to work fulltime during pregnancy, and then take three months off from work after the baby's birth. Jaelyn enjoys her career and finds satisfaction in her job as an attorney. Jaelyn and David are financially secure and have close emotional relationships with their parents; however, both sets of grandparents live on the other side of the country from where Jaelyn and David live.

APPLYING THE STRENGTHS MODEL—THE CASE OF JULIETTE

Significant Individual, Infant, Family, Societal, and Cultural Factors

- Juliette became pregnant as a teenager unintentionally.
- She is experiencing symptoms of anxiety and depression.
- She is experiencing the medical complication of Hyperemesis Gravidarum.

Treatment Barriers

- Financial barriers to access treatment due to lack of health insurance.
- Not able to physically travel to a provider due to bedrest order.
- Familial approach to mental health concerns does not include seeing services.

Risk Factors

- Juliette was 17 years old when she became pregnant.
- Juliette comes from a low SES background.
- Juliette is experiencing a medical complication of pregnancy that interferes with her education and quality of life.

Enlisting Support from Family, the Community, and Medical Professionals

- Consult with Juliette's mother to discuss treatment options.
- Work with community agencies to determine what treatments may be available to Juliette.
- Explore federal/state resources available to pregnant women and provide this information to Juliette.

Noticeable Symptoms, Severity, & DSM-5-TR Diagnosis OR Needs Identified by Family & Treatment Team

- Juliette is having anxiety that is interfering with her sleep.
- Juliette is having difficulty concentrating on schoolwork.
- She expresses that she is feeling hopeless about the future.

Goals Identified by Family

- Address Juliette's anxiety and help her sleep better.
- Help her refocus on schoolwork prior to the baby's arrival.
- Increase her feelings of hope for the future.

Treatment Recommendations

- Conduct a complete assessment for depression, anxiety, and suicidality.
- Coordinate care with her OB/GYN to discuss the Hyperemesis Gravidarum diagnosis and how to support her mental health.

- Address Juliette's anxiety and depressive symptoms through Interpersonal Therapy.

Helpful, Protective, and Resilience Factors

- Juliette's mother is emotionally supportive.
- Juliette has a track record of academic success.
- Nate and his parents are supportive of Juliette and the baby.

Self-Care & Wellness

- Juliette has an emotionally supportive mother.
- Juliette cares about her academic and career progress.
- Juliette could be supported in engaging with friendships again in way that feels meaningful to her.

APPLYING THE STRENGTHS MODEL—THE CASE OF JAELYN

Significant Individual, Infant, Family, Societal, and Cultural Factors

- Jaelyn has experienced two previous miscarriages.
- Jaelyn has a history of depression and suicide attempt.
- Jaelyn is experiencing anxiety about her current pregnancy.

Treatment Barriers

- Jaelyn has stopped taking previously prescribed medication due to concerns about the health of her baby.
- Jaelyn is African American, a cultural group that may have less trust in the mental health care system.
- Jaelyn may need telehealth services and childcare to successfully engage in treatment after her baby's birth.

Risk Factors

- Jaelyn has had two previous miscarriages.
- Jaelyn has a history of depression and suicide attempt.
- Jaelyn is over age 35.

Enlisting Support from Family, the Community, and Medical Professionals

- Jaelyn's husband David is supportive and wants her to seek treatment.
- A referral to a psychiatrist to assess her current concerns about medication and how she is coping without being on her previous medication.
- Coordinating care with her OB/GYN to address Jaelyn's concerns about the pregnancy.

Noticeable Symptoms, Severity, & DSM-5-TR Diagnosis OR Needs Identified by Family & Treatment Team

- Jaelyn is having anxiety about her pregnancy and the health of her baby.
- Jaelyn has stopped participating in activities she previously enjoyed (e.g., gardening, Zumba).
- Jaelyn has been crying frequently, is feeling down, has a lack of energy and is withdrawing from friends (outside of her paid employment).

Goals Identified by Family

- Get treatment for Jaelyn so that she can start to feel better.
- Discuss whether restarting medication may be helpful to her.
- Decrease her anxiety about the pregnancy.

Treatment Recommendations

- Assess Jaelyn's current anxiety and depressive symptoms.
- Conduct a comprehensive suicide risk assessment considering Jaelyn's history of a suicide attempt while she was in college.
- Address trauma from previous miscarriages.
- Incorporate Behavioral Activation approaches to help Jaelyn begin engaging in previously enjoyable activities.

Helpful, Protective, and Resilience Factors

- Jaelyn is intelligent and high achieving and enjoys her career.
- Jaelyn and her husband David have a positive, supportive relationship.
- Their extended family is supportive.

Self-Care & Wellness

- Jaelyn cares about her health and pregnancy.

- Jaelyn has a supportive partner.
- Jaelyn has self-care activities that she previously enjoyed.

REFERENCES

American Psychiatric Association (APA). (2022). *Diagnostic and statistical manual of mental disorders* (5th ed.; text revision).

Andres, E., Baird, S., Bingenheimer, J. B., & Markus, A. R. (2016). Maternity leave access and health: A systematic narrative review and conceptual framework development. *Maternal and Child Health Journal, 20*, 1178–1192. doi:10.1007/s10995-015-1905-9

Baker, L., Cross, S., Greaver, L., Wei, G., Lewis, R., & Healthy Start CORPS (2005). Prevalence of postpartum depression in a Native American Population. *Maternal and Child Health Journal, 9*, 21–25. doi:10.1007/s10995-005-2448-2

Banker, J. E., & LaCoursiere, D. Y. (2014). Postpartum depression: risks, protective factors, and the couple's relationship. *Issues in Mental Health Nursing, 35*(7), 503–508. doi:10.3109/01612840.2014.888603

Bina, R. (2008). The impact of cultural factors upon postpartum depression: A literature review. *Health Care for Women International, 29*, 568–592. doi:10.1080/07399330802089149

Bingol, F. B., & Bal, M. D. (2020). The risk factors for postpartum posttraumatic stress disorder and depression. *Perspectives in Psychiatric Care, 56*(4), 851–857.

Bloch, M., Rotenberg, N., Koren, D., & Klein, E. (2005). Risk factors associated with the development of postpartum mood disorders. *Journal of Affective Disorders, 88*(1), 9–18. doi:10.1016/j.jad.2005.04.007

Blue Cross Blue Shield. (BCBS). (n.d.). *Pediatricians screen new moms for postpartum depression*. Retrieved February 14, 2022, from https://www.bcbs.com/the-health-of-america/articles/pediatricians-screen-new-moms-postpartum-depression

Bodnar-Deren, S., Klipstein, K., Fersh, M., Shemesh, E., & Howell, E. A. (2016). Suicidal ideation during the postpartum period. *Journal of Women's Health, 25*(12), 1219–1224. doi:10.1089/jwh.2015.5346

Borra, C., Iacovou, M., & Sevilla, A. (2015). New evidence on breastfeeding and postpartum depression: The importance of understanding women's intentions. *Maternal and Child Health Journal, 19*(4), 897–907. doi:10.1007/s10995-014-1591-z

Bray, B. (2019, April). Bundle of joy? *Counseling Today, 61*(10), 30–35. https://ct.counseling.org/2019/03/bundle-of-joy/

Centers for Disease Control and Prevention (CDC). (n.d.). *Reproductive health: Depression among women*. https://www.cdc.gov/reproductivehealth/depression/index.htm#Postpartum

Cox, J. L., Holden, J. M., & Sagovsky, R. (1987). Detection of postnatal depression: Development of the 10-item Edinburgh Postnatal Depression Scale. *British Journal of Psychiatry, 150*, 782–786. https://uwm.edu/mcwp/wp-content/uploads/sites/337/2015/11/Tip-Sheet-EPDS_updated.pdf

Dagher, R. K., Bruckheim, H. E., Colpe, L. J., Edwards, E., & White, D. B. (2021). Perinatal depression: Challenges and opportunities. *Journal of Women's Health, 30*(2), 154–159. doi:10.1089/jwh.2020.8862

Davey, H. L., Tough, S. C., Adair, C. E., & Benzies, K. M. (2011). Risk factors for sub-clinical and major postpartum depression among a community cohort of Canadian women. *Maternal and Child Health Journal, 15*(7), 866–875. doi:10.1007/s10995-008-0314-8

De Sousa Machado, T., Chur-Hansen, A., & Due, C. (2020). First-time mothers' perceptions of social support: Recommendations for best practice. *Health Psychology Open*. doi:10.1177/2055102919898611

Dekel, S., Ein-Dor, T., Berman, Z., Barsoumian, I. S., Agarwal, S., & Pitman, R. K. (2019). Delivery mode is associated with maternal mental health following childbirth. *Archives of Women's Mental Health, 22*, 817–824. doi:10.1007/s00737-019-00968-2

Dembosky, A. (2021). A humane approach to caring for new mothers in psychiatric crisis. *Health Affairs, 40*(10), 1528–1533. doi:10.1377/hlthaff.2021.01288

Figueiredo, B., Canario, C., & Field, T. (2014). Breastfeeding is negatively affected by prenatal depression and reduces postpartum depression. *Psychological Medicine, 44*(5), 927–936. doi:10.1017/S0033291713001530

García-Blanco, A., Monferrer, A., Grimaldos, J., Hervás, D., Balanzá-Martínez, V., Diago, V., Vento, M., & Cháfer-Pericás, C. (2017). A preliminary study to assess the impact of maternal age on stress-related variables in healthy nulliparous women. *Psychoneuroendocrinology, 78*, 97–104. doi:10.1016/j.psyneuen.2017.01.018

Gartner, L. M., Morton, J., Lawrence, R. A., Naylor, A. J., O'Hare, D., Schanler, R. J., et al. (2005). Breastfeeding and the use of human milk. *Pediatrics, 115*, 496–506. doi:10.1542/peds.2004-2491

Gastaldon, C., Solmi, M., Correll, C. U., Barbui, C., & Schoretsanitis, G. (2022). Risk factors of postpartum depression and depressive symptoms: Umbrella review of current evidence from systematic reviews and meta-analyses of observational studies. *The British Journal of Psychiatry, 221*(4), 591–602. doi:10.1192/bjp.2021.222

Gray, A., & Barnett, J. (2021). Welcoming new life under lockdown: Exploring the experiences of first-time mothers who gave birth during the COVID-19 pandemic. *The British Journal of Health Psychology*, 1–19. doi:10.1111/bjhp.12561

Gjerdingen, D., Katon, W., & Rich, D. E. (2008). Stepped care treatment of postpartum depression A primary care-based management model. *Women's Health Issues, 18*(1), 44–52. doi:10.1016/j.whi.2007.09.001

Gressier, F., Guillard, V., Cazas, O., Falissard, B., Glangeaud-Freudenthald, N. M-C., & Sutter-Dallaye, A.-L. (2017). Risk factors for suicide attempt in pregnancy and the post-partum period in women with serious mental illnesses. *Journal of Psychiatric Research, 84*, 284–291. doi:10.1016/j.jpsychires.2016.10.009

Hahn-Holbrook, J., Haselton, M. G., Schetter, C. D., & Glynn, L. M. (2013). Does breastfeeding offer protection against maternal depressive symptomatology? A prospective study from pregnancy to 2 years after birth. *Archives of Women's Mental Health, 16*(5), 411–422. doi:10.1007/s00737-013-0348-9

Hain, S., Oddo-Sommerfeld, S., Bahlmann, F., Louwen, F., & Schermelleh-Engel, K. (2016). Risk and protective factors for antepartum and postpartum depression: A prospective study. *Journal of Psychosomatic Obstetrics & Gynecology, 37*(4), 119–129. doi:10.1080/0167482X.2016.1197904

Harrington, B. (2014). *The new dad: Take your leave*. [Powerpoint]. Boston College Center for Work and Family, Boston, MA. https://www.bc.edu/content/dam/files/centers/cwf/research/publications/researchreports/The%20New%20Dad-%20Take%20Your%20Leave%20June%202014%20-%20June%205.pdf

Hassert, S., & Kurpius, S. E. (2011). Latinas and postpartum depression: Role of partner relationship, additional children, and breastfeeding. *Journal of Multicultural Counseling and Development, 39*(2), 90–100. doi:10.1002/j.2161-1912.2011.tb00143.x

Hauck, Y. L., Fenwick, J., Dhaliwal, S. S., & Butt, J. (2011). A Western Australian Survey of Breastfeeding Initiation, Prevalence and Early Cessation Patterns. *Maternal and Child Health Journal, 15*(2), 260–268. doi:10.1007/s10995-009-0554-2

Holmes, T. H., & Rahe, R. H. (1967). The Social Readjustment Rating Scale. *Journal of Psychosomatic Research, 11*(2), 213–218. https://doi.org/10.1016/0022-3999(67)90010-4

Johnson, K. A. (2017). *The fourth trimester: A postpartum guide to healing your body, balancing your emotions and restoring your vitality*. Shambhala Publications. https://www.shambhala.com/wp/wp-content/uploads/2018/05/Sanctuary-PDF.pdf

Kettunen, P. & Hintikka, J. (2017). Psychosocial risk factors and treatment of new onset and recurrent depression during the post-partum period. *Nordic Journal of Psychiatry, 71*(5), 355–361. doi:10.1080/08039488.2017.1300324

Kim, T., Connolly, J., & Tamim, H. (2014). The effect of social support around pregnancy on postpartum depression among Canadian teen mothers and adult mothers in the maternity experiences survey. *BMC Pregnancy and Childbirth*. doi:10.1186/1471-2393-14-162.

Kleiman, K. R., & Raskin, V. D. (2013). *This isn't what I expected: Overcoming postpartum depression*. De Capo Press.

Kroenke, K., Spitzer, R. L., & Williams, J. B. W. (1999). *Patient Health Questionnaire-9*. doi:10.1037/t06165-000

La Leche League (LLL) (n.d.). La Leche League USA. https://lllusa.org/

Lagarto, A. & Duaso, M. J. (2021). Fathers' experiences of fetal attachment: A qualitative study. *Infant Mental Health Journal*, 1–12. doi:10.1002/imhj.21965

Martini, J., Bauer, M., Lewitzka, U., Voss, C., Pfennig, A., Ritter, D., & Wittchen, H.-U. (2019). Predictors and outcomes of suicidal ideation during peripartum period. *Journal of Affective Disorders, 257*, 518–526. doi:10.1016/j.jad.2019.07.040

Meeussen, L., & Van Laar, C. (2018). Feeling pressure to be a perfect mother relates to parental burnout and career ambitions. *Frontiers in Psychology, 9*. doi:10.3389/fpsyg.2018.02113

Meltzer-Brody, S., Maegbaek, M. L., Medland, S. E., Miller, W. C., Sullivan, C. P., & Munk-Olsen, T. (2017). Obstetrical, pregnancy and socio-economic predictors for new-onset severe postpartum psychiatric disorders in primiparous women. *Psychological Medicine, 47*, 1427–1441. doi:10.1017/S0033291716003020

Mezzacappa, E. S. (2004). Breastfeeding and maternal stress response and health. *Nutrition Reviews, 62*(7), 261–268. doi:10.1111/j.1753-4887.2004.tb00050.x

Mohrbacher, N., & Kendall-Tackett, K. (2010). *Breastfeeding made simple: Seven natural laws for nursing mothers* (2nd ed.). New Harbinger Publications.

Murakami, K., Turale, S., Skirton, H., Doris, F., Tsujino, K., Ito, M., & Kutsunugi, S. (2016). Experiences regarding maternal age-specific risks and prenatal testing of women of advanced maternal age in Japan. *Nursing and Health Sciences, 18*, 8–14. doi:10.1111/nhs.12209

Myers, J. E., & Sweeney, T. J. (2005). The Indivisible Self: An evidenced-based model of Wellness (reprint). *The Journal of Individual Psychology, 61*(1), 269–279.

Negron, R., Martin, A., Almog, M., Balbierz, A., & Howell, E. A. (2012). Social support during the postpartum period: Mothers' views on needs, expectations, and mobilization of support. *Maternal and Child Health Journal, 17*(4), 616–623. doi:10.1007/s10995-012-1037-4

Peacock-Chambers, E., Dicks, K., Sarathy, L., Brown, A. A., & Boynton-Jarrett, R. (2017). Perceived maternal behavioral control, infant behavior, and milk supply: A qualitative study. *Journal of Developmental and Behavioral Pediatrics, 38*(6), 401–408. doi:10.1097/DBP.0000000000000455

Perrin, E. C., Hurley, S. M., Mattern, K., Flavin, L., & Pinderhughes, E. E. (2019). Barriers and stigma experienced by gay fathers and their children. *Pediatrics, 143*(2), 1–9.

Postpartum Support International (PSI) (n.d.-a). *Postpartum support international—psi*. Retrieved 2019 from https://www.postpartum.net/

Postpartum Support International (PSI) (n.d.-b). Postpartum psychosis. Retrieved March 28, 2022, from https://www.postpartum.net/learn-more/postpartum-psychosis/

Roubinov, D. S., Luecken, L. J., Crnic, K. A., & Gonzales, N. A. (2014). Postnatal depression in Mexican American fathers: Demographic, cultural, and familial predictors. *Journal of Affective Disorders, 152*, 360–368. doi:10.1016/j.jad.2013.09.038

Rudman, A., & Waldenström, U. (2007). Critical views on postpartum care expressed by new mothers. *BMC Health Services Research, 7*(1). doi:10.1186/1472-6963-7-178-F

Scheyer, K., & Urizar, Jr., G. G. (2016). Altered stress patterns and increased risk for postpartum depression among low-income pregnant women. *Archive of Women's Mental Health, 19*, 317–328. doi:10.1007/s00737-015-0563-7

Silverman, M., Reichenberg, A., Savitz, D., Cnattingius, S., Lichtenstein, P., Hultman, C., Larsson, H., & Sandin, S. (2017). The risk factors for postpartum depression: A population-based study. *Depression and Anxiety, 34*(2), 178–187. doi:10.1002/da.22597

Sherbourne, C. D., & Stewart, A. L. (1991). The MOS social support survey. *Social Science & Medicine, 32*(6), 705-714.

Skovholt, T. M. (2001). *The resilient practitioner: Burnout prevention and self-care strategies for counselors, therapists, teachers, and health professionals.* Taylor & Francis.

Skovholt, T. M., & Trotter-Mathison, M. (2011). *The resilient practitioner: Burnout prevention and self-care strategies for counselors, therapists, teachers, and health professionals* (2nd ed.). Taylor & Francis. doi:10.4324/9780203893326

Spinelli, M. (2018). Infanticide and American criminal justice (1980–2018). *Archives of Women's Mental Health.* doi:10.1007/s00737-018-0873-7

Tebeka, S., Le Strat, Y., & Dubertret, C. (2016). Developmental trajectories of pregnant and postpartum depression in an epidemiologic survey. *Journal of Affective Disorders, 203*, 62–68. doi:10.1016/j.jad.2016.05.058

Thompson, K. (2020, January 10). *It's time to retire the phrase "breast is best" once and ...* Retrieved from https://www.todaysparent.com/baby/breastfeeding/yes-breast-is-best-but-its-time-to-retire-that-phrase-once-and-for-all/

United States Department of Labor. (n.d.). *Paid parental leave.* Retrieved February 14, 2022, from https://www.dol.gov/general/jobs/benefits/paid-parental-leave

5

Conception, Pregnancy, and Birth

Isabel A. Thompson

Personal Narrative

We were a family of three, excited to bring our second daughter into the world. My first pregnancy wasn't bad, aside from developing preeclampsia at 38 weeks and having to be induced four days later, delivering my first daughter via emergency C-section. During my second pregnancy, I developed gestational diabetes at 27 weeks, which tripled my chances of getting preeclampsia again. At 37 weeks, my blood pressure was dangerously high, and I was sent to labor and delivery to have my C-section. The surgery went great, but my recovery was a nightmare. The nurses noticed some bleeding coming from my incision, and instead of calling my doctor, they put some glue over it and told the doctor the next morning. Since the bleeding didn't stop, I had steri-strips over my incision to stop the bleeding. Unfortunately, blood clots formed, and I had to wear a wound vac for two weeks, going in every other day to have it removed, cleaned, and replaced. Stitches were put in afterwards, but my incision was still leaking and would not close. My doctor and I agreed that it would be best to just keep the area clean and dry and let the healing process happen naturally. Six and a half months passed before my incision was fully healed. I found myself sinking into a dark hole that I couldn't quite crawl out of. I felt useless, like I had no purpose or meaning. I would lie in bed and beg God to just let me die so my misery would end. I felt so many emotions at once, yet I felt empty inside. Numb. I wanted nothing more than to enjoy life with my precious family, but every day felt like a new burden. I had no motivation to clean or shower or even eat. I just laid there, nursed the baby, and laid there some more. My husband kept pushing me to seek help because he didn't know how to help me, but I felt hopeless. I felt like it wasn't even worth anyone else's time or effort to fix me. I had officially hit rock bottom, an all-time low. I tried everything I could to overcome the feeling of doom and dread. I tried meditation, prayer, spending time alone, spending time with friends and family. Nothing helped. Nothing took away the pain I felt inside for what seemed like no reason at all. I eventually had to schedule an appointment with my doctor. My youngest is nearly two, and I still take my antidepressants. I was ashamed at first, but I know that those pills help me be the mom my kids deserve. That is more important to me than battling the demons that had consumed me before.

—*Anonymous*

DOI: 10.4324/9780429440892-5

The experiences of conception, pregnancy, and childbirth are life altering in the best of circumstances and can be traumatic if a woman experienced trauma during childbirth (Furuta et al., 2018). It is crucial to help the mother, her partner, and family feel safe enough to share their story with their clinician. This chapter explores the experiences of conception, pregnancy, and birth and presents useful information for clinicians working with pregnant and new mothers, and families. Furthermore, pregnant women, especially first-time mothers, may experience some level of anxiety during pregnancy (Huizink et al., 2014), and anxiety disorders are also common during pregnancy (Viswasama et al., 2019), so clinicians should be prepared to address mood symptoms even if their client does not have, or develop, peripartum depression (PPD) or another maternal mood disorder.

Depression, anxiety, or post-traumatic stress disorder (PTSD) during pregnancy increases the risk of postpartum psychiatric disorders (Nillni et al., 2018). Maternal mood disorders are also associated with consequent risks to maternal and infant health and wellbeing. For instance, maternal PTSD has a negative impact on the bonding between mother and infant (Muzik et al., 2016), and maternal depression and anxiety are associated with mother–infant bonding problems (Nolvi, Karlsson, Bridgett, Pajulo et al., 2016). Difficulties with maternal–infant bonding can cause other developmental problems, including delays in language and motor skill development (Boyd et al., 2006).

While previous diagnostic definitions of postpartum depression focused on depression after the birth of the baby (APA, 2000), the DSM-5-TR recognizes that peripartum depression can begin in pregnancy (APA, 2022). Regarding the use of antidepressants for pregnant women experiencing PPD, the risks of psychotropic medication must be weighed against the risks of having PPD during pregnancy without psychotropic treatment (Mitchell & Goodman, 2018). This diagnostic timeframe is important for clinicians to consider, as they may work with those who are pregnant or trying to conceive. Clinical awareness that mood disturbances can start during pregnancy increases clinical sensitivity to clients' presenting concerns and treatment options.

In the case study example, Jesse begins to struggle emotionally during pregnancy and feels isolated, especially due to her experience of pregnancy during the COVID-19 pandemic. As you read Jesse's case study, consider how you could address her distress using the STRENGTHS model and what treatment approaches you would implement.

Case Study: Jesse

Jesse became pregnant easily and her experience of pregnancy was smooth in that she did not experience any medical complications during pregnancy. However, she struggled emotionally with feelings of isolation, primarily due to the COVID-19 pandemic. She felt that she missed out on in-person activities with other pregnant mothers, such as prenatal yoga classes. Her vision of pregnancy as a time of communal activities connecting with other pregnant women was not realized, as she spent time at home working remotely. She developed a good relationship with her midwife. Overall, she was excited to give birth and her birth plan was to give birth at a birth center. She started her labor process by going to the birth center. However, her son was in a breech position and there were some concerns about continuing to pursue a natural birth at the birth center. Jesse conferred with her husband and midwife and decided to transfer to a hospital setting, even though that was not her preference. Because she was giving birth in an area that had been severely impacted by the COVID-19 pandemic, her partner was not allowed to join her in the labor and delivery area. She struggled with strong physical pain during labor and did not have the emotional support that she needed. She ended up having an emergency C-section as her infant's heart rate was slowing down too much. In the days and weeks following the birth, Jesse expressed grief that the birth experience had not been what she had hoped for. She struggled with sadness and frequent crying spells. While she loved her baby, Jayden, she found herself not feeling connected to her infant son as much as she thought she would.

Reflection Questions for Clinicians

- What aspects of Jesse's birth story would you want to explore if you were her counselor/mental health provider?
- What aspects of Jesse's story may connect with DSM-5-TR criteria for PPD, or mood symptoms, or the potential development of such symptoms?
- Are there any aspects of her story that are personally triggering for you? Are there any aspects of her story that you connect with strongly or feel disconnected from?
- If you were working as her counselor/mental health provider, what support, training, or resources would you need to be most effective with her?

Case Study: Marisela

Marisela wanted to have a vaginal birth with as few interventions as possible. She had had a cesarean birth for her first birth and wanted to have as natural a birth as possible for the birth of her second child. Therefore, she researched potential care providers in her area and had found a midwife with whom she felt very comfortable and who supported her plan to have a VBAC (vaginal birth after cesarean). She had identified both her partner and birth doula as support people to assist her during labor. She completed an extensive birth education program prior to going into labor, studying natural ways for coping with the physical intensity of labor. She also did prenatal yoga and attended birth education classes with her partner. Although she was nervous about a home birth, she decided to pursue one, especially due to COVID-19 restrictions in the hospital setting which would not allow both her partner and her birth doula to attend the birth. During the birth, she was able to have her doula and partner and midwife present. Her main challenges were with managing her older daughter's needs in the postpartum, as her daughter struggled to adjust to the birth of her brother and the time and energy he demanded from her mother. Her older daughter began experiencing sleep difficulties and regressed with her toilet training. Marisela felt guilty that she could not attend to her older daughter in the way that she was used to before the birth of her son.

Reflection Questions for Clinicians

- What aspects of Marisela's birth story would you want to follow-up with if you were counselor/mental health provider?
- What aspects of Marisela's story may connect with the DSM-5-TR criteria for PPD, or mood symptoms, or the potential development of such symptoms?
- Are there any aspects of Marisela's story that are personally triggering for you? Are there any aspects of her story that you connect with strongly or feel disconnected from?

As these two case studies illustrate, each mother's experience of conception, pregnancy, and birth is unique. Furthermore, each father/partner and family navigates the stressors inherent in the experience of pregnancy differently.

CONCEPTION

Conception refers to the physiological process of successful fertilization of an ovum and subsequent implantation of the embryo (Newman & Newman, 2018). For some couples, conception happens readily when they decide to have a baby. For others, the journey to conception is complicated and lengthy. As counselors, we must be attuned to how prospective parents (or a prospective parent) pursuing conception may face experiences of marginalization and discrimination, especially those who are same sex (Tsfati & Ben-Ari, 2019) or gender non-binary (Fischer, 2021).

INFERTILITY

For heterosexual couples experiencing infertility, conception may include costly and invasive infertility treatments. If a person or couple you are working with experienced infertility in their journey to conception, it is valuable to gather information about their experiences. Infertility impacts approximately 12 percent of women in the United States of childbearing age (15–44 years) (Newman & Newman, 2018). Infertility has been defined as "the inability to conceive" (Newman & Newman, 2018, p. 93). It can be the result of "problems in the reproductive system of the man, the woman, or both" (Newman & Newman, p. 93, 2018). Secondary infertility refers to a couple experiencing infertility or the inability to carry a baby to term after previously giving birth (Mayo Clinic, n.d.).

ASSESSING CONCEPTION-RELATED RISK FACTORS

When assessing for conception-related risk factors, understanding pregnancy intention is important, as unintended pregnancy is associated with development of PPD (Gastaldon et al., 2022). Further, a challenging and stressful conception should be addressed in treatment, as maternal stress during pregnancy can have negative effects on their baby's emotional reactivity (Nolvi, Karlsson, Bridgett, Korja et al., 2016). The questions below can be helpful as a starting point for assessment of pregnancy intention.

Sample Assessment Questions: Pregnancy Intention

- Was this a planned/intended pregnancy?
- Tell me about your planning process.
- Was this pregnancy unexpected? If so, how are the mother and/or couple experiencing pregnancy?
- How does the father or partner feel about this pregnancy?
- Did both members of the couple desire to pursue having a baby with equal enthusiasm? Was one member of the couple more enthusiastic and the other member of the couple accommodated their desire to have a child (or additional children)? (If working with a couple.)
- What do other extended family members think and feel about this pregnancy? How are their thoughts/feelings impacting you? (If applicable.)

These assessment questions lay a foundation to discuss a client's full experience of pregnancy in further depth, which is crucial for accurate assessment, as complications experienced during pregnancy or childbirth are associated with double the risk of developing PPD (Tebeka et al., 2016, p. 66).

THE ADJUSTMENTS OF PREGNANCY

Pregnancy is a period of adjustment that is experienced differently by each family. Pregnancy has many dimensions, including the physical development of the baby (or babies), the concurrent hormonal and physical changes that the mother experiences, and the accompanying psychological, emotional, social, and role changes (Newman & Newman, 2018). Expectant fathers/partners, grandparents, and extended family members also go through changes as they prepare for the birth (Newman & Newman, 2018).

Pregnancy can also be marked by spiritual changes as expectant mothers and their partners consider the meaning and purpose of the pregnancy. Counselors who demonstrate insight and empathy for the changes that pregnant people experience will be able to serve them effectively. Pregnancy is a vulnerable time, both physically and socially. Physically, a woman's immune system operates differently while pregnant to support the developing fetus (Digitale, 2017). Pregnant women and their developing babies are more likely to develop severe outcomes if they contract contagious viruses like COVID-19 (CDC, 2021). Pregnant women and the developing fetus are sensitive to ingested substances like drugs or alcohol and environmental toxins, in addition to maternal stress, all of which can negatively impact the fetus (Newman & Newman, 2018). Socially, pregnant woman can be subject to discrimination and bias. Pregnant women experiencing depression or other mood symptoms benefit from treatment to help them manage pregnancy and care effectively for their unborn baby and their own wellbeing.

UNDERSTANDING THE IMPACT OF MEDICAL COMPLICATIONS OF PREGNANCY

Women who have medical complications during pregnancy experience additional stressors, which can contribute to psychological distress. They may also have accompanying worries and fears about the health of their developing baby. Therefore, it is important for clinicians to understand a woman's perception of her pregnancy, the complications experienced, and her perception of her coping ability.

Although studies do not suggest a consistent direct link between medical complications and the development of psychiatric disorders, the following specific medical complications have been associated with increased risk for the development of PPD: hyperemesis gravidarum (HG), gestational hypertension, preeclampsia, and C-section (Meltzer-Brody et al., 2017, p. 1428). Given the risks associated with these conditions and the possible development of PPD, understanding the medical complications of pregnancy as well as obstetrical complications can help clinicians be more aware of issues impacting pregnant clients. It is incumbent upon clinicians to obtain a comprehensive medical history, including medical complications of pregnancy (see Table 5.1), to develop treatment plans that address a pregnant person's unique needs.

Table 5.1
Medical Complications of Pregnancy

Category of Medical Complication	Medical Complication	Prevalence Rate	Symptoms During Pregnancy	Risk of PPD/ Acute Stress
Hypertensive Disorders of Pregnancy	Preeclampsia	5–8% (Simkin et al., 2010)	Multi-organ condition, may lead to hypertension and protein in urine (Simkin et al., 2010).	Associated with risk of acute stress and PPD (Meltzer-Brody, 2017).
Hypertensive Disorders of Pregnancy	Chronic Hypertension Gestational Hypertension	5–10% (Thombre et al., 2015)	High blood pressure prior to pregnancy that continues. High blood pressure during pregnancy (Thombre et al., 2015).	Both conditions associated with risk of PPD (Strapasson et al., 2018).
	Gestational Diabetes	3–5% (Simkin et al., 2010)	Elevated blood sugar levels that must be monitored (Simkin et al., 2010).	Associated with risk of acute stress (Meltzer-Brody, 2017).
	Hyperemesis Gravidarum	0.3–2% (Kramer et al., 2013)	Severe nausea and vomiting resulting in dehydration and body weight loss (>5%). May require hospitalization (Kramer et al., 2013).	Associated with risk of PPD (Meltzer-Brody, 2017).

There are numerous medical complications that pregnant mothers may experience, including hypertensive disorders of pregnancy, which includes chronic hypertension, gestational hypertension, and preeclampsia (Thombre et al., 2015). Women experiencing hypertensive disorders of pregnancy are more likely to experience depression symptoms (Strapasson et al., 2018). Experiencing preeclampsia during pregnancy is associated with "PPD and onset of an acute stress reaction" (Meltzer-Brody, 2017, p. 1435). Both gestational hypertension and gestational diabetes are associated with increased risk of psychiatric disorders: Gestational hypertension is associated with increased rates of PPD and gestational diabetes is associated with increased risk of acute stress in the postpartum period (Meltzer-Brody, 2017, pp. 1436–1437). Therefore, clinicians working with pregnant women should be aware of these associations and closely monitor and screen their pregnant clients and clients who have recently given birth for these associated mental health and psychosocial concerns.

Most women experience nausea and vomiting during early pregnancy. It typically resolves by week 20 of pregnancy and can range from mild nausea without vomiting, to more moderate nausea with vomiting (Kramer et al., 2013). Women with hyperemesis gravidarum (HG) experience severe nausea and persistent vomiting (Abramowitz et al., 2017). This medical complication is associated with a higher risk of PPD (Meltzer-Brody, 2017).

Counselors can provide psychoeducation and screening with pregnant clients who are experiencing medical complications of pregnancy, such as providing general information about how medical complications of pregnancy relate to maternal mental health and ensuring a pregnant person is getting care from their healthcare provider, while also providing emotional validation. Counselors can encourage clients to be attuned to their own emotional and mental state and to talk about any concerns or symptoms that worsen. In addition, counselors can advocate and provide interprofessional training for healthcare professionals, especially OB/GYNs and midwives, about the increased risk of PPD associated with these medical complications.

CHANGING BODIES, BODY IMAGE, AND SELF-ACCEPTANCE

Women's bodies physically change to accommodate and nourish the developing fetus. These changes can impact their body image and sense of themselves (Newman & Newman, 2018). How a woman experiences these changes varies greatly and is associated with many factors including the impact of the pregnancy changes on her mental and physical wellbeing. While some women may feel energized during pregnancy, many struggle with fatigue and various physical and emotional discomforts. Moreover, women who experience depression while pregnant may struggle more than other pregnant women with sustaining health promoting behaviors and following the guidelines for health for pregnancy (Newman & Newman, 2018).

BIRTH

Birth is a major life transition, both for the baby (or babies in the case of twins or multiples) being born and the mother and her partner/family. While the birth experience can be a highlight in many people's lives, it can also be a traumatic experience if the mother did not have the birth experience she had hoped for, or if there were birth complications. Given the high rates of Cesarean section in the United States, approximately one third of women are now experiencing birth by C-section (Martin et al., 2018). Further, hospitalization of the mother or baby beyond the typical stay after birth should be addressed when working with mothers, partners, and families. As you are reading this section, we invite you to reflect on your own birth culture, what you were raised to believe about birth, birthing mothers, and newborns, and what beliefs you currently have, personal experiences of giving birth or witnessing birth, and how these could impact your work with clients who may have similar or different beliefs about birth. If your beliefs around birth are so strong that you might have difficulty working with a client who has different beliefs or practices related to birth, we recommend you seek additional training, supervision, or consultation. Furthermore, if you find that unresolved feelings from your own experiences related to birth contribute to a secondary traumatic stress reaction, we strongly recommend you seek support for yourself.

THE PROCESS OF BIRTH

Having a basic knowledge of the physical process of birth and the emotional states that frequently accompany it is helpful for counselors and other mental health professionals. Birth is a multidimensional process that includes both physical action and accompanying feelings and psychological and role changes. Physically, "Birth is initiated by involuntary contractions of the uterine muscles, commonly referred to as labor" (Newman & Newman, 2018, p. 102). When someone describes going into labor, they are referring to this involuntary process of physical contractions which typically become more intense as labor progresses. As shown in Table 5.2, the process of birth is described in three stages medically and five stages psychologically (Newman & Newman, 2018). Psychologically, transition is when the intensity of physical sensations increases; this is not a medical stage but a significant shift for the birthing person (Newman & Newman, 2018).

Table 5.2

Medical and Psychological Stages of Birth

Medical Stage of Birth	Characteristics	Psychological Stage of Birth	Sensations	Needs of Birthing Person
		First Stage	Initial signs that labor will begin soon (e.g., water breaking, contractions).	Instrumental support and emotional validation.
First Stage	"Begins with the onset of uterine contractions and ends with the full dilation of the cervix."	Second Stage	Intensity of contractions increases—a birthing person may contact their midwife or go to the hospital for birth during this stage.	Emotional and physical support to manage intense and painful sensations.

(Continued)

Table 5.2 (Continued)
Medical and Psychological Stages of Birth

Medical Stage of Birth	Characteristics	Psychological Stage of Birth	Sensations	Needs of Birthing Person
		Transition/ Third Stage	Intense physical sensations/ pain— intensity of contractions increases, pause between contractions decreases.	Support and encouragement to cope with intense physical sensations.
Second Stage	"Begins at full dilation and ends with delivery of the baby."	Fourth Stage	The birth itself.	Connection to the baby during birth.
Third Stage	"Begins with delivery and ends with expulsion of the placenta."	Fifth Stage	Immediate postpartum and returning home from birthing location (if outside the home).	Skin-to-skin contact with baby (Mohrbacher & Kendall-Tackett, 2010). Breastfeeding support (if intending to breastfeed).

Note: Information about medical and psychological stages of birth and associated characteristics/sensations is from Newman & Newman, 2018, p. 102.

After a vaginal delivery that is relatively uncomplicated, and with a healthy newborn, the mother and baby can interact and have skin-to-skin time together immediately, which facilitates bonding and breastfeeding initiation (Mohrbacher & Kendall-Tackett, 2010). After surgical births such as C-sections or when the baby is showing signs of distress, the mother may not have this immediate bonding time after birth. Skin-to-skin contact very soon after delivery may be possible after surgical births provided mother and baby are doing well medically. Assisting expectant parents to advocate for skin-to-skin contact after birth can be helpful. Further, discussing a mother's perception of birth and the immediate postpartum is helpful to determine if they perceived it as positive, neutral, or traumatic.

BIRTH CULTURE

Birth culture refers to worldview factors that influence the way in which society and culture shape our experiences of birth and in effect provide a role for the pregnant woman to play (Newman & Newman, 2018). In the United States and Canada, a dominant approach is to medicalize birth (Shaw, 2013), with the accompanying cultural norm that mothers should give birth in a hospital. Concurrently practiced alternative approaches such as birth center births, home births, and midwifery care, tend to be perceived as outside the cultural norm in the United States. In cultures around the world and subcultures within the United States, approaches to birth can vary greatly, as do expectations about where to give birth and who should attend to a woman's medical and emotional needs during birth. When working with a woman and her family, it is helpful to get a sense of the cultural norms they may have regarding pregnancy and childbirth and reflect on your own beliefs to avoid imposing them on your client.

HEALTHCARE AND BIRTH ATTENDANTS

Mothers have many choices about who they will entrust with their medical care during the perinatal period in the immediate postpartum and beyond. While most pregnant women in the United States choose an obstetrician/gynecologist (OB/GYN) to provide their care, approximately 13 percent of women choose midwives to serve as their primary caregivers during pregnancy and after the birth (Weisband et al., 2018). Expectant mothers can elect to include their partners and/or trained birth attendants such as birth doulas in their pregnancy and postpartum experience.

In the United States, it has become more common for fathers or partners to be involved in the birth process (Newman & Newman, 2018). Fathers/partners may complete training about the stages of birth and birthing mothers' needs. An example is the Mindfulness-Based Childbirth and Parenting (MBCP) course, developed for expectant parents, which focuses on mindfulness practices for coping with pain during childbirth and for the adjustments of having a newborn (Bardacke, 2012).

There is a growing body of evidence that having a birth doula, who is a trained non-medical birth attendant, reduces the risk of unneeded medical interventions and increases a mother's comfort during birth (Newman & Newman, 2018). Doulas attend to the mother's (and partner's) needs, especially focusing on the mother's physical and emotional comfort. They can aid with non-medical support, such as providing cool water or snacks to the laboring mother, massage, suggesting pain-relieving movement, and offering verbal encouragement and agreed-upon relaxation cues, such as music or soft lighting (Newman & Newman, 2018). Doulas are trained both in the childbirth process and to provide support to the mother and her partner as they experience labor and birth (Steel et al., 2015).

Birth doulas can help to normalize a woman's bodily sensations during childbirth and assist with agreed-upon non-medical pain management approaches such as massage. They also help the woman and her partner advocate for their needs and preferences in the childbirth process and "protect the birth space from unwanted interruptions while aiming to complement the midwife or obstetrician in their clinical role" (Steel et al., 2015, p. 226). Birth doulas are trained to honor a birthing person's wishes and advocate for them and their partners. For example, if the mother is giving birth in a hospital setting but wants to avoid continuous fetal monitoring (which entails having a monitor strapped to her body that limits her movements), the doula can assist in communicating this to medical staff. When unexpected medical situations arise, birth doulas can help support the birthing parent and their partner.

Some clients may feel a cultural clash as they navigate pregnancy and prepare for birth, as they receive contradictory messages about pregnancy and birth from the mainstream culture and from their family of origin and/or cultural group membership. When mental health clinicians have knowledge about diverse birth cultures, they can most effectively aid their clients. For example, if a pregnant woman shared that she wanted to give birth at home with a midwife and doula, how would you respond? As with other elements in a client's life, it is important to understand our own cultural perspective regarding pregnancy and birth.

BIRTH TRAUMA AND OBSTETRICAL COMPLICATIONS

While childbirth can be a safe and fulfilling experience for some women, for others, childbirth is traumatic (Beck & Watson, 2019). Some researchers define traumatic birth as meeting DSM criteria for a traumatic event (Ayers, 2017). Women who experience birth trauma believed "that their lives or their baby's lives were in danger, or that their physical and emotional well-being was at risk" during birth (Garbes, 2018, p. 125). Understanding the mother's subjective experience and perception is essential and consistent with other definitions of trauma, which emphasize the person's perception of the event as traumatic.

The following risks factors during birth are associated with the development of PTSD: "a negative subjective birth experience, having an operative birth (i.e. assisted vaginal or caesarean section), lack of support during birth, and dissociation" (Ayers et al., 2016 as cited in Ayers, 2017, p. 427). A woman's perception of birth and support during labor matters, which reinforces the importance of continuous labor support, from birth doulas, partners, or other healthcare professionals. Mental health professionals who are aware of the risks of traumatic birth, and the impact on mothers, can help pregnant women identify support people to help them during the birth process.

Researchers are also examining preventative and positive factors that influence a woman's experience of birth and increase her resilience even in the face of some of the risk factors listed above (Ayers, 2017). Researchers have begun examining post-traumatic growth among perinatal women (Ayers, 2017). "Post-traumatic growth refers to experiencing positive changes in beliefs or functioning as a result of challenging life events or circumstances" (Ayers, 2017, p. 428). Some mothers who have experienced trauma in childbirth may experience post-traumatic growth responses (Sawyer & Ayers, 2009). Clinical mental health counselors and other mental health professionals working with women who have experienced traumatic birth can help them to process and integrate these experiences. Using a post-traumatic growth framework, a counselor can highlight a mother's resilience and focus on empowering her to consider meaning and purpose after a traumatic birth experience.

Preterm Birth and Neonatal Intensive Care

Preterm birth is defined as giving birth to a live baby who is less than 37 weeks of gestational age (WHO, n.d.). Preterm births can be very stressful for mother and baby, depending on the gestational age of the baby and their condition at birth. Some preterm babies may require a hospital stay in the Neonatal Intensive Care Unit (NICU) to assess their condition and/or provide needed medical treatment for them.

C-Section

In the United States, giving birth by cesarean section, or what is often termed a C-section, is quite common (Newman & Newman, 2018). A C-section is a surgical delivery that involves an incision into the mother's abdomen to deliver the baby. C-sections are necessary when complications during labor, or the condition of the mother or baby, preclude a safe vaginal delivery. C-section births can be either planned or unplanned (Newman & Newman, 2018). The rate of cesarean delivery was 31.9 percent in 2016 (Martin et al., 2018) and the United States has one of the highest rates in the world of C-section births (Nagle & Samari, 2021). Many C-section births in the United States may not be necessary (in other words, it would have been safe for the mother to deliver vaginally) (Newman & Newman, 2018).

Postpartum Hemorrhage

Postpartum hemorrhage (PPH) is a complication of birth and the immediate postpartum. Women naturally lose blood during the birthing process, as they birth the baby and then the placenta. However, some women experience postpartum or maternal hemorrhage, which is "defined as a cumulative blood loss or greater than or equal to 1,000 ML or blood loss accompanied by signs or symptoms of hypovolemia within 24 hours after the birth process, [and] remains the leading cause of maternal mortality worldwide" (ACOG, n.d.; hypovolemia refers to lack of blood volume). Experiencing postpartum hemorrhage may increase a mother's risk of developing PPD, so women who have experienced PPH should be screened for depression symptoms (Wang et al., 2022).

Maternal Mortality

Mothers and families may have moments of bliss after the birth of their baby, but some may feel unsupported and immensely stressed during this period of intense adjustment. Others may be left with intense fear and trauma if their baby is in a critical condition or if the mother herself is in a critical condition. Beyond experiencing adverse health outcomes, some mothers die during childbirth or shortly after giving birth. Maternal mortality rates in the United States have been rising in recent years, especially among Black mothers (Hoyert, 2022). Counselors should be aware of the risks for mothers, especially Black mothers, during pregnancy, birth, and the postpartum to help them advocate for their healthcare needs.

CHALLENGES OF THE IMMEDIATE AND EARLY POSTPARTUM

The immediate postpartum period in the hours, days, and weeks after a new baby is born can be experienced very differently by different mothers and families. A commonality is that all mothers who have given birth have experienced a significant physiological event and have emotional and psychological adjustment.

The significance of the first hour after birth is highlighted by the term "the golden hour" (Shaw, 2017). Neczypor and Holley (2017) describe the evidence-based "Golden Hour Protocol" which emphasizes the importance of the mother and baby having uninterrupted skin-to-skin contact for a least one hour after birth, early establishment of breastfeeding, and includes delaying umbilical cord clamping. However, when medically uncomplicated births occur in many Westernized medical settings, medical routines and procedures can unnecessarily interrupt mother–infant bonding, such as whisking the baby away from the mother to be wiped off and/or bathed (Mohrbacher & Kendall-Tackett, 2010), which can be unnecessary at best or even harmful for mother–infant bonding. Skin-to-skin contact between mother and baby immediately after birth is beneficial to facilitate both bonding and breastfeeding (Mohrbacher, & Kendall-Tackett, 2010; Neczypor & Holly, 2017). This can allow the baby to "crawl" to the breast and latch on if the mother intends to breastfeed her infant. If a mother had a C-section delivery, skin-to-skin contact immediately after birth can still be possible if the mother is in a stable condition and has expressed her wishes to her medical team.

In the immediate postpartum period, a mother's body goes through numerous changes. After the birth of the baby, the placenta is delivered. This process can be painful, as healthcare attendants may need to push on the mother's stomach to assist with placenta delivery. The umbilical cord that connected her to her baby is cut. Depending on the birth environment, delayed cord cutting may be possible, allowing for more of the umbilical blood to pass to the baby.

The time right after birth is one of intense physical, emotional, and psychological adjustment for mothers (Mohrbacher & Kendall-Tackett, 2010). A woman loses a lot of blood right after the birth and may wish to rest. However, for many women in Western culture, the mother is thrust immediately into the role of caring for her newborn while simultaneously attempting to attend to her own postpartum physical needs. Newborns' circadian rhythms are not yet developed, so their sleeping hours do not conform to the 24-hour day (Simkin et al., 2010), which means that tired mothers who have just given birth are also likely dealing with sleep disruption and deprivation. However, lactation consultants can support a mother who wants to breastfeed in approaches such as nursing while lying down to help a mother get needed rest while breastfeeding (Mohrbacher & Kendall-Tackett, 2010).

Counselors need to be aware of how sociocultural factors impact a mother and her family. After the birth of the baby, mothers and parents who have greater sense of community and greater instrumental support from community members or extended family may have a reduced likelihood of experiencing distress and peripartum depression. For new mothers there is typically a heightened stress and greater demand in the immediate postpartum as compared with their partners, as infants naturally bond with their primary caregiver who is often a tired mother who just gave birth.

Postpartum doulas may provide a powerful buffer for mothers and reduce their stress in the postpartum period, especially mothers who are navigating the postpartum period without adequate support from family or community. Postpartum doulas are trained to attend to new mothers' physical and emotional needs and support nourishing calm to her baby (or babies). Counselors who are aware of these adjunctive resources can provide their clients with information about them, although socioeconomic factors impact the feasibility of hiring a postpartum doula.

Reflection Questions for Clinicians

- Consider your familial/cultural/personal beliefs about conception, pregnancy, birth, and parenting.
- What cultural norms or practices regarding pregnancy, birth, or parenting were you taught?
- If you have personally experienced pregnancy and/or birth (either your own or a partner's), how has this experience impacted your beliefs?
- Are there any clinical issues related to conception, pregnancy, or birth that might be sensitive or triggering for you?

We encourage clinicians to reflect on their own experiences with birth and to seek support for themselves (if needed) in the form of counseling, supervision, consultation, and/or further training.

MULTIPLE PERSPECTIVES: FATHER/PARTNER AND FAMILY RELATIONSHIPS

Expectant fathers/partners go through changes in how they see themselves and are seen by others. Expectant grandparents and extended family also go through changes as they prepare for their new family member (Newman & Newman, 2018). First-time fathers/partners are marking a shift from not being parents to becoming parents, which is a major life role change.

Expectant fathers want to be involved in their partners' pregnancy, and their partners generally want them to be involved as well, but expectant fathers may struggle with how to engage and may have a sense of "paddling upstream" as they encounter barriers to involvement (Widarsson et al., 2015, p. 1059). For example, a father who accompanied their pregnant partner to a midwifery appointment still felt excluded, as the healthcare provider only directed comments to the mother (Widarsson et al., 2015). This sort of exclusion exacerbates a partner's feeling left out even when they make proactive attempts to be involved. Healthcare providers and counselors should be sure to use inclusive language, clearly invite both parents to appointments, and direct comments to both parents (when both are present).

Fathers and partners may also experience difficulties with the adjustment to pregnancy, and their mental health and emotional needs should be addressed. Although more likely to develop after a baby's birth, paternal depression may develop during a partner's pregnancy, and risk factors for the development of paternal depression during pregnancy include the father's level of stress and ill health (Underwood et al., 2017). We need to address the needs of fathers/partners by including them in appointments, being attuned to risk factors, and screening for symptoms of paternal depression.

Family relationships change during pregnancy as well, especially in the case of a first pregnancy in an extended family, when the couple's parents are about to become grandparents for the first time and their siblings are going to become first-time aunts and uncles (Newman & Newman, 2018). Expectations about the role that the grandparents and extended family will play in the new baby's life vary according to familial and cultural traditions. Exploring a client's familial relationships and the expectations around pregnancy and birth can be beneficial to clinical work during the peripartum.

MULTICULTURAL CONSIDERATIONS

Understanding broader cultural narratives around conception, pregnancy, and birth is essential as well. Expectations around family formation, conception, pregnancy, and birth are socio-culturally grounded. Gaining a clear understanding of a mother's experiences and whether they felt nourished and supported by the dominant narratives in their story or if they felt disempowered, invisible, or marginalized during the conception, pregnancy, and birth process is crucial.

Mainstream narratives of conception, pregnancy, and birth tend to privilege the stories of White, cisgender, non-disabled women and perpetuate conventional gender roles based on heterosexual norms. Furthermore, the intersection of misogyny, sexism, heterosexism, ableism, and other forms of bias is often highlighted during the process of conception, pregnancy, and birth. "Women of color, lesbian and queer people, as well people who do not fall within a gender binary, understand that our full personhood or womanhood is still considered conditional" (Garbes, 2018, p. 78). This sense of conditionality or marginality can be exacerbated by cultural narratives of pregnancy. Counselors should avoid exacerbating this sense of exclusion by directly inviting clients to share their identities and the experiences they have had while pregnant.

The way others perceive an expectant mother often reflects the norms and values of the society in which they are embedded; norms about who should become pregnant, when, where, with whom, at what age, and under what circumstances. For example, pregnant mothers who are teenagers may face judgment from others. On the other hand, pregnant mothers who are older than 35 may also face judgments, though the percentage of women delaying pregnancy has increased greatly (Murakami et al., 2016). We can help expectant mothers who are over age 35 both by highlighting their strengths, and by normalizing pregnancy over age 35.

Conception and Pregnancy for LGBTQ+ Couples

For some mothers and parents, especially same-sex or gender non-binary parents/couples, conception may include many decisions and steps, as well as dealing with societal perceptions and prejudices as they make decisions about their family and how to conceive. Conception for same-sex couples involves a series of decisions after the initial intention to conceive is established, such as how to conceive, whose genetic material will be used, as well as who will carry the baby (Markus et al., 2010). Gay male couples may face choices about who would serve as a surrogate for their pregnancy, and how they would go about this (Tsfati & Ben-Ari, 2019) or they may decide to pursue adoption to become parents.

Lesbian couples seeking to become parents have many choices with regards to how to do so, including becoming pregnant through a previous opposite-sex relationship, serving as foster parents, adopting, becoming a stepparent, or through donor insemination (DI) (Markus et al., 2010, p. 124). Lesbian couples choosing DI face decisions regarding which member of the couple would become pregnant, which donor sperm (whether from a known or unknown donor) to use, as well as insemination options (Markus et al., 2010). Moreover, lesbian women who are pregnant and seeking prenatal medical care also face decisions about whether, when, or how to 'come out' to their healthcare provider if this person does not already know their sexual orientation identity (Markus et al., 2010).

Decisions about conception, pregnancy, birth, and parenting also impact single women, bisexual women, and transgender individuals, who also have distinct life experiences and needs (Markus et al., 2010). Single women who want to become mothers face decisions about how to conceive, and whether to use a donor process. Individuals who identify as non-binary also face unique challenges, such as biases imposed by other people (including healthcare providers) and choices about when or how to address their identity with others.

Some individuals and families seeking to conceive and become parents challenge societal norms about what a family is (or should be). Polygamists and polyamorous families who want to become parents also face decisions surrounding how to proceed with conception and parenting and legal barriers around who will be considered the legal parents (Solomon, 2021). We recommend that you examine your beliefs, life experiences, and expectations about conception, pregnancy, parenting, and family, to root out sexist, ageist, ableist, racist, heterosexist, or other biases, as clinicians need to be multiculturally competent to avoid causing harm to clients (ACA, 2014).

APPLICATIONS TO COUNSELING

Since PPD can (and often does) develop during pregnancy, it is crucial that clinicians and healthcare providers screen pregnant women for it. Screenings during pregnancy should be increased to aid in the prevention and early intervention of PPD (Kleiman & Raskin, 2013). Further, many women may feel reluctant to share the depth of their depressive symptoms with their doctors (Kleiman & Raskin, 2013). While pregnancy is often a joyous time, it can also be one fraught with anxiety about the baby and its development, how to care for the baby, and the transition for the mother, couple, or family when the new baby arrives (Simkin et al., 2010). First-time mothers are experiencing the huge transition to becoming parents responsible for the survival and loving care of their new baby and the accompanying lifestyle changes that curtail the time they used to have to pursue their own self-care or interests. Mothers with an older child or children have already experienced the transition to motherhood and have been through birth before but may experience anxiety about how they will meet their new baby's needs, along with those of their older child or children, let alone their own self-care needs and household responsibilities. Mothers who have experienced a previous traumatic birth or previous PPD may have heightened anxiety when compared with a first-time mother. Thus, understanding your client's experience is essential and exploring how they perceive *this* pregnancy, the upcoming birth, and their fears can be beneficial. Coupling this with a positive asset search to explore the strengths and resources pregnant mothers bring to the table can be very useful.

Pregnant women who may not meet the criteria for PPD or have not been in contact with a mental health provider can still experience symptoms of anxiety and depression or may have an undiagnosed mood disorder. For instance, in a qualitative study with 14 pregnant women, experience of stress and depressive symptoms was a common factor in the pursuit of prenatal yoga (Kinser & Masho, 2015). Therefore, counselors who partner with prenatal yoga teachers to provide psychoeducation around PPD could be a useful preventative community service.

ADDRESSING CONCEPTION, PREGNANCY, AND BIRTH IN TREATMENT

The take-home message we want to emphasize is to be intentional and use your attentive listening skills and caring attitude to convey to the mother/birthing parent and partner/spouse that you care about how they experienced the process of conception. Follow-up with this aspect of their story if it has relevance to the current presenting problem. For example, if a mother is currently experiencing acute stress and marital conflict and has a history of infertility treatments, this should be addressed. Sometimes we may become focused on current symptoms and miss a key aspect of the broader context; attending to the story of the conception itself can provide useful clues as we piece together the picture of the mother who is sharing her story with us. When a person shares their story, it can be a healing factor to help them identify their strengths. A counselor can help reframe the story in such a way that they/she can experience themselves as strong and can integrate the painful elements of their story in a cohesive and meaningful narrative. Counselors may use a narrative approach, especially with clients who experienced perinatal loss (Romney et al., 2021). A narrative approach can help identify disheartening narratives and strengthen empowering narratives to integrate any trauma associated with conception, pregnancy, or birth, within a meaningful framework.

Birth Narratives: What Is Your Birth Story?

As illustrated in the case studies in this chapter, women's experiences of birth can be markedly different. The nuances of each person's and family's story may hold clues to their current symptoms and distress, as well as their recovery and healing process. In addition to inviting mothers and families to share their current birth story, inviting them to share about previous pregnancy and birth experiences, including experiences of perinatal loss (Hutti et al., 2013), is helpful, as these experiences can impact a current pregnancy and birth experience. We recommend that clinicians take time to understand each mother and each family's unique story of conception, pregnancy, and birth. When a mother experiences significant challenges or stressors in the peripartum, this increases their overall perceived stress level, which is connected to the development of mood symptoms, whether during pregnancy or after birth (Meltzer-Brody et al., 2017). Further, mothers who experience complications during pregnancy or childbirth have a two-fold increased risk of peripartum depression (Tebeka et al., 2016). Therefore, inviting mothers to share their story can aid in comprehensive case conceptualization, accurate diagnosis, and effective tailored treatment. As discussed earlier, it is crucial for counselors to examine our own birth cultural beliefs to avoid imposing our own beliefs and/or projecting our experiences onto our clients.

ASSESSING SUBSTANCE USE DURING PREGNANCY

Another significant clinical consideration during pregnancy is the mother's use of substances such as nicotine, alcohol, marijuana, and other drugs as these can impact the developing fetus by harming the "fetal environment" (Newman & Newman, 2018, p. 109). Many substances are teratogens during pregnancy and can negatively impact the developing baby (Newman & Newman, 2018). A pregnant woman's use of prescribed medications, supplements, vitamins, and over-the-counter medications can also impact the fetal environment. While the focus here is on the mother's use of substances, it should be noted that male-mediated effects of drugs on the sperm can then impact the fetus also (Newman & Newman, 2018).

ASSESSING HISTORY OF SEXUAL ABUSE AND/OR SEXUAL ASSAULT

Pregnant people/women who have a history of sexual abuse and/or sexual assault experience added dimensions of stress and/or trauma during pregnancy. The process of pregnancy and birth sometimes can trigger trauma related to an expectant person's history of sexual abuse or sexual assault. An expectant mother's history of childhood sexual abuse is associated to adverse outcomes during pregnancy and birth, and it is recommended that clinicians focus on "early identification of women with a child abuse history as such women require trauma-sensitive care and consideration" (Brunton & Dryer, 2021, p. 1). Counselors and other mental health professionals working with pregnant women and new mothers are advised to gather a sexual abuse history early in treatment and be attuned to the potential impact of this trauma during the peripartum.

ASSESSING INTIMATE PARTNER VIOLENCE DURING PREGNANCY

While estimates of intimate partner violence (IPV) in pregnancy vary, between 3 percent and 9 percent of pregnant women experience IPV; factors such as being single, being an ethnic/racial minority, and experiencing poverty increase the risk of experiencing IPV (Alhusen et al., 2015). It is also likely that these prevalence rates are underestimates (Deshpande & Lewis-O'Conner, 2015). Intimate partner violence has been defined as "a pattern of coercive control of one intimate partner by the other that includes physical and sexual violence, threats of physical or sexual violence, and emotional abuse in the context of physical and sexual violence" (Alhusen et al., 2015 p. 100). In the cases of sexual assault or coercive sexual encounters in which a woman did not want to become pregnant, but the partner refused to use birth control (such as condoms), IPV can directly lead to pregnancy (Deshpande & Lewis-O'Conner, 2013). Screening pregnant clients for experience of IPV is essential, as it can negatively impact maternal and neonatal health (Alhusen et al., 2015) and violent experiences during pregnancy are a risk factor for developing PPD (Gastaldon et al., 2022). Experiencing poverty during pregnancy can increase the likelihood of an expectant mother undergoing a variety of these negative life experiences and exposures to harmful substances or stressors, including IPV (Newman & Newman, 2018).

BIOPSYCHOSOCIAL THEORETICAL MODEL

Conception, pregnancy, and birth are impacted by the macrosystem, exosystem, mesosystem, microsystem, and chronosystem (Bronfenbrenner, 1979). Many challenges couples encounter during conception, pregnancy, and birth have biopsychosocial components or can be viewed from a biopsychosocial lens. For example, infertility has been conceptualized as a biopsychosocial crisis for couples (Thompson, 2021). Macrosystem factors such as healthcare systems and public policy have a major impact on a person's and family's experience of conception and pregnancy. For instance, in the case of infertility, health insurance may not cover fertility interventions or the use of assistive reproductive technology. Even for people who do not experience infertility, when a person lives in a country without a nationally socialized healthcare system, concern about the out-of-pocket cost of birth can create added stress during pregnancy. Furthermore, the lack of paid maternal/paternal/parental leave in the United States has an impact on the experience of pregnancy and birth. Exosystemic factors including institutional norms and hospital policies exert influence on a woman's experience of pregnancy and birth. This factor was highlighted during the COVID-19 pandemic, when birthing mothers faced COVID restrictions about who could be present with them during birth. The microsystem of a woman's family, friend, and healthcare providers exerts strong influence on the experience of pregnancy and birth and whether/how an expectant mother experiences support. The mesosystem and interactions between these microsystems are also influential, as when a mother senses that communication is smooth between her partner/family and chosen healthcare provider, she may experience more harmony. Prevailing norms and expectations for conception, pregnancy, and birth change through time with generational, social, and cultural factors.

ETHICAL AND LEGAL CONSIDERATIONS

In the United States, the federal right to abortion ended in June of 2022 when the U.S. Supreme Court overturned *Roe V. Wade* (Jaffe, 2022). This has changed the landscape of maternal healthcare, particularly for those residing in states that ban or restrict abortion access (Jaffe, 2022). Some pregnant women/people may have fears about what this change means for them.

Multicultural competence is an essential aspect of clinical competence (ACA, 2014). As counselors, we have an ethical responsibility to avoid causing harm at a minimum and to be of benefit to our clients whenever possible (ACA, 2014). Imposing our own biases and judgments on a pregnant client is harmful, so seeking supervision and consultation can be helpful when struggling with imposing our own values onto clients.

One of the primary considerations ethically and legally is protecting the health and safety of the mother and infant and their family. Clinicians must be trained to accurately screen and assess suicidality. Furthermore, clinicians must be aware of the risks of infanticide associated with postpartum psychosis, assess for infanticidal thoughts, and be prepared to take immediate action to protect the safety the mother and infant (or infants in the case of twins or multiple births). In Chapter 6, we describe assessment tools and instruments for screening.

BARRIERS TO TREATMENT

A major challenge to implementing the recommendations discussed in this chapter to effectively treat pregnant women is difficulties associated with the screening and referral of pregnant women at risk of developing PPD or who may already be experiencing depression (Feeley et al., 2016). Many pregnant women have regular appointments with their chosen pregnancy healthcare provider (whether OB/GYN, family doctor, or midwife). Moreover, awareness of women's peripartum mental health needs and that mood disorders may begin during pregnancy itself is more recent. Because emotional disorders are the most common complication of childbirth one would imagine that such screening is routinely occurring and that women feel safe disclosing their distress to their doctors (Kleiman & Raskin, 2013). However, this may not be the case, as mothers may fear the stigma and judgment associated with having PPD or other mood symptoms. For these reasons, many suicidal pregnant individuals and mothers may remain fearful to reveal the depth of their distress to their doctors (Kleiman & Raskin, 2013). Even if a healthcare provider screened appropriately and provided a referral to a mental health provider, would a woman feel safe to follow-up on a mental health referral? Part of the advocacy effort that we can do as a profession is to reduce the stigma associated with mental health issues during pregnancy (and after birth) and help encourage expectant and new mothers to seek treatment. Community outreach efforts and preventative psychoeducational programs are one way that counselors can both offer expertise and information and reduce the stigma associated with mental health issues, especially during pregnancy.

Pregnant women experiencing stress and depressive symptoms may be seeking support in places outside of their doctor, healthcare provider, or the counseling office. In a qualitative study exploring women's experiences of prenatal yoga, the researchers' findings indicated that "pregnant women seek out prenatal yoga to deal with feelings of stress and depressive symptoms" (Kinser & Masho, 2015, p. 323). While yoga practice is often a very effective complement to mental health services, for women experiencing PPD it is not a substitute for mental health treatment. Mental health professionals could do a more effective job in reaching potential clients who are pregnant and engaged in prenatal activities. For example, doing outreach at prenatal yoga classes could be an effective way of connecting with pregnant women to provide psychoeducation regarding maternal mental health as well as resources for those women who would benefit from additional support such as therapy.

While complementary approaches to self-manage symptoms like prenatal yoga can be a powerful adjunct to treatment, they should not take the place of talking to a counselor or other qualified mental health professional when a person's symptoms are interfering with their daily life or are distressing. Counselors and other mental health professionals can also link their pregnant clients to competent psychiatric care for assessment. Because pregnant women receiving appropriate medical care frequently attend appointments with their OB/GYN or midwife, we recommend, when feasible, partnering with local OB/GYN or midwifery practices to support pregnant women and make treatment as accessible as possible.

IMPACT OF THE COVID-19 PANDEMIC

Understanding the contextual factors that influence and impact a woman and her family is essential. For example, does this woman have access to healthcare that she feels confident in? In the current post-COVID era, understanding the broader contextual factors that a mother and family are dealing with is also crucial. Has a mother experienced additional stress due to the pandemic situation? Did she alter her birth plan due to the pandemic? Many women giving birth at a hospital during the COVID-19 pandemic experienced restrictions and could only have one support person during childbirth. This limitation can increase stress if a birthing mother wants to have more than one support person during this challenging time. For example, if a birthing mother wanted to have both her husband and her mother with her, but was forced to choose between them, this could create stress and additional tension on top of the expected stresses of giving birth. Mental health counselors should be attuned to the impact of COVID-19, if applicable, as the COVID-19 pandemic impacted pregnant mothers and their partners and families. For instance, researchers found that experiencing the COVID-19 pandemic had negative impacts on maternal–infant bonding for Portuguese mothers (Fernandes et al., 2021). The following questions can be useful to explore as you are gathering a person's history with regards to COVID-19.

> **Sample Assessment Questions: COVID-19 Experiences**
>
> - Have you or a family member experienced illness due to COVID-19?
> - Was your experience of pregnancy impacted by the COVID-19 pandemic? If so, how?
> - Did a COVID-19 diagnosis during pregnancy or at delivery (either for mother or infant) impact your ability to spend time bonding with your baby after birth?

LOOKING FORWARD: IMPROVING SCREENING AND INTERVENTION DURING PREGNANCY

Given the importance of maternal mental health during pregnancy and the adverse consequences to both mother and baby that are associated with maternal mental health disorders during pregnancy (Nillni et al., 2018), it is imperative for clinicians to be trained to accurately screen, assess, diagnose, and treat pregnant women. Despite this urgent need, graduate training programs in psychology and counseling do not have existing curriculum standards regarding peripartum mental health. We recommend that change is needed, starting in education and advocating for professional training and curriculum standards that address maternal mental health. Furthermore, we also recommend clinicians who are licensed, and practicing, pursue training opportunities in the areas of maternal and infant mental health. We also recommend continuing research focusing on a strengths-based and wellness approach to early intervention and treatment, which may help women and families as they grapple with challenges such as PPD.

CONCLUSION

In this chapter, we provided an overview of conception, pregnancy, and birth and discussed birth culture. We also provided self-reflection questions for clinicians to consider their own values and beliefs surrounding conception, pregnancy, and birth. We discussed counseling applications to effectively work with clinical issues related to conception, pregnancy, and birth.

APPLYING THE STRENGTHS MODEL—THE CASE OF JESSE

Significant Individual, Infant, Family, Societal, and Cultural Factors

- Unplanned emergency C-section surgical birth.
- Felt emotionally isolated while pregnant during COVID-19 pandemic.

Treatment Barriers

- Difficulty with accessing in-person treatment due to COVID-19 pandemic.
- Needing childcare support to be able to focus on counseling/therapy sessions.

Risk Factors

- Experience of pregnancy and birth did not match her expectations.
- Felt emotionally isolated during pregnancy and during birth as her partner could not be with her.

Enlisting Support from Family, the Community, and Medical Professionals

- Helping her partner to support her in her recovery.
- Involving her midwife to help her connect with a counselor.

Noticeable Symptoms, Severity, & DSM-5-TR Diagnosis OR Needs Identified by Family & Treatment Team

- Crying spells.
- Difficulty bonding with her baby.

Goals Identified by Family
- Help Jesse process the C-section birth.
- Alleviate her feelings of sadness and crying spells.

Treatment Recommendations
- Counseling to address birth experience and allow her to share her birth narrative.
- IPT to strengthen her relationships.

Helpful, Protective, and Resilience Factors
- Jesse has a positive relationship with her partner.
- Jesse is open to seeking treatment.

Self-Care & Wellness
- Support Jesse's interest in yoga and connect with postnatal yoga classes.
- Help her connect with other mothers, either online or in-person.

REFERENCES

Abramowitz, A., Miller E. S., & Wisner, K. L. (2017). Treatment options for hyperemesis gravidarum. *Archive of Women's Mental Health, 20*, 363–372. doi:10.1007/s00737-016-0707-4

Alhusen, J. L., Ray, E., Sharps, P., & Bullock, L. (2015). Intimate partner violence during pregnancy: Maternal and neonatal outcomes. *Journal of Women's Health, 24*(1), 100–106. doi:10.1089/jwh.2014.4872

American Counseling Association. (ACA). (2014). *Code of Ethics.* https://www.counseling.org/resources/aca-code-of-ethics.pdf

American Psychiatric Association (APA). (2000). *Diagnostic and statistical manual of mental disorders* (4th ed.; text revision).

American Psychiatric Association (APA). (2022). *Diagnostic and statistical manual of mental disorders* (5th ed.; text revision).

Ayers, S. (2017). Birth trauma and post-traumatic stress disorder: The importance of risk and resilience. *Journal of Reproductive and Infant Psychology, 35*(5), 427–430. doi:10.1080/02646838.2017.1386874

Bardacke, N. (2012). *Mindful birthing: Training the mind, body, and heart for childbirth and beyond.* Harper Collins.

Beck, C. T., & Watson, S. (2019). Mothers' experiences interacting with infants after traumatic childbirth. *MCN, American Journal of Maternal Child Nursing, 44*, 338–344. doi:10.1097/NMC.0000000000000565

Boyd, R. C., Zayas, L. H. & McKee, M. D. (2006). Mother–infant interaction, life events and prenatal and postpartum depressive symptoms among urban minority women in primary care. *Maternal and Child Health Journal, 10*, 139. doi:10.1007/s10995-005-0042-2

Bronfenbrenner, U. (1979). *The ecology of human development: Experiments by nature and design*. Harvard University Press.

Brunton, R., & Dryer, R. (2021). Child sexual abuse and pregnancy: A systematic review of the literature. *Child Abuse & Neglect, 111*. doi:10.1016/j.chiabu.2020.104802

Center for Disease Control and Prevention. (CDC). (2021, August). Pregnant and recently pregnant people at risk of severe illness from Covid-19. https://www.cdc.gov/coronavirus/2019-ncov/need-extra-precautions/pregnant-people.html

Deshpande, N. A., & Lewis-O'Connor, A. (2013). Screening for Intimate Partner Violence during pregnancy. *Reviews in Obstetrics & Gynecology, 6*(3/4): 141–148. PMID: 24920977

Digitale, E. (2017). Immune system changes during pregnancy are precisely timed. https://med.stanford.edu/news/all-news/2017/09/immune-system-changes-during-pregnancy-are-precisely-timed.html

Feeley, N., Bell, L., Hayton, B., Zelkowitz, P., & Carrier, M. (2016). Care for Postpartum Depression: What do women and their partners prefer? *Perspectives in Psychiatric Care, 52*, 120–130. doi:10.1111/ppc.12107

Fernandes, D. V., Canavarro, M. C., & Moreira, H. (2021). Postpartum during COVID-19 pandemic: Portuguese mothers' mental health, mindful parenting, and mother–infant bonding. *Journal of Clinical Psychology, 77*, 1997–2010. doi:10.1002/jclp.23130

Fischer, O. J. (2021). Non-binary reproduction: Stories of conception, pregnancy, and birth, *International Journal of Transgender Health, 22*(1/2), 77–88. doi:10.1080/26895269.2020.1838392

Furuta, M., Horsch, A., Ng, E. S. W., Bick, D., Spain, D., & Sin, J. (2018). Effectiveness of trauma-focused psychological therapies for treating post-traumatic stress disorder symptoms in women following childbirth: A systematic review and meta-analysis. *Frontiers in Psychiatry, 9*(Article 591). doi:10.3389/fpsyt.2018.00591

Gastaldon, C., Solmi, M., Correll, C. U., Barbui, C., & Schoretsanitis, G. (2022). Risk factors of postpartum depression and depressive symptoms: Umbrella review of current evidence from systematic reviews and meta-analyses of observational studies. *The British Journal of Psychiatry, 221*(4), 591–602. doi:10.1192/bjp.2021.222

Garbes, A. (2018). *Like a mother: A feminist journey through the science and culture of pregnancy*. Harper Wave.

Hoyert, D. L. (2022). Maternal mortality rates in the United States, 2020. Division of Vital Statistics. doi:10.15620/cdc:103855.

Huizink, A. C., Menting, B., Oosterman, M., Verhage, M. L., Kunseler, F. C. & Schuengel, C. (2014). The interrelationship between pregnancy-specific anxiety and general anxiety across pregnancy: A longitudinal study. *Journal of Psychosomatic Obstetrics and Gynaecology, 35*(3), 92–100. doi:10.3109/0167482X.2014.944498

Hutti, M. H., Armstrong, D. S., & Myers, J. (2013). Evaluation of the Perinatal Grief Intensity Scale in the subsequent pregnancy after perinatal loss. *Journal of Obstetrics, Gynecologic, and Neonatal Nursing, 42*, 697–706. doi:10.1111/1552-6909.12249

Jaffe, S. (2022). Federal abortion rights end, but not legal challenges. *The Lancet, 400*(10345), 13–14. doi:10.1016/S0140-6736(22)01236-3

Kinser, P., & Masho, S. (2015). "Yoga was my saving grace": The experience of women who practice prenatal yoga. *Journal of the American Psychiatric Nurses Association, 21*(5), 319–326. doi:10.1177/1078390315610554

Kleiman, K. R., & Raskin, V. D. (2013). *This isn't what I expected: Overcoming postpartum depression*. De Capo Press.

Kramer, J., Bowen, A., Stewart, N., & Muhajarine, N. (2013). Nausea and vomiting of pregnancy: Prevalence, severity and relation to psychosocial health. *MCN, The American Journal of Maternal/Child Nursing, 38*(1), 21–27. doi:10.1097/NMC.0b013e3182748489

Markus, E., Weingarten, A., Duplessi, Y., & Jones, J. (2010). Lesbian couples seeking pregnancy with donor insemination. *Journal of Midwifery & Women's Health, 55*(2), 124–132. doi:10.1016/j.jmwh.2009.09.014

Martin, J. A., Hamilton, B, E., Osterman, M. J. K., Driscoll, A. K., & Drake, P. & National Center for Health Statistics (U.S.) (2018). Births: Final data for 2016. *National Vital Statistics Reports 67*(1); DHHS publication; no. (PHS) 2018-1120. Retrieved from: https://stacks.cdc.gov/view/cdc/51199

Mayo Clinic (n.d.). Secondary infertility: Why does it happen? Retrieved from https://www.mayoclinic.org/diseases-conditions/infertility/expert-answers/secondary-infertility/faq-20058272

Meltzer-Brody, S., Maegbaek, M. L., Medland, S. E., Miller, W. C., Sullivan, P., & Munk-Olsen, T. (2017). Obstetrical, pregnancy and socio-economic predictors for new-onset severe postpartum psychiatric disorders in primiparous women. *Psychological Medicine, 47*, 1427–1441. doi:10.1017/S0033291716003020

Mitchell, J. & Goodman, J. (2018). Comparative effects of antidepressant medications and untreated major depression on pregnancy outcomes: A systemic review. *Archives of Women's Mental Health, 21*, 505–516. doi:10.1007/s00737-018-0844-z

Mohrbacher, N., & Kendall-Tackett, K. (2010). *Breastfeeding made simple: Seven laws for nursing mothers* (2nd ed.). New Harbinger Publications.

Murakami, K., Turale, S., Skirton, H., Doris, F., Tsujino, K., Ito, M., & Kutsunugi, S. (2016). Experiences regarding maternal age-specific risks and prenatal testing of women of advanced maternal age in Japan. *Nursing and Health Sciences, 18*, 8. doi:10.1111/nhs.12209

Muzik, M., McGinnis, E. W., Bocknek, E., Morelen, D., Rosenblum, K. L., et al. (2016). PTSD symptoms across pregnancy and early postpartum among women with lifetime PTSD diagnosis. Depression *and Anxiety, 33*(7), 584–591. doi:10.1002/da.22465

Nagle, A., & Samari, G. (2021). State-level structural sexism and cesarean sections in the United States. *Social Science & Medicine, 289*, 1–7. doi:10.1016/j.socscimed.2021.114406

Newman, B. M., & Newman, P. R. (2018). *Development through life: A psychosocial approach.* (13th ed.). Cengage Learning.

Neczypor, J. L., & Holley, S. L. (2017). Providing evidence-based care during the golden hour. *Nursing for Women's Health, 21*(6), 462–472. doi:10.1016/j.nwh.2017.10.011.

Nillni, Y. I., Mehralizade, A., Mayer, L., & Milanovic S. (2018). Treatment of depression, anxiety, and trauma-related disorders during the perinatal period: A systematic review. *Clinical Psychology Review, 66*, 136–148. doi:10.1016/j.cpr.2018.06.004

Nolvi, S., Karlsson, L., Bridgett, D. J., Korja, R., Huizink, A. C., Kataja, E., & Karlsson, H. (2016). Maternal prenatal stress and infant emotional reactivity six months postpartum. *Journal of Affective Disorders, 199*, 163–170. doi:10.1016/j.jad.2016.04.020

Nolvi, S., Karlsson, L., Bridgett, D. J., Pajulo, M., Tolvanen, M., & Karlsson, H. (2016). Maternal postnatal psychiatric symptoms and infant temperament affect early mother–infant bonding. *Infant Behavior & Development, 43*, 13–23. doi:10.1016/j.infbeh.2016.03.003

Romney, J., Fife, S. T., Sanders, D., & Behrens, S. (2021). Treatment of couples experiencing pregnancy loss: Reauthoring loss from a narrative perspective. *International Journal of Systemic Therapy, 32*(2), 134–152. doi:10.1080/2692398X.2020.1855621

Sawyer, A., & Ayers, S. (2009). Post-traumatic growth in women after childbirth. *Psychology and Health, 24*(4), 457–471. https://doi.org/10.1080/08870440701864520

Sharma, D. (2017). Golden hour of neonatal life: Need of the hour. *Maternal Health, Neonatology and Perinatology, 3*, article 16. doi:10.1186/s40748-017-0057-x

Shaw, J. C. A. (2013). The medicalization of birth and midwifery as resistance. *Health Care for Women International, 34*(6), 522–536. https://doi.org/10.1080/07399332.2012.736569

Simkin, P., Whalley J., Keppler, A. et al. (2010). *Pregnancy, childbirth, and the newborn: The complete guide* (4th ed.). Meadowbrook Press.

Solomon, A. (2021, March). How polyamorists and polygamists are challenging family norms. *The New Yorker*. https://www.newyorker.com/magazine/2021/03/22/how-polyamorists-and-polygamists-are-challenging-family-norms

Steel, A., Frawley, J., Adams, J. & Diezel, H. (2015). Trained or professional doulas in the support and care of pregnant and birthing women: A critical integrative review. *Health and Social Care in the Community, 23*(3), 225–241. doi:10.1111/hsc.12112

Strapasson, M. R., Ferreira, C. F., & Ramos, J. G. L. (2018). Obstetrics Associations between postpartum depression and hypertensive disorders of pregnancy. *International Journal of Gynecology and Obstetrics, 143*, 367–373. https://doi.org/10.1002/ijgo.12665

Tebeka, S., Le Strat, Y., & Dubertret, C. (2016). Developmental trajectories of pregnant and postpartum depression in an epidemiologic survey. *Journal of Affective Disorders, 203*, 62–68. doi:10.1016/j.jad.2016.05.058.

The American College of Obstetricians and Gynecologists (ACOG, n.d.). Postpartum hemorrhage practice bulletins. https://www.acog.org/clinical/clinical-guidance/practice-bulletin/articles/2017/10/postpartum-hemorrhage

Thombre, M. K., Talge, N. M., & Holzman, C. (2015). Association between pre-pregnancy depression/anxiety symptoms and hypertensive disorders of pregnancy. *Journal of Women's Health, 24*(3), 228–236. doi:10.1089/jwh.2014.4902

Thompson, J. (2021). The effectiveness of couple therapy on psychological and relational variables and pregnancy rates in couples with infertility: A systematic review. *Australian and New Zealand Journal of Family Therapy, 42*, 120–144. doi:10.1002/anzf.1446

Tsfati, M. & Ben-Ari, A. (2019). Between the social and the personal: Israeli male gay parents, surrogacy and socio-political concepts of parenthood and gender, *Journal of GLBT Family Studies, 15*(1), 42–57. doi:10.1080/1550428X.2017.1413475

Underwood L., Waldie K. E., Peterson E., D'Souza, S., Verbiest, M., McDaid, F., & Susan Morton, S. (2017). Paternal depression symptoms during pregnancy and after childbirth among participants in the Growing Up in New Zealand study. *JAMA Psychiatry, 74*(4), 360–369. doi:10.1001/jamapsychiatry.2016.4234

Viswasama, K., Eslick, G. D., & Starcevic, V. (2019). Prevalence, onset and course of anxiety disorders during pregnancy: A systematic review and meta analysis. *Journal of Affective Disorders, 255*, 27–40. doi:10.1016/j.jad.2019.05.016

Wang, K., Qiu, J., Meng, L., Lai, X., Yao, Z., & Peng, S. (2022). Postpartum hemorrhage and postpartum depressive symptoms: A retrospective cohort study. *Depression and Anxiety, 39*(3), 246–253. doi:10.1002/da.23245

Weisband, Y. K., Gallo, M. F., Klebanoff, M., Shoben, A., & Norris, A. H. (2018). Who uses a midwife for prenatal care and for birth in the United States? A secondary analysis of Listening to Mothers III. *Women's Health Issues, 28*(1), 89–96. doi:10.1016/j.whi.2017.07.004

Widarsson, M., Engstrom, G., Tyden, T., Lundberg, T., & Hammar, L. M. (2015). "Paddling upstream": Fathers' involvement during pregnancy as described by expectant fathers and mothers. *Journal of Clinical Nursing, 24*, 1059–1068. doi:10.1111/jocn.12784

World Health Organization. (WHO). (n.d.). Preterm Birth Fact Sheet. Retrieved July 16, 2021 from https://www.who.int/news-room/fact-sheets/detail/preterm-birth

6

Screening and Diagnosis of Peripartum Depression and Related Disorders

Vanessa Beatriz Teixeira

Personal Narrative

I gave birth to my third son right before the COVID-19 pandemic and while I was ecstatic, I couldn't help but feel sad and cry all the time. I talked to my OB and she prescribed Zoloft with a one-month follow up. Within one month, I was feeling better. She prescribed another month of medications and said, "if you feel better, you can stop taking them, otherwise call for another appointment." I felt better so I stopped cold turkey. A month and a half later, the depression came back with a vengeance. I called my doctor and was told, "it is a controlled substance, so we have to see you in person which we aren't doing due to Covid." I called three more times and was turned away each time. I thought I was strong enough and could push through until I tried to drown myself in the bathtub thinking I was doing my family a favor. I don't know if I had any suicidal ideation before the act. I knew I felt like a failure. I knew I felt I was letting everyone down. It wasn't until I was in the tub underwater that I realized how bad off I was. While I laid there I kept telling myself it was for the best. What pulled me up is I knew if I didn't leave a note for my kids, they would blame themselves one day. I actually wrote my note that night before my husband called 9-1-1. I ended up Baker Acted and finally received the help I needed. I was angry that my doctor let me down, but I'm thankful for the emergency resources that allowed me the help I so desperately needed in uncertain times.

— *Anonymous*

As described in the anonymous personal narrative above, symptoms of PPD can be overwhelming and lead to suicidal thoughts and actions. Women experiencing PPD that is untreated are at higher risk for negative outcomes, such as the suicide attempt described in this anonymous personal narrative. In this chapter, we explore the urgent need for screening for PPD and suicidal ideation to protect women, babies, and their families.

This comprehensive chapter focuses on the complexities of screening women who may present with symptoms of PPD and accurately diagnosing clients with PPD. Evaluating peripartum women with suicidal or homicidal ideation is also highlighted,

DOI: 10.4324/9780429440892-6

and how clinicians can prepare to intervene appropriately to protect mother and baby if these critical issues are present. Other significant counseling issues that clinicians may face when working with women and families are also explored, including paternal peripartum depression, adoptive depression, and perinatal loss.

SCREENING AND SUICIDE PREVENTION

The brief personal narrative at the beginning of this chapter showcases complex and serious symptoms of PPD. Typical symptoms many women experience during pregnancy and after giving birth can look very similar to symptoms of depression, including fatigue, lack of energy, difficulty sleeping, and feeling sad. It is crucial for clinicians to be aware that hormone levels change drastically during pregnancy and after birth, which could trigger less alarming symptoms that can look like "baby blues." Many women experience "baby blues" as a normal part of postpartum adjustment, with an estimate of 50–80 percent of women experiencing symptoms associated with "baby blues" shortly after birth (Buist, 1996). "Baby blues" symptoms can include feelings of sadness, tension, irritability, headaches, confusion and forgetfulness, which can look very similar to PPD (Brockington & Kumar, 1982; Inwood, 1985). These symptoms are short-lived and do not generally persist after three weeks of delivery (Inwood, 1985). Studies have demonstrated, however, that women who experience these symptoms are at increased risk for PPD (APA, 2022). Symptoms of PPD are more pervasive and debilitating than the "baby blues" and can lead to more severe symptomology including maternal suicide and infanticide.

Preventing maternal suicide should be a primary concern for both mental health and healthcare professionals when screening women for PPD in pregnancy and postpartum. Maternal suicide is the most common cause of pregnancy-associated mortality, with most of these women dying by suicide after giving birth (Metz et al., 2016). Several research studies have found similar characteristics associated with maternal suicide. Maternal suicide most often occurs during the first year after giving birth, typically when the infant is 9–12 months of age. This spike in deaths could be attributed to the lack of support mothers experience after the first few months of delivery, as well as women going back to work as their children are nearly 12 months of age, in this study conducted in Australia where maternity leave is usually 12 months (Thornton et al., 2013). Many women go back to work well before their baby is 12 months old, especially in the United States, as maternity leave is frequently 6–12 weeks or less. Studies have also found that postpartum women who are suicidal use more lethal means of suicide such as hanging or jumping to complete suicide. Lastly, most women who die by suicide in pregnancy and postpartum have experienced a previous mood or anxiety disorder (Gold et al., 2012; Grigoriadis et al., 2017; Thornton et al., 2013). These alarming research findings are important for mental health counselors to be aware of in order to help prevent maternal suicide and to provide effective treatment to women experiencing suicidal ideation and intention.

While mental health professionals are typically trained to screen and assess for suicidal ideation in men and women, less training is available for assessing postpartum psychosis and infanticide, which is defined as killing an infant within the first year of birth (Spinelli, 2019). While infanticide is rare, with estimates of 1–2 out of 1,000 deliveries, it is a crucial topic for clinicians to be aware of and to be comfortable assessing (Rehman, St Clair, & Platz, 1990; Kumar, 1994). This topic is often taboo and can make both clients and clinicians feel apprehensive about assessing and openly discussing postpartum psychosis. Infanticide is often precipitated by a psychotic episode that can include command hallucinations that repeatedly tell the mother to kill her infant. Delusions can also be present and may distort the mother's thinking into believing that her infant is possessed and therefore must be killed (APA, 2022). Clinicians should be aware of the strong connection between postpartum psychosis and a diagnosis of bipolar disorder. Evidence suggests that up to 50 percent of women with a personal or family history of bipolar disorder develop postpartum psychosis that is triggered by pregnancy (APA, 2022; Brockington, 1996; Jones & Craddock, 2002).

Screening women for PPD is an important preventative measure during pregnancy and after birth so that prevention and early intervention measures can be taken quickly to avoid any potentially serious and dangerous symptoms, including psychosis, or suicidal and homicidal ideation. Findings from the United States Preventive Services Task Force (Siu et al., 2016) sparked numerous professional organizations to now require practitioners to screen pregnant and postpartum women for PPD, including the American Academy of Pediatrics, the American College of Obstetrics and Gynecology (ACOG, 2016), and the American Medical Association.

Numerous validated and evidence-based assessment instruments are available for clinicians to screen women for mild to severe PPD symptoms such as depression, anxiety, psychosis, suicidality, and homicidality. Table 6.1 includes most of the readily available assessments that clinicians can use to screen PPD symptoms, along with some detailed information about each instrument's number of items, estimated time to complete, cost to the client, and languages available. These instruments include the Edinburgh Postnatal Depression Screen (EPDS; Cox, Holden, & Sagovsky, 1987), Patient Health Questionnaire-9 (PHQ-9; Kroenke, Spitzer, & Williams, 1999), Postpartum Distress Measure (PDM; Allison et al., 2011), and the Postpartum Depression Screening Scale (PDSS; Beck & Gable, 2000). The Perinatal Anxiety Screening Scale (PASS; Somerville et al., 2014) can be used for assessing symptoms of anxiety. These assessments are typically at no cost, self-administered, short to complete, and available in several languages. Clinicians can also utilize various other widely used validated assessment instruments that are not specifically created for PPD but can assess for depression, anxiety, psychosis, suicidality, and homicidality. These include the Beck Depression Inventory (BDI; Beck et al., 1961), Self-Rating Depression Scale (SDS; Zung, 1965), State-Trait Anxiety Inventory for Adults (STAI-AD; Spielberger, 1983), Beck Anxiety Inventory (BAI; Beck et al., 1988), Scale for Suicidal Ideation (SSI; Beck et al., 1979), and the Ask Suicide-Screening Questions (ASQ) Tool (NIMH, 2020).

Table 6.1
PPD Screening Tools

Screening Tool	Number of Questions	Estimated Time to Complete	Languages Available	Cost
Edinburgh Postnatal Depression Screen (EPDS)	10	Less than 5 minutes	English Spanish	No
Patient Health Questionnaire (PHQ-9)	9	Less than 5 minutes	English Spanish	No
Postpartum Distress Measure (PDM)	10	Less than 5 minutes	English	No
Postpartum Depression Screening Scale (PDSS)	35	5–10 minutes	English Spanish	Yes
Perinatal Anxiety Screening Scale (PASS)	31	Less than 5 minutes	English	No
The PPSC Suicide Assessment (PPSC)	17	Less than 5 minutes	English	No

While there are many available assessments to screen women with PPD symptoms, clinicians should choose the assessment that better matches their client's specific needs and that will be the most comprehensive, especially if more severe symptoms of suicidal and/or homicidal ideation are present. After the screening process is complete, it is essential for health professionals to clearly explain the screening results and complete a mental health counseling referral to begin treatment for the presenting symptoms associated with PPD (ACOG, 2016).

DIAGNOSIS OF PERIPARTUM DEPRESSION AND RELATED DISORDERS

While various symptoms associated with PPD are quite common in women during pregnancy and after birth, the clinical diagnosis of PPD is less common. Statistical evidence of PPD has been gathered for decades, showing that between 7 percent and 9 percent of women experience a major depressive episode during pregnancy and postpartum, with 50 percent of these episodes beginning while the woman is still pregnant (APA, 2022). For women who experience PPD with psychotic features, the risk of once again developing these symptoms is between 30 percent and 50 percent (APA, 2022). Due to the seriousness and potential lethality of PPD symptoms, accurate diagnosis is essential for effective treatment. The DSM-5-TR gives a brief, yet clear, description of the criteria clients must present to be diagnosed with this disorder. While the DSM-5-TR does not classify PPD as a separate disorder, it is classified as a specifier, labeled 'with peripartum onset' in four separate diagnoses: major depressive disorder (MDD), bipolar I and II disorders, and brief psychotic disorder (APA, 2022). The 'with peripartum onset' specifier can be applied to a current or most recent episode of major depression in MDD as well as mania, hypomania, or major depression in bipolar I or bipolar II disorder.

A diagnosis of MDD requires five or more symptoms during a two-week period including depressed mood most of the day, significant weight loss or weight gain, insomnia or hypersomnia, psychomotor agitation or retardation, fatigue or loss of energy, feelings of worthlessness or excessive guilt, difficulty with concentration or indecisiveness, and recurrent thoughts of death or suicidal ideation (APA, 2022). Depressive symptoms can manifest in different ways. In new mothers, depression can look like very poor hygiene or an overly messy house, difficulty bonding with the baby or not wanting to play or care for the baby, forgetting important tasks like feeding or changing the baby, or sleeping too much or an inability to sleep at all.

For women experiencing symptoms of mania or hypomania for more than one week, such as inflated self-esteem or grandiosity, a reduced need for sleep, flight of ideas, being more talkative and goal oriented, or engaging in impulsive behaviors, a diagnosis of bipolar I or II disorder *with peripartum onset* would be more appropriate. If symptoms of PPD are present and the client does not appear to meet the criteria for MDD or bipolar disorders, counselors can also rule out other DSM-5-TR diagnoses, including brief psychotic disorder, substance-related disorders, or disorders that may be induced by medications or other medical illnesses.

When treating co-occurring substance-related disorders, some clinicians might find that they are unsure which comes first, the substance-related diagnosis or a co-occurring diagnosis such as MDD. Mothers who use substances can be challenging to work with from a clinical perspective due to the physical and emotional problems caused by drugs and addiction to both mothers and infants (Pajulo et al., 2012). According to the Substance Abuse and Mental Health Services Administration, among pregnant women ages 15–44, illicit drug and alcohol use average 5 percent to 9 percent. In contrast, drug and alcohol use drastically increased with mothers who recently gave birth, with an average of 10 percent to 30 percent (SAMHSA, 2014). Therefore, screening for substance abuse and dependence should be a routine part of the treatment process.

Counselors may find the following screening instruments helpful when assessing for substance use and dependence during the peripartum period, as these instruments are self-administered and developed and tested for use with pregnant women: The T-ACE Screening Tool, the TWEAK, the Alcohol Use Disorders Identification Test-Concise (AUDIT-C), the 4Ps Plus, and CRAFFT (Jordan, Farley, & Grace, 2018). The TWEAK assessment is designed for use in adults and the name is an acronym that stands for tolerance, worried, eye-opener, amnesia, and k/cut down, which are the aspects of problematic alcohol use it assesses (Russell, 1994). The 4Ps Plus is a validated screening instrument designed to assess substance abuse during pregnancy. The name stands for Parents, Partner, Past, and Pregnancy, which are dimensions assessed (Chasnoff et al., 2007). Sample questions include: "Did either of your parents ever have a problem with alcohol or drugs?" and "In the month before you knew you were pregnant, how many beers/how much wine/how much liquor did you drink?" (Chasnoff et al., 2007, p. 745). CRAFFT stands for the key words of the six items in the second section of the assessment—Car, Relax, Alone, Forget, Friends, Trouble—which are also dimensions that the instrument assesses. This assessment is designed for an adolescent/young adult population, so it is recommended for use when working with people aged 21 or younger (Knight et al., 1999).

During the process of finding an accurate diagnosis for clients, clinicians often face a major challenge; differential diagnoses that can mirror symptoms of PPD. Many pregnant and postpartum women experience varying symptoms of DSM-5-TR disorders, including postpartum anxiety (PPA), postpartum OCD (obsessive-compulsive disorder), and postpartum PTSD (post-traumatic stress disorder). Pregnancy and hormone changes can trigger mental health diagnoses such as the ones noted above. Postpartum anxiety is frequently experienced by women during the peripartum period and is one of the most diagnosed postpartum clinical disorders (Reck et al., 2008). In fact, 30 percent of women who recently gave birth reported symptoms of generalized anxiety (Wenzel et al., 2003). Mothers with PPA have indicated significant difficulty bonding with their babies compared with mothers without a clinical diagnosis (Tietz et al., 2014). While postpartum anxiety is common, the DSM-5-TR does not have the 'with peripartum onset' specifier for any anxiety disorder. Nevertheless, counselors can utilize screening tools to accurately diagnose anxiety disorders such as the PROMIS Emotional Distress—Anxiety—Short Form, Beck Anxiety Inventory (BAI; Beck et al., 1988), and the Perinatal Anxiety Screening Scale (PASS) (Somerville et al., 2014). Clinicians can also use their clinical judgment with regards to treatment addressing the peripartum onset of anxiety.

In addition to experiencing postpartum anxiety, women during the postpartum period are also at an increased risk for developing postpartum PTSD. Research has indicated that PPA has been associated with postpartum PTSD (Polachek et al., 2014). Postpartum PTSD has been linked to women who experience high risk pregnancies, emotional crises during pregnancy, a fear of childbirth, and women who expect to feel severe pain during childbirth (Polachek et al., 2016). Three screening tools for accurate diagnosis of PTSD among pregnant and postpartum women have been developed, including the Traumatic Event Scale (Wijma et al., 1997), the Perinatal PTSD Questionnaire (PPQ; Hynan, 1998), and the City Birth Trauma Scale (Ayers et al., 2018). Counselors should be attuned to how pregnant women and new mothers describe their pregnancy and birth experience and use these screening tools if a mother experienced trauma (or possible trauma) during pregnancy or delivery or is presenting with symptoms of PTSD. One final consideration should be given to women who develop OCD during pregnancy or the postpartum, as the peripartum period can initiate or exacerbate this severe diagnosis (Russell et al., 2013). When OCD in the postpartum period is left undiagnosed and untreated, symptoms can lead to several challenges to both baby and mother, including disrupting the mother–infant bond and negative cognitive-behavioral development in the newborn (Brandes et al., 2004). OCD in the peripartum period is a serious diagnosis with debilitating symptoms for clients and their families. OCD symptoms can include unwanted, obsessive, and intrusive thoughts or compulsions to complete an activity numerous times to reduce fears and obsessions (APA, 2022). Among peripartum women, these obsessions and compulsions could be related to an unborn child, the infant, or the mothering role. Three screening tools have been developed for assessing OCD among peripartum women: the Perinatal Obsessive-Compulsive Scale (POCS), the Parental Thoughts and Behaviors Checklist (PTBC), and the Postpartum Distress Measure (Abramowitz et al., 2006; Allison et al., 2011; Lord et al., 2011).

POSTADOPTION DEPRESSION (PAD)

Parental postadoption depression (PAD) has not received much attention in clinical research and the media (Payne et al., 2010). Since peripartum depression (PPD) is mostly associated with giving birth, adoptive parents may feel stigmatized when experiencing PPD symptoms following the placement of an adoptive child. Similar to the societal expectations of pregnancy and childbirth as a happy time for the new mother and father/partner, parents of adoptive children are often expected to feel happy and blissful during and after the adoption process. While pregnancy, childbirth, and adoption can be stressful events, the adoptive process oftentimes contains additional stressors such as infertility, financial issues, as well as a formal parental evaluation (Payne et al., 2010). While adoptive mothers experience less anxiety than postpartum mothers (Mott et al., 2011), rates of depression among these women have been found to be similar to rates of PPD in biological mothers, ranging from 15 percent to 28 percent (Foli et al., 2012; Mott et al., 2011; Payne et al., 2010; Senecky et al., 2009). These findings suggest that PPD may not solely result from the hormonal and physical changes related to pregnancy and delivery (Senecky et al., 2009). Clinicians can consider other social and situational stressors and factors related to welcoming a child into the family that are more strongly associated with PPD.

When working with adoptive parents either before, during, or after the placement of an adoptive child, counselors should be aware of and pay close attention to potential risk factors and resilience factors for PAD. In a longitudinal study, researchers found that adoptive parents who report a lower sense of parental competency tend to experience higher levels of stress and emotional arousal. In contrast, parents who report a higher sense of parental competency experienced fewer depressive symptoms (Anthony et al., 2019). Another study found several risk factors associated with PAD, including lack of family and friend support and higher levels of stress within romantic partner relationships. In contrast, higher levels of optimism and life satisfaction appear to decrease depressive symptoms (Foli et al., 2016). Other risk factors for depression in adoptive mothers during the first year following an adoption include lack of sleep, history of infertility, mental health diagnoses, and marital dissatisfaction (Mott et al., 2011). Most notably, adoptive parents are at higher risk for PAD when they have high expectations of the adoption process, including unrealistic and oftentimes unmet expectations of themselves as parents, the child they are adopting, close friends, family and society (Foli, 2010; Foli et al., 2016).

Figure 6.1
Middle Range Theory of Parental Postadoption Depression

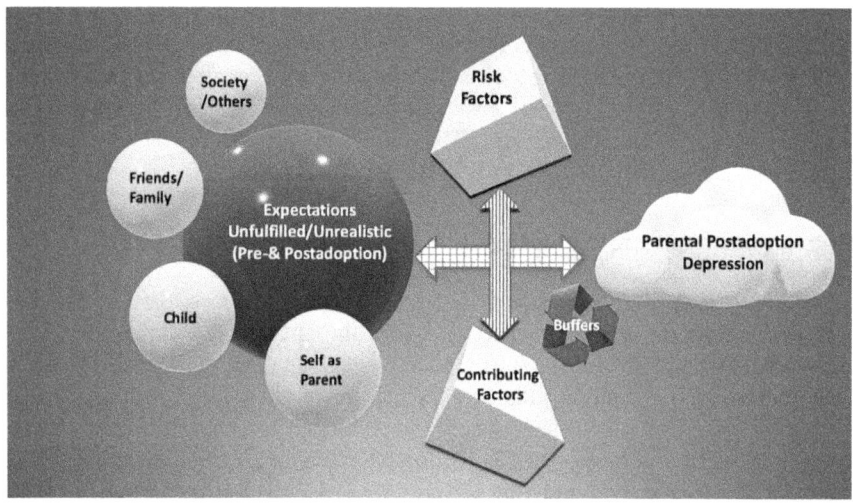

Copyright 2019 Karen J. Foli. Reprinted with permission.

Figure 6.1 illustrates the middle range theory of parental postadoption depression model. Both adoptive mothers and fathers can struggle with depression during the adoption process. Numerous research studies mentioned in this book detail the negative impact parental depression has on the entire family, including children. Hence, counselors are encouraged to advocate for regular depression screening for adoptive mothers and fathers. This could facilitate prevention, early interventions, and treatment of PAD (Foli & Gibson, 2011).

PERINATAL LOSS

Perinatal loss, which is defined as the loss of a child during pregnancy, birth, or after birth, can be a form of disenfranchised grief because there is a lack of culturally and socially sanctioned rituals for parents enduring such grief (Markin & Zilcha-Mano, 2018). For instance, many couples experiencing the loss of miscarriage before 12 weeks of pregnancy may not have yet shared that they were pregnant and feel isolated as they experience miscarriage. Even if parents do share about a miscarriage or stillbirth, others may not understand the depth of their pain and suffering. This could be the most isolating form of grief, because it is least understood and there is a lack of empathy. Further, women and families with a history of perinatal loss may be especially anxious during another pregnancy and may need extra support (Simkin et al., 2010).

Perinatal loss can be a difficult and sensitive topic for counselors to approach with clients. While there is no consistent or widely recognized definition or time frame for perinatal loss, the loss of a child before, during, or after birth can be complex and traumatic for all family members. Clients can experience perinatal grief in numerous situations when loss occurs, including miscarriage, a pre-term baby, a child with a disability or impairment, stillbirth, neonatal death, death of a twin, and giving the child for adoption (Wallerstedt & Higgins, 1996). Studies have shown that perinatal loss can increase the rates of anxiety and depression for both parents during subsequent pregnancies (Hunter et al., 2017). A large-scale epidemiological study found that women who lost a child had four times higher depression rates and seven times higher PTSD rates compared with those of nonbereaved parents (Gold et al., 2016). When approaching the topic of perinatal loss, counselors must be aware of the unique grief process experienced by mothers and fathers.

Parents who face a perinatal loss oftentimes experience disenfranchised grief due to the nontraditional, or ambiguous, type of death of an unborn or newly born child (Lang et al., 2011). Grieving mothers generally express concern about social support from hospital staff, family members, and society after stillbirth (Cacciatore, 2010). While parents are suffering a tremendous loss, they are often met with unintentionally dismissive or minimizing reactions from family members, friends, healthcare professionals, and society as a whole. Examples include healthcare providers treating pregnancy loss as not significant or important, lack of acknowledgment by friends and family of the deceased baby's birthday or anniversary of death, and a lack of solemn rituals for mourning the death of a child, such as having a funeral. The dismissive attitude of society toward this type of loss makes mourning more complicated, isolating, and painful for parents (Lang et al., 2011). Consequently, counselors should pay special attention to validating and supporting this unique grief process.

Another important factor to consider with perinatal loss is the physiological impact it has on women. The death of a child inside or outside of the womb can be a devastating and traumatic experience, both mentally and physically. For instance, women may continue to lactate and experience other intrusive biological and hormonal changes in their body, with no baby to care for or take home (Dickens, 2020). Women who gave birth to a baby who did not survive may also have to deal with painful labor healing and recovery. These physical changes to a woman's body can be a painful reminder of the baby's death.

Additionally, women who experience a stillbirth are often overwhelmed by the trauma of losing a child before they are born. This grief can feel isolating since other family members may not have interacted with the baby prior to its death (Cacciatore, 2010). For women, this complex grief can symbolize a loss of maternal identity, which is not recognized by society (Gaudet et al., 2010). Furthermore, conceiving and getting pregnant after perinatal loss has its own set of complex physical and psychological factors. Women who become pregnant shortly after perinatal loss tend to experience more grief symptoms, higher anxiety, and difficulty with prenatal attachment. Other risk factors for experiencing intense grief symptoms include the number of losses and a perinatal loss later in the pregnancy (Gaudet et al., 2010).

Multiple Perspectives: Paternal PPD

Both mothers and fathers are vulnerable to experiencing depression and PPD symptoms during the peripartum period (Nazareth, 2011). The topic of paternal PPD has limited research and attention in clinical practice and research, especially when compared with maternal PPD. Nevertheless, paternal PPD is a significant problem for families and has shown negative effects for infants. Not surprisingly, maternal PPD is the strongest predictor of paternal PPD. The incidence rate for fathers who *did not* have a spouse with PPD ranged from 1 percent to 25 percent. In comparison, the incidence rate drastically increased for fathers who did have a spouse struggling with PPD, ranging from 24 percent to 50 percent (Goodman, 2004). Research indicates that more than half of mothers with PPD begin experiencing depressive symptoms during the first six weeks after childbirth (Stowe et al., 2005). Conversely, fathers experience paternal PPD later than mothers with PPD, usually within the first 12 months of the infant's life, with highest rates of symptoms between three and six months postpartum (Davis et al., 2011; Paulson & Bazemore, 2010).

Fathers with paternal PPD may often be reluctant to seek help from doctors or mental health counselors for their PPD symptoms (Nazareth, 2011). In general, men seek mental health counseling services less often than women, especially when they feel uncomfortable disclosing personal concerns, experience self-stigma about seeking counseling, and have negative attitudes about therapy (Pederson & Vogel, 2007). This lack of help-seeking behavior is a significant concern for clinicians, especially knowing how depressive symptoms experienced by the father negatively impact children and the family unit. Studies have found numerous negative effects for young children with fathers experiencing depression, including negative parenting behavior, an increase in fathers spanking infants, and a decrease in fathers reading to their children (Davis et al., 2011). Paternal PPD is also associated with more severe and long-term consequences in children, including increased risk of social, emotional, and behavior problems, as well as an increase in DSM-5 disorders, such as oppositional defiant disorder and conduct disorder (Ramchandani, Stein, et al., 2008; Ramchandani, O'Connor, et al., 2008). It is important for clinicians to be aware of the immense negative toll related to paternal PPD. It not only impacts both parents, but all the children in the home as well.

Perinatal Death—Family Members and Siblings

Depending on the type of perinatal death, family members will experience grief in different ways. While giving special attention to the mother's experience of perinatal loss is essential, counselors must also consider other family members, including the mother's partner and other children in the home. Consideration should be given to the potential change in romantic relationships after perinatal loss, as grief is experienced differently by each partner. Men may grieve differently after the loss of a child, and counselors should encourage healthy and open conversations between partners to bring awareness of how grief is unique and can look and feel different for each person

(Costin & McMurrich, 2013). Fathers who experience stillbirth often report feeling ignored and invalidated in their grief. Acknowledging a man's fatherhood and validating his unique grief experience is essential (Cacciatore et al., 2013; Lang et al., 2011). Lastly, surviving children are also significantly impacted by perinatal loss, and may not be able to process their grief due to grieving parents (Cacciatore, 2010). These children should also be provided with support, education, and debriefing about the loss of their sibling (Cacciatore et al., 2009).

Multicultural Considerations: Perinatal Loss

Counselors working with families who have experienced perinatal loss must be aware of and reflect on cultural implications, biases, and attitudes toward this type of grieving process (Markin & Zilcha-Mano, 2018). Special attention should be given to using validating language when discussing the loss with family members (Costin & McMurrich, 2013). It is also important for counselors to recognize there is no timeline for grief, and depression and perinatal grief symptoms can be long-lasting. Clinicians can help parents have a more positive grief process by allowing parents to share the painful perinatal death experience and normalizing their intense and unique bereavement. Positive and adaptive coping skills such as positive reframing, emotional support, and acceptance have been associated with lower levels of perinatal grief in women who have lost a child (Lafarge et al., 2017). Spiritual beliefs, faith, and religious values can also mediate the bereavement process following perinatal loss (Wright, 2020). Paying close attention to how each family member experiences and copes with this grieving process is essential. Counselors should adapt their treatment and therapeutic approach based on the individualized needs of grieving families. Table 6.2 has useful suggestions for professionals to help family members through their bereavement period (Costin & McMurrich, 2013).

Table 6.2
Support for Bereaved Parents

Engage with the mother or couple to find out about who their baby is.
Ask about the pregnancy and about the hopes and dreams the parents had for the child.
Find out the names that were considered and why the baby's particular name was chosen.
Ask about whether there was a nursery, or plans for one.
Record the baby's measurements.
Make a hand and footprint of the baby if possible.
Ask the parents if they would like a lock of hair from the baby.
Take pictures of the baby and hold them for the parents in the event they regret not taking pictures themselves.

Copyright © Costin & McMurrich (2013). Reprinted with permission.

APPLICATIONS TO COUNSELING

Clinicians should be well prepared for both assessing and intervening with any client who is an imminent threat to themselves or others. Safety of the mother and infant should be a top priority for all clinicians. Hence, knowing how and when to handle imminent harm to the mother, infant, or other family members is essential. Gliatto and Rai (1999) recommend simple and concrete guidelines when working with clients with imminent threat of harm, including assessing for a history of mental health issues, screening for substance use, completing a mental status exam, and asking the client to detail any plans for harm, including access to lethal means. Hospitalizing clients should be reserved for those with a specific plan to commit harm, reasonable access to lethal means, recent life stressors, and symptoms of psychosis. Family members should be part of any transition to inpatient care. Table 6.3 introduces the *Assess, Intervene and Monitor for Suicide Prevention* (AIM-SP) model, which provides a helpful step-by-step guide for assessing, intervening, and monitoring clients with suicidal ideation (Brodsky et al., 2018). This model can be slightly modified and applied when working with clients who present with homicidal ideation. Counselors should also seek supervision and work collaboratively with clients and family members when imminent threat of harm is present.

Table 6.3

The AIM-SP Model's Ten Steps for Applying Best Suicide Prevention Practices to Everyday Clinical Care

Assess	Step 1: Inquire explicitly about suicide ideation and behavior, past and present.
	Step 2: Identify risk factors in addition to suicidal ideation and behavior.
	Step 3: Implement and maintain continued focus on safety.
Intervene	Step 4: Introduce and develop a collaborative safety plan intervention for managing suicidality, including lethal means restriction.
	Step 5: Initiate coping strategies and supports.
	Step 6: Integrate suicide-specific treatment targets in treatment planning process.
Monitor	Step 7: Increase flexibility and contact availability.
	Step 8: Initiate increased monitoring during periods of highest risk.
	Step 9: Involve family and other social supports.
	Step 10: Invoke clinicians' peer support and consultation.

Copyright © 2018 Brodsky, Spruch-Feiner, and Stanley. Reprinted with permission.

After evaluating clients for risk of harm, safety planning is an essential part of working with mothers who may be at risk of harming themselves or their babies. This structured process focuses on assisting clients with identifying and outlining ways they can maintain their safety and the safety of others. Safety plans often detail individualized and specific information such as the mother's triggers for harm, positive coping skills, helpful people and places to reach out to for help, and reasons for living. The sample safety plan in Figure 6.2 was created by Stanley and Brown

(2008) and provides a six-step process for safety planning with at-risk clients. The authors of this book strongly suggest using a safety plan similar to this when working with mothers. Some additional helpful suicide prevention resources for working with mothers and their families are outlined in Table 6.4.

Figure 6.2
Stanley-Brown Safety Plan

STANLEY - BROWN SAFETY PLAN

STEP 1: WARNING SIGNS:
1.
2.
3.

STEP 2: INTERNAL COPING STRATEGIES – THINGS I CAN DO TO TAKE MY MIND OFF MY PROBLEMS WITHOUT CONTACTING ANOTHER PERSON:
1.
2.
3.

STEP 3: PEOPLE AND SOCIAL SETTINGS THAT PROVIDE DISTRACTION:
1. Name: _____ Contact: _____
2. Name: _____ Contact: _____
3. Place: _____ 4. Place: _____

STEP 4: PEOPLE WHOM I CAN ASK FOR HELP DURING A CRISIS:
1. Name: _____ Contact: _____
2. Name: _____ Contact: _____
3. Name: _____ Contact: _____

STEP 5: PROFESSIONALS OR AGENCIES I CAN CONTACT DURING A CRISIS:
1. Clinician/Agency Name: _____ Phone: _____
   Emergency Contact : _____
2. Clinician/Agency Name: _____ Phone: _____
   Emergency Contact : _____
3. Local Emergency Department: _____
   Emergency Department Address: _____
   Emergency Department Phone : _____
4. Suicide Prevention Lifeline Phone: 1-800-273-TALK (8255)

STEP 6: MAKING THE ENVIRONMENT SAFER (PLAN FOR LETHAL MEANS SAFETY):
1.
2.

The Stanley-Brown Safety Plan is copyrighted by Barbara Stanley, PhD & Gregory K. Brown, PhD (2008, 2021). Individual use of the Stanley-Brown Safety Plan form is permitted. Written permission from the authors is required for any changes to this form or use of this form in the electronic medical record. Additional resources are available from www.suicidesafetyplan.com

Copyright © Stanley & Brown, 2008, 2021. Image permitted for individual use.

Table 6.4
Suicide Prevention Resources

Suicide Prevention Organization	Website/Contact Information
American Foundation for Suicide Prevention	https://afsp.org/
Zero Suicide: A detailed guide to Zero Suicide implementation and strategy	https://zerosuicide.edc.org/
Suicide Safety Plan: Free phone application	https://www.suicidesafetyplan.app/
20/20 Mom: Maternal suicide awareness campaign	https://www.2020mom.org/
988 Suicide & Crisis Lifeline	https://988lifeline.org/
Crisis Text Line	https://www.crisistextline.org/ or Text HOME to 741741

Figure 6.3
988 Suicide & Crisis Lifeline

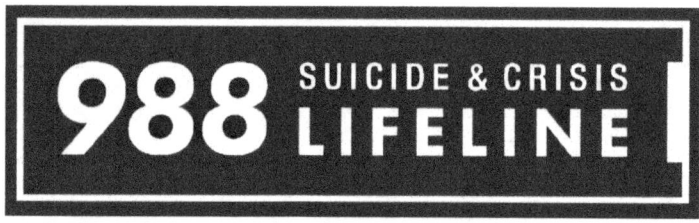

Copyright © 988 Suicide & Crisis Lifeline.

Treating Paternal Peripartum Depression

Clinicians can be creative and collaborative with treatment options for paternal PPD. Freitas and Fox (2015) suggested eight effective steps and interventions that can be used when treating fathers for PPD. First, clinicians can provide a safe therapeutic space to help fathers verbally and openly express vulnerable emotions and experiences. Developing the emotional language skills that many fathers lack is an important first step. Second, clinicians should focus on the father's experience of becoming a parent. Asking questions while also assessing for depressive symptoms can be helpful. Third, clinicians can identify paternal role models as well as personal goals for fatherhood. Identifying past and/or present positive and negative paternal role models can aid in the process of aligning paternal behaviors with personal goals for the demanding task of fatherhood.

The fourth step suggested by Freitas and Fox (2015) in the treatment of paternal PPD involves exploring the social construct of fatherhood. In other words, clinicians can help the father understand what it means to be a father by exploring the messages he has received throughout his life about the expectations of this new role. These messages about the meaning of fatherhood are often received from immediate or distant family members, social media, the community, church teachings, and/or the father's current family unit. The next step invites the father to "jump in" and bond with his baby frequently. Clinicians should encourage both the father and mother to create various and frequent opportunities for bonding to increase the father's skill set for properly taking care of the baby on his own. The sixth step involves creating a community for the father and building a network of like-minded fathers. The clinician can help with this task by helping search for local resources focused on helping new fathers in the complex transition to fatherhood.

The final two steps in treating paternal PPD include collaborating with healthcare providers and practicing reflexivity (Freitas & Fox, 2015). Acknowledging that depression is a medical problem, clinicians and clients benefit from a collaborative approach with medical providers. This collaborative approach is especially helpful when medications are prescribed for severe depressive symptoms. Further, a collaborative approach could also assist with outreach to fathers with PPD who may not approach a mental health professional without support and/or referral from a medical provider. Lastly, practicing reflexivity centers on the clinician's need to check their own bias and potential countertransference that may present itself when treating paternal PPD. Reflexivity is especially important when looking at gender norms and the clinician's attitudes toward men and fathers as well as personal expectations and beliefs of the father role.

ETHICAL AND LEGAL CONSIDERATIONS

Clinicians have ethical and legal responsibilities to assess their clients for safety risks and take immediate actions to protect their clients and identifiable targets from harm (Tarasoff v. Regents of the University of California, 1976). Accurate assessment of suicide risk, including assessing for suicidal ideation, intent, and means, is a significant ethical consideration when working with people who present with symptoms of peripartum PPD or other maternal mood disorders, as suicidal ideation is associated with depression and other psychiatric disorders (Eggleston et al., 2009). Maternal suicide is a leading cause of mortality during the peripartum period (Gressier et al., 2017). Assessing for previous suicide attempts is essential, as a previous suicide attempt is a risk factor for future suicide attempts (Bostwick, et al., 2016). As described earlier in this chapter, mothers who are experiencing depression or anxiety should be assessed for suicidality as well. Clinicians should also assess for other risk factors related to maternal suicide, including limited social support, substance abuse, interpersonal violence, and a history of abuse (Chin et al., 2022). Clinicians should also assess mothers for any infanticidal thoughts and intentions, as research suggests frequent missed opportunities for effective screening and intervention by health professionals that could prevent infant deaths by their mothers (Van Rensburg et al., 2020).

BARRIERS TO TREATMENT

Correctly diagnosing PPD can be difficult for some clinicians, especially since symptoms associated with hormonal fluctuations during pregnancy and postpartum "baby blues" can mimic symptoms of PPD (Brockington & Kumar, 1982; Inwood, 1985). While feeling fatigued, experiencing low energy, and having bouts of sadness can be related to hormonal changes or "baby blues," clinicians can closely monitor and assess pregnant and postpartum women as part of early prevention, since their symptoms can quickly become severe enough to warrant a clinical diagnosis of PPD.

Another barrier to treatment includes mothers not seeking therapy when they are experiencing symptoms of depression during pregnancy and postpartum. Many mothers fear judgment, being labeled, or even having their children taken from them if they seek therapy and admit to the severity of their PPD symptoms (Sampson et al., 2014; Sampson et al., 2021). Counselors can take an advocacy role and normalize symptoms of PPD with women, families, and healthcare providers to reduce the stigma of seeking mental health treatment.

IMPACT OF THE COVID-19 PANDEMIC

Studies conducted during the COVID-19 pandemic have reported a negative and often detrimental impact on maternal mental health, including an increase in symptoms of depression during pregnancy and the postpartum period (Bérard et al., 2022; Koyucu & Karaca, 2021). Specifically, depression, anxiety, and stress were reported as highest in the third trimester (28–40 weeks) of women's pregnancies during the pandemic (Bérard et al., 2022). Financial worries, frequent exposure to news outlets about the pandemic, and difficulties related to isolating at home with children contributed to an increase in anxiety and stress. This higher rate of mental health symptoms is concerning, as mental disorders during pregnancy can lead to an increase in obstetric and maternal complications (Koyucu & Karaca, 2021).

CONCLUSION

Mental health counselors face numerous complex issues when working with women and families struggling with PPD. The process of screening and accurately diagnosing PPD and other mental health concerns such as PTSD and OCD in the peripartum period can be a challenge. Maintaining the safety of women and their babies by evaluating for suicidal and/or homicidal ideation is a top priority for counselors. As mandated reporters, counselors must be prepared to quickly intervene when the safety of family members is in jeopardy. In addition, various significant, rarely discussed clinical issues were explored in this chapter, including paternal peripartum depression, adoptive depression, and perinatal loss. The more awareness and understanding counselors have about these critical counseling issues, the better they can help clients and their families navigate the peripartum experience.

Case Study: Johanna

Johanna is a 39-year-old Haitian woman with a history of multiple miscarriages in the past ten years. After several rounds of IVF treatments, Johanna became pregnant with twin boys and was finally able to carry the pregnancy to full term last year. During her pregnancy, Johanna reported that she and her husband felt extremely anxious that she would have another miscarriage. During the delivery, Johanna had a major birth complication that left one of the twins without oxygen and he passed away. While the other baby was healthy, Johanna and her husband were devastated and had limited family support, as most of their family reside in Haiti. They both experienced severe anxiety and worry about their surviving infant dying after bringing him home from the hospital. Johanna was unable to sleep or function due to her fears. When her surviving son was six weeks old, Johanna was admitted to the hospital for suicidal ideation. She was prescribed medication for depression and anxiety and has not reported any thoughts of suicide since leaving the hospital. During the baby's one year check-up with the pediatrician, Johanna reported that she still experiences symptoms of anxiety and depression related to her baby's death last year. Her husband still experiences nightmares of the birth, where he watched his son pass away. He still regrets not holding the baby or organizing a funeral service for him, as is traditional in Haitian culture. Johanna often feels overwhelmed with sadness about the death of her son, and guilt over not feeling more grateful about the baby who is still alive. Johanna and her husband are both having a great deal of difficulty planning for her son's first birthday party and asked the pediatrician for any resources or support groups to help during this difficult time.

APPLYING THE STRENGTHS MODEL—THE CASE OF JOHANNA

Significant Individual, Infant, Family, Societal, and Cultural Factors

- History of several miscarriages and one stillbirth in the past 12 months.
- History of anxiety during pregnancy as well as postpartum anxiety, depression, and suicidal ideation.

- Current symptoms of anxiety, depression, and grief.
- Spouse experiencing current symptoms of anxiety and grief.
- Haitian culture and funeral rituals not honored with infant's death.

Treatment Barriers

- Haitian culture could impact stigma of mental health counseling treatment.
- Limited family support, with family residing in Haiti.

Risk Factors

- History of anxiety during pregnancy.
- Limited family support.
- Complications during birth with death of infant.
- History of hospitalization for suicidal ideation.

Enlisting Support from Family, the Community, and Medical Professionals

- Family supports via virtual platforms such as video calls.
- Social supports via culturally diverse Haitian groups, virtual or local.
- Community supports and resources for grieving parents via virtual or local groups.
- Mental health counseling services for both parents related to grief, anxiety, and depression.

Noticeable Symptoms, Severity, & DSM-5-TR Diagnosis OR Needs Identified by Family & Treatment Team

- Mother reports current symptoms of anxiety, depression, and grief.
- Father reports current symptoms of anxiety and grief.
- Need for psychological support and sharing of experiences with other grieving parents.
- Potential DSM-5-TR diagnosis: F43.8 Prolonged Grief Disorder.

Goals Identified by Family

- Resources and increase in supports for grieving parents, including support groups.

- Reduction in anxiety and depressive symptoms related to baby's death.
- Reduction in feelings of guilt and increase in positive feelings.
- Explore ways to honor infant's death through cultural rituals.

Treatment Recommendations
- CBT therapy for dealing with trauma and grief symptoms (for both parents).
- CBT therapy for dealing with anxiety and depressive symptoms.
- "Baby and me" sessions with mother and baby to increase positive feelings about surviving child.
- Referral for potential pharmacological treatment interventions for anxiety.
- Create or review safety plan for any potential current or future suicidal ideation.

Helpful, Protective, and Resilience Factors
- Spousal support and understanding related to grief experiences.
- Actively seeking resources and supports from medical professionals.
- Connection to Haitian culture and rituals.

Self-Care & Wellness
- Psychological self-care by attending mental health counseling treatment and/or grief support groups.
- Emotional self-care by prioritizing emotional needs related to grief, anxiety, and depression.
- Personal self-care by reaching out to and fostering family and social supports.
- Spiritual self-care by exploring ways to honor infant's death.

REFERENCES

Abramowitz, J. S., Khandker, M., Nelson, C. A., Deacon, B. J., & Rygwall R. (2006). The role of cognitive factors in the pathogenesis of obsessive-compulsive symptoms: A prospective study. *Behaviour Research and Therapy*, 44(9), 1361–1374.

Allison, K. C., Wenzel, A., Kleiman, K., & Sarwer, D. B. (2011). *Postpartum Distress Measure*. doi:10.1037/t35682-000

American College of Obstetrics and Gynecology (ACOG). (2016). Screening for Perinatal Depression. https://www.acog.org/Resources-And-Publications/Committee-Opinions/Committee-on-Obstetric-Practice/Screening-for-Perinatal-Depression

American Psychiatric Association (APA). (2022). *Diagnostic and statistical manual of mental disorders* (5th ed.; text revision).

Anthony, R. E., Paine, A. L., & Shelton, K. H. (2019). Depression and anxiety symptoms of British adoptive parents: A prospective four-wave longitudinal study. *International Journal of Environmental Research and Public Health*, *16*(24). doi:10.3390/ijerph16245153

Ayers, S., Wright, D. B., & Thornton, A. (2018). Development of a measure of postpartum PTSD: The City Birth Trauma Scale. *Frontiers of Psychiatry*, *9*, 409. doi: 10.3389/fpsyt.2018.00409

Beck, A. T., Kovacs, M., & Weissman, A. (1979). *Scale for Suicide Ideation* [Beck Scale for Suicide Ideation]. APA PsycTests. doi:10.1037/t01299-000

Beck, A. T., Epstein, N., Brown, G., & Steer, R. (1988). *Beck Anxiety Inventory*. APA PsycTests. doi:10.1037/t02025-000

Beck, A. T., Ward, C. H., Mendelson, M., Mock, J., & Erbauch, J. (1961). *Beck Depression Inventory*. APA PsycTests. doi:10.1037/t00741-000

Beck, C. T., & Gable, R. K. (2000). *Postpartum Depression Screening Scale*. APA PsycTests. doi:10.1037/t42726-000

Bérard, A., Gorgui, J., Tchuente, V., Lacasse, A., Gomez, Y.-H., Côté, S., King, S., Muanda, F., Mufike, Y., Boucoiran, I., Nuyt, A. M., Quach, C., Ferreira, E., Kaul, P., Winquist, B., O'Donnell, K. J., Eltonsy, S., Chateau, D., Zhao, J.-P., … Zaphiratos, V. (2022). The COVID-19 pandemic impacted maternal mental health differently depending on pregnancy status and trimester of gestation. *International Journal of Environmental Research and Public Health*, *19*(5). doi:10.3390/ijerph19052926

Bostwick, J. M., Pabbati, C., Geske, J. R., & McKean, A. J. (2016). Suicide attempt as a risk factor for completed suicide: Even more lethal than we knew. *American Journal of Psychiatry*, *173*(11), 1094–1100. doi:10.1176/appi.ajp.2016.15070854

Brandes, M., Soares, C. N., & Cohen, L. S. (2004). Postpartum onset obsessive-compulsive disorder: Diagnosis and management. *Archives of Women's Mental Health*, *7*(2), 99–110. doi:10.1007/s00737-003-0035-3

Brockington, I. (1996). *Motherhood and mental health*. Oxford: Oxford University Press.

Brockington, I. F., & Kumar R. (Eds.). (1982). *Motherhood and mental illness*. Grune and Stratton.

Brodsky, B. S., Spruch-Feiner, A., & Stanley, B. (2018). The Zero Suicide Model: Applying evidence-based suicide prevention practices to clinical care. *Frontiers in Psychiatry*, *9*(33). doi:10.3389/fpsyt.2018.00033

Buist, A. (1996). *Psychiatric disorders associated with childbirth: A guide to management*. McGraw Hill.

Cacciatore, J. (2010) The unique experiences of women and their families after the death of a baby. *Social Work in Health Care*, *49*(2), 134–148. doi:10.1080/00981380903158078

Cacciatore, J., Erlandsson, K., & Rådestad, I. (2013). Fatherhood and suffering: A qualitative exploration of Swedish men's experiences of care after the death of a baby. *International Journal of Nursing Studies*, *50*(5), 664–670. doi:10.1016/j.ijnurstu.2012.10.014

Cacciatore, J., Schnebly, S., & Froen J., F. (2009). The effects of social support on maternal anxiety and depression after stillbirth. *Health & Social Care in the Community*, *17*(2), 167–176. doi:10.1111/j.1365-2524.2008.00814.x

Chasnoff, I. J., Wells, A. M., McGourty, R. F., & Bailey L. K. (2007). Validation of the 4P's Plus screen for substance use in pregnancy validation of the 4P's Plus. *Journal of Perinatology*, *27*, 744–748.

Chin, K., Wendt, A., Bennett, I. M., & Bhat, A. (2022). Suicide and maternal mortality. *Current Psychiatry Reports*, *24*(4), 239–275. doi:10.1007/s11920-022-01334-3

Costin, A., & McMurrich, C. A. (2013). A discussion of parental validation following stillbirth using transforming counseling and education. *International Journal of Childbirth Education*, *28*(3), 71–74.

Cox, J. L., Holden, J. M., & Sagovsky, R. (1987). *Edinburgh Postnatal Depression Scale*. doi:10.1037/t01756-000

Davis, R. N., Davis, M. M., Freed, G. L., & Clark, S. J. (2011). Fathers' depression related to positive and negative parenting behaviors with 1-year-old children. *Pediatrics, 127*, 612–618. doi:10.1542/peds.2010-1779

Dickens, J. (2020). Lactation after loss: Supporting women's decision-making following perinatal death. *British Journal of Midwifery*. doi:10.12968/bjom.2020.28.7.442

Eggleston, A. M., Calhoun, P. S., Svikis, D. S., Tuten, M., Chisolm, M. S., & Jones, H. E. (2009). Suicidality, aggression, and other treatment considerations among pregnant, substance-dependent women with posttraumatic stress disorder. *Comprehensive Psychiatry, 50*(5), 415–423.

Foli, K. J. (2010). Depression in adoptive parents: A model of understanding through grounded theory. *Western Journal of Nursing Research, 32*(3), 379–400. doi:10.1177/0193945909351299

Foli, K. J., & Gibson, G. C. (2011). Sad adoptive dads: Paternal depression in the post-adoption period. *International Journal of Men's Health, 10*(2), 153–162. doi:10.3149/jmh.1002.153

Foli, K. J., South S. C., & Lim E. (2012). Rates and predictors of depression in adoptive mothers: Moving toward theory. *Advances in Nursing Science, 35*, 51–63.

Foli, K. J., South S. C., Lim E., & Hebdon, M. (2016). Longitudinal course of risk for parental postadoption depression. *Journal of Obstetric, Gynecologic & Neonatal Nursing, 45*(2), 210–226.

Freitas, C. J., & Fox, C. A. (2015). Fathers matter: Family therapy's role in the treatment of paternal peripartum depression. *Contemporary Family Therapy, 37*, 417–425. doi:10.1007/s10591-015-9347-5

Gaudet, C., Sejourne, N., Camborieux, L., Rogers, R., & Chabrol, H. (2010). Pregnancy after perinatal loss: Association of grief, anxiety and attachment. *Journal of Reproductive and Infant Psychology, 28*(3), 240–251.

Gliatto, M. F., & Rai, A. K. (1999). Evaluation and treatment of patients with suicidal ideation. *American Family Physician, 6*, 1500.

Gold, K. J., Leon, I., Boggs, M. E., & Sen, A. (2016). Depression and posttraumatic stress symptoms after perinatal loss in a population-based sample. *Journal of Women's Health, 25*(3), 263–269. doi:10.1089/jwh.2015.5284

Gold, K. J., Singh, V., Marcus, S. M., & Palladino, C. L. (2012). Mental health, substance use and intimate partner problems among pregnant and postpartum suicide victims in the National Violent Death Reporting System. *General Hospital Psychiatry, 34*(2), 139–145. doi:10.1016/j.genhosppsych.2011.09.017

Goodman, J. H. (2004). Paternal postpartum depression, its relationship to maternal postpartum depression, and implications for family health. *Journal of Advanced Nursing, 45*(1), 26–35. doi:10.1046/j.1365-2648.2003.02857.x

Gressier, F., Guillard, V., Cazas, O., Falissard, B., Glangeaud-Freudenthal, N. M., & Sutter-Dallay, A. L. (2017). Risk factors for suicide attempt in pregnancy and the post-partum period in women with serious mental illnesses. *Journal of Psychiatric Research, 84*, 284–291. doi:10.1016/j.jpsychires.2016.10.009

Grigoriadis, S., Wilton, A. S., Kurdyak, P. A., Rhodes, A. E., VonderPorten, E. H., Levitt, A., ... Vigod, S. N. (2017). Perinatal suicide in Ontario, Canada: A 15-year population-based study. *Canadian Medical Association journal, 189*(34), e1085–e1092. doi:10.1503/cmaj.170088

Hunter, A., Tussis, L., & MacBeth, A. (2017). The presence of anxiety, depression and stress in women and their partners during pregnancies following perinatal loss: A meta-analysis. *Journal of Affective Disorders, 223*, 153–164. doi:10.1016/j.jad.2017.07.004

Hynan, M. (1998). The perinatal posttraumatic stress disorder (PTSD) questionnaire (PPQ). In Zalaquett, C. & Wood, R. (Eds.), *Evaluating stress: A book of resources* (pp. 199–200). Scarecrow Press.

Inwood, D. G. (Ed.). (1985). *Recent advances in postpartum psychiatric disorders*. American Psychiatric Press.

Jones I., & Craddock N. (2002) Do puerperal psychotic episodes identify a more familial subtype of bipolar disorder? Results of a family history study. *Psychiatric Genetics, 2*, 177–180.

Jordan, R. G., Farley, C. L., Grace, K. T. (Eds.). (2018). *Prenatal and Postnatal Care: A Woman-Centered Approach*. Wiley.

Knight, J. R., Shrier, L. A., Bravender, T. D., Farrell, M., Vander Bilt, J., & Shaffer, H. J. (1999). A brief new screen for adolescent substance abuse. *Archives of Pediatric and Adolescent Medicine, 153*(6), 591–596.

Koyucu, R. G., & Karaca, P. P. (2021). The Covid 19 outbreak: Maternal mental health and associated factors. *Midwifery, 99*, 103013. doi:10.1016/j.midw.2021.103013

Kroenke, K., Spitzer, R. L., & Williams, J. B. W. (1999). *Patient Health Questionnaire-9*. doi:10.1037/t06165-000

Kumar, R. (1994) Postnatal mental illness: A transcultural perspective. *Social Psychiatry and Psychiatric Epidemiology, 29*, 250–264.

Lafarge, C., Mitchell, K., & Fox, P. (2017). Posttraumatic growth following pregnancy termination for fetal abnormality: The predictive role of coping strategies and perinatal grief. *Anxiety, Stress, and Coping, 30*(5), 536–550.

Lang, A., Fleiszer, A. R., Duhamel, F., Sword, W., Gilbert, K. R., & Corsini-Munt, S. (2011). Perinatal loss and parental grief: The challenge of ambiguity and disenfranchised grief. *OMEGA, 63*(2), 183–196.

Lord, C., Rieder, A., Hall, G.B., Soares, C.N., & Steiner, M. (2011). Piloting the Perinatal Obsessive-Compulsive Scale (POCS): Development and validation. *Journal of Anxiety Disorders, 25*(8), 1079–1084.

Markin, R. D., & Zilcha-Mano, S. (2018). Cultural processes in psychotherapy for perinatal loss: Breaking the cultural taboo against perinatal grief. *Psychotherapy, 55*(1), 20–26. doi:10.1037/pst0000122

Metz, T. D., Rovner, P., Hoffman, M. C., Allshouse, A. A., Beckwith, K. M., & Binswanger, I. A. (2016). Maternal deaths from suicide and overdose in Colorado, 2004–2012. *Obstetrics & Gynecology, 128*, 1233–1240.

Mott, S. L., Schiller, C. E., Richards, J. G., O'Hara, M. W., & Stuart, S. (2011). Depression and anxiety among postpartum and adoptive mothers. *Archive of Women's Mental Health, 14*(4), 335–343. doi:10.1007/s00737-011-0227-1

National Institute of Mental Health. (NIMH). (2020). Ask Suicide-Screening Questions (ASQ) Toolkit. https://www.nimh.nih.gov/research/research-conducted-at-nimh/asq-toolkit-materials

Nazareth I. (2011). Should men be screened and treated for postnatal depression? *Expert Review of Neurotherapeutics, 11*(1), 1–3. doi:10.1586/ern.10.183

Pajulo, M., Pyykkonen, N., Kalland, M., Helenius, H., Punamaki, R. L. & Suchman, N. (2012). Substance-abusing mothers in residential treatment with their babies: Importance of pre-and postnatal maternal reflective functioning. *Infant Mental Health Journal, 33*, 70–81.

Paulson J. F., & Bazemore S. D. (2010). Prenatal and postpartum depression in fathers and its association with maternal depression: A meta-analysis. *JAMA, 303*(19), 1961–1969. doi:10.1001/jama.2010.605

Payne, J. L., Fields, E. S., Meuchel, J. M., Jaffe, C. J., & Jha, M. (2010). Post adoption depression. *Archives of Women's Mental Health, 13*(2), 147–151. doi:10.1007/s00737-009-0137-7

Pederson, E. L., & Vogel, D. L. (2007). Male gender role conflict and willingness to seek counseling: Testing a mediation model on college-aged men. *Journal of Counseling Psychology, 54*(4), 373–384. doi:10.1037/0022-0167.54.4.373

Polachek, I. S., Dulitzky, M., Margolis-Dorfman, L., & Simchen, M. J. (2016). A simple model for prediction postpartum PTSD in high-risk pregnancies. *Archives of Women's Mental Health, 19*(3), 483–490. doi:10.1007/s00737-015-0582-4

Polachek, I. S., Harari, L. H., Baum, M., & Strous, R. D. (2014). Postpartum anxiety in a cohort of women from the general population: Risk factors and association with depression during last week of pregnancy, postpartum depression and postpartum PTSD. *The Israel Journal of Psychiatry and Related Sciences, 51*(2), 128–134. ProQuest document ID 1777659232.

Ramchandani, P., Stein, A., O'Connor, T., Heron, J., Murray, L., & Evans, J. (2008). Depression in men in the postnatal period and later child psychopathology: A population cohort study. *Journal of American Academy of Child Adolescent Psychiatry, 47*(4), 390–398.

Ramchandani, P., O'Connor, T. O., Evans, J., Heron, J., Murray, L., & Stein, A. (2008). The effects of pre- and postnatal depression in fathers: A natural experiment comparing the effects of exposure to depression in offspring. *The Journal of Child Psychology and Psychiatry, 49*(10), 1069–1078.

Reck, C., Struben, K., Backenstrass, M., Stefenelli, U., Reinig, K., Fuchs, T., ... Mundt, C. (2008). Prevalence, onset and comorbidity of postpartum anxiety and depressive disorders. *Acta Psychiatrica Scandinavica, 118*(6), 459–468. doi:10.1111/j.1600-0447.2008.01264.x

Rehman, A. U., St Clair, D., & Platz, C. (1990). Puerperal insanity in the 19th and 20th centuries. *British Journal of Psychiatry, 156,* 861–865.

Russell, E. J., Fawcett, J. M., & Mazmanian D. (2013). Risk of obsessive-compulsive disorder in pregnant and postpartum women: A meta-analysis. *Journal of Clinical Psychiatry, 74*(4), 377–385.

Russell, M. (1994). New assessment tools for drinking in pregnancy: T-ACE, TWEAK, and others. *Alcohol Health and Research World, 18*(1), 55–61.

Sampson, M., Duron, J. F., Maldonado Torres, M. I., & Davidson, M. R. (2014). A disease you just caught: Low-income African American mothers' cultural beliefs about postpartum depression. *Women's Healthcare: A Clinical Journal for NPs, 2*(4), 44–50.

Sampson, M., Yu, M., Mauldin, R., Mayorga, A., & Gonzalez, L. G. (2021). "You withhold what you are feeling so you can have a family": Latinas' perceptions on community values and postpartum depression. *Family Medicine and Community Health, 9*(3), e000504. doi.10.1136/fmch-2020-000504

Senecky, Y., Agassi, H., Inbar, D., Horesh, N., Diamond, G., Bergman, Y. S., & Apter, A. (2009). Post-adoption depression among adoptive mothers. *Journal of Affective Disorders, 115*(1/2), 62–68. doi:10.1016/j.jad.2008.09.002

Simkin, P., Whalley, J., Keppler, A., Durham, J., & Bolding, A. (2010). Common changes and concerns in pregnancy. Chapter 3 in *Pregnancy, childbirth and the newborn: The complete guide* (pp. 32–61). Meadowbrook Press.

Siu, A. L., Bibbins-Domingo, K., Grossman, D. C., Baumann, L. C., Davidson, K.W., Ebell, M., et al. (2016). Screening for depression in adults: US Preventive Services Task Force Recommendation Statement. US Preventive Services Task Force (USPSTF). *JAMA, 315,* 380–387.

Spielberger, C. D. (1983). *State-Trait Anxiety Inventory for Adults* [STAI Form Y]. Mind Garden. doi:10.1037/t06496-000

Spinelli, M. (2019). Infanticide and American criminal justice (1980–2018). *Archives of Women's Mental Health, 22*(1), 173–177. doi:10.1007/s00737-018-0873-7

Somerville, S., Dedman, K., Hagan, R., Oxnam, E., Wettinger, M., Byrne, S., Coo, S., Doherty, D., & Page, A. C. (2014). *Perinatal Anxiety Screening Scale*. APA PsycTests. doi:10.1037/t70429-000

Stanley, B., & Brown, G. K. (2008). Safety Plan Treatment Manual to Reduce Suicide Risk: Veteran Version. https://sefbhn.org/assets/zero-suicide-recommended-evaluation-tools/safety-plans/stanley-brown-safety-manual.pdf

Stowe, Z. N., Hostetter, A. L., & Newport, D. J. (2005). The onset of postpartum depression: Implications for clinical screening in obstetrical and primary care. *American Journal of Obstetrics and Gynecology, 192*(2), 522–526. doi:10.1016/j.ajog.2004.07.054

Substance Abuse and Mental Health Services Administration. (SAMHSA). (2014). Results from the 2013 National Survey on Drug Use and Health: Summary of National Findings, NSDUH Series H-48, HHS Publication No. (SMA) 14-4863. Rockville, MD.

Tarasoff v. Regents of the University of California, 131 Cal. Rptr. 14 (Cal. 1976).

Thornton, C., Schmied, V., Dennis, C., Barnett, B., & Dahlen, H. G. (2013). Maternal deaths in NSW (2000–2006) from nonmedical causes (suicide and trauma) in the first year following birth. *Biomed Research International*, 1–6. doi:10.1155/2013/623743

Tietz, A., Zietlow, A., & Reck, C. (2014). Maternal bonding in mothers with postpartum anxiety disorder: The crucial role of subclinical depressive symptoms and maternal avoidance behaviour. *Archives of Women's Mental Health, 17*(5), 433–442. doi:10.1007/s00737-014-0423-x

Van Rensburg, N. J., Spies, R., & Malan, L. (2020). Infanticide and its relationship with postpartum psychosis: A critical interpretive synthesis. *Journal of Criminal Psychology, 10*(4), 293–310. doi:10.1108/JCP-05-2020-0018

Wallerstedt, C., & Higgins, P. (1996). Facilitating perinatal grieving between the mother and the father. *Journal of Obstetric, Gynecologic, and Neonatal Nursing, 25*(5), 389–394. doi:10.1111/j.1552-6909.1996.tb02442.x

Wenzel, A., Haugen, E. N., Jackson, L. C., & Robinson, K. (2003). Prevalence of generalized anxiety at eight weeks postpartum. *Archives of Women's Mental Health, 6*(1), 43–49. doi:10.1007/s00737-002-0154-2

Wijma, K., Soderquist, J., & Wijma, B. (1997). Posttraumatic stress disorder after childbirth: A cross sectional study. *Journal of Anxiety Disorders, 11*(6), 587–597. doi:10.1016/s0887-6185(97)00041-8

Wright, P. M. (2020). Perinatal loss and spirituality: A metasynthesis of qualitative research. *Illness, Crisis & Loss, 28*(2), 99–118. doi:10.1177/1054137317698660

Zung, W. W. K. (1965). *Self-Rating Depression Scale [Zung Self-Rating Depression Scale; Index of Potential Suicide; Zung Index of Potential Suicide]*. doi:10.1037/t04095-000

7

Multiple Routes to Motherhood
Role and Identity Changes and Clinical Implications

Isabel A. Thompson
with contributor Carly Paro-Tompkins

Personal Narrative

As a 24-year-old mother of two girls under the age of 2, I went through an immense amount of lifestyle change in a short amount of time. This, coupled with the traumatic nature of the birth of my children, has taken an immense toll on my mental health. With my first birth, my epidural failed, they couldn't properly monitor the baby's heartbeat, and they took me in for an emergency C-section. The last thing I remember is shrieking in pain because I felt the doctor cut into me as the anesthesiologist hastily put me under general anesthesia. I was not okay afterward. At my six-week checkup I filled out their questionnaire. "No, I don't feel like harming myself or my baby. No, I'm not sleeping. No, I don't have an appetite. No, I have no interest in anything I used to enjoy." I could've spoken out and let my doctor know how I was feeling, but I was supposed to deal with it, wasn't I? How was I supposed to know what I was feeling wasn't "normal"? It took over a year of feeling hopeless and like a failure for my husband to finally ask me why I was acting the way I was. Then I looked up and realized I was spending over seven hours a day on my phone, my house was a disaster, and I had let my business fizzle out. I was also six months pregnant with my second child. I felt like a shell of my former self, just going through the motions and trying to put on the facade of the mother I was trying to be. At my next prenatal appointment, I got a diagnosis of PTSD and Postpartum Depression. I started on medication and saw a light at the end of the tunnel. I planned a beautiful unmedicated VBAC for my second baby and thought that things were finally going to get better. At my 38-week appointment, the baby's heart rate was irregular and was fluctuating too much, and they sent me in for a repeat C-section. I laid on the OR table sobbing and begging the anesthesiologist to put me out. I was petrified of feeling them cut into me again and horrified at the thought of my sporadic breathing and lack of oxygen intake affecting my baby. I was hyperventilating and shaking violently, unable to control myself. My husband was beside my head trying desperately to calm me down. Another birth I wasn't able to fully experience or enjoy. Now, four months later, I'm pursuing treatment. After calling office after office,

> I have finally opted for an online therapy service and am looking forward to my first appointment soon. I'm hopeful that this will be beneficial for me and that I can begin to fulfill my own expectations as a wife and a mother.
> —Anonymous

In this chapter, we focus on the multiple routes to motherhood/parenthood, examining role and identity changes people experience when becoming parents for the first time, and address the adjustment associated with welcoming another child (or children) into the family. As described in the personal narrative above, becoming a mother involves profound changes and these can impact a mother's mental health and wellbeing. For first-time biological mothers, the birth of the baby marks a profound before and after moment, from being an independent agent to becoming a mother, responsible 24/7 for their new baby. Mothers of multiples, such as those who birth twins or triplets, have unique stressors, which we explore in this chapter. Non-biological mothers, including adoptive and stepmothers, experience role and identity changes, which we also explore in this chapter. Men who become fathers and non-binary/transgender individuals who become parents also experience role and identity changes. Partner, family, and friend dynamics all change when a baby arrives or is welcomed through marriage or adoption.

Parents who already have children also experience changes when welcoming additional children; however, they have already made the identity shift of becoming parents. When a mother or parent experiences PPD, as described in the narrative above, this makes adjusting to these changes more complex for everyone, so we will provide clinical recommendations to address adjustment and coping that are tailored to parents' unique needs and their journey to parenthood. Our intention is to include and acknowledge diverse family constellations, dynamics, and individual experiences to aid in efficacious treatment. Many of the applications to counseling that we describe in this chapter can be adapted to meet the specific individual or cultural needs of your current clients.

THE ADJUSTMENT TO MOTHERHOOD

Every person's journey to motherhood is different, whether it is by adoption, in vitro, a surprise or planned pregnancy, surrogacy, or marriage, but there is a shared experience of transitioning into the role of being a mother. Some parents' journeys are fraught with difficult twists and turns, while others seem to slide more seamlessly into parenthood. First-time mothers, making a life change to becoming mothers, are prone to doubt their parenting, and some may feel significant anxiety about the new tasks demanded by parenting (Chavis, 2016). Regardless of their feelings about the journey, once their baby, babies, child, or children arrive, they accommodate and adjust to this new role.

Some people adapt to the parent role by expanding their identity and others by extinguishing old parts of themselves. Laney et al. (2015) suggest that women "incorporated their children into their identities through a process of self-loss, identity fracturing, and redefinition" (p. 139). This self-loss process can be painful but marks an opportunity for redefinition of self to motherhood. Mothers' identities expand and benefit personal relationships with increased empathy for others and investment in future generations, while increasing career commitment (Laney et al., 2013).

In a qualitative study with 30 first-time mothers, researchers found three core themes in their data analysis: 1) fragmented identities (creating space for their firstborn child); 2) new identity boundaries (expanded to incorporate children); 3) life as a mother (deepening effect on their personality and identity) (Laney et al., 2015). First-time mothers may lose a sense of identity as they "give up their own needs and wants to care for the infant" (Laney et al., 2015, p. 132). Participants spoke of motherhood as transformative to their identity and sense of self, viewing their children as part of themselves, with some sharing that they could not fathom their lives or identities independently from motherhood (Laney et al., 2015). These findings point to the significance of motherhood for a person's identity, the way they see themselves, and their sense of meaning in life.

FIRST-TIME BIOLOGICAL MOTHERS

First-time biological mothers (who carry their baby during pregnancy) experience the physical changes associated with pregnancy, sometimes almost immediately. For instance, one of the first indicators of pregnancy can be nausea in the first trimester. Pregnancy impacts expectant mothers in diverse ways, depending on their life history. Expectant first-time mothers who have experienced a previous pregnancy loss can have more intense reactions to pregnancy. The role of motherhood can be thought of as beginning during pregnancy, as an expectant mother's body is creating life, particularly once the expectant mother is aware of her developing baby. The anticipation of birth is part of pregnancy as a mother readies her body and mind to welcome her child. When a first-time mother carries to term and gives birth, they experience the full role transition into motherhood with a newborn requiring near constant attention. Life changes that women go through, such as pregnancy and parenting, have been associated with increased anxiety (Chavis, 2016). In a study of 86 first-time mothers, higher levels of perceived social support and competence were associated with lower levels of reported anxiety (Chavis, 2016), which suggests that family, friend, and significant other support, coupled with self-efficacy, can reduce maternal anxiety.

PPD and First-Time Mothers

As described above, becoming a mother is a huge identity shift. PPD can complicate a mother's adjustment to motherhood and integrating her new role (Sockol et al., 2014). In two studies examining the relationship between the attitudes of first-time mothers about motherhood and their levels of emotional distress during pregnancy and the postpartum, there was an association between a mother's attitudes and anxiety and depression symptoms during the transition to parenthood (Sockol et al., 2014). In the first study, researchers developed and validated the Attitudes toward Motherhood Scale (AToM), which assesses "beliefs related to others' judgment," with items including: "If I make a mistake, people will think I am a bad mother" and "Seeking help with my baby from other people makes me feel incompetent" (Sockol et al., 2014, p. 204). The AToM scale also assesses "beliefs related to maternal responsibility" with items including: "If I love my baby, I should want to be with him/her all the time" (Sockol et al., 2014, p. 204). When you hear a client expressing these or similar statements about their beliefs about motherhood, administering the AToM could be a helpful assessment tool to further assess their beliefs and address them in treatment.

Whether a mother already has a baby/child or is a first-time mother also seems to impact the relationship between breastfeeding and PPD. While breastfeeding has been associated with lower rates of PPD overall, first-time breastfeeding mothers experience greater depressive symptoms than other mothers (Mezzacappa & Endicott, 2007). Mezzacappa and Endicott (2007) found that parity (i.e., number of births) mediated the association between breastfeeding and PPD, such that women with more than one birth had a significantly lower risk of developing PPD with breastfeeding compared with first-time breastfeeding mothers. This suggests that with each birth mothers gain confidence in parenting or practice breastfeeding and, consequently, depression rates decrease.

Surrogacy

A subset of biological mothers do not experience pregnancy directly but become mothers through gestational surrogacy. For heterosexual couples who become parents using a gestational surrogate, their child shares their DNA, but the mother did not physically carry or give birth to the child (Golombok et al., 2011). In the case of traditional surrogacy for heterosexual couples, "the surrogate mother and the commissioning father are the genetic parents of the child" (Golombok et al., 2011, p. 1579).

Gestational surrogacy is also a reproductive option for gay male couples; one father is a genetic parent, an egg donor the genetic mother and a gestational surrogate who carries and births the baby (Golombok et al., 2018). Gestational surrogacy is also a reproductive option for lesbian couples for whom donor insemination and pregnancy are not viable (Rubio et al., 2020).

MOTHERS OF MULTIPLES

The percentage of multiple births has increased throughout the world (Prino et al., 2016). This is in part due to the higher use of artificial reproduction technology (ART) such as in vitro fertilization, which increases the chance of having monozygotic twins by about 60 percent as compared with natural conception (Parazzini et al., 2016).

Multiple births can also occur spontaneously without the use of ART and can include twins, which can be monozygotic (identical) or dizygotic (fraternal), as well as triplets and higher multiples (Newman & Newman, 2018). Mothers of twins, triplets, and higher multiples care for two or more infants at once while still trying to take care of themselves and their relationships. Because there are practical demands of taking care of the needs of two or more infants, this can negatively impact the mother/parents emotionally, physically, and financially.

The relationship between a baby and caregiver can be impacted when the baby is one of a set of twins or one of higher multiples such as triplets. For instance, the presence of more than one infant may impact the parent–infant synchrony, which "refers to a close match between the parent's and the infant's affective behavior that is sensitive to microshifts in the infant's state and signal" (Feldman & Eidelman, 2004, p. 1134). Triplets may be at an especial disadvantage, due to the presence of three infants vying for their parents' attention.

When parenting stress, anxiety, and maternal depression of first-time mothers of twins were compared with parenting stress, anxiety, and maternal depression of first-time mothers of singleton babies, Riva Crugnola et al. (2020) reported that the mothers of twins had "significantly higher state anxiety" and higher reported stress levels, but maternal depression levels were not significantly different (p. 665). When considering the stressors of mothers of twins or higher multiples, it is important to consider the mother's/family's perceived resources and supports. When internal and/or external resources are lacking, a family with twins may experience more stress and need mental health intervention. If parents of twins have supportive internal resources (attachment style) and supportive external resources (perceived support from grandmothers), having twins could be a normative life event on par with having a singleton baby (Taubman-Ben-Ari et al., 2008). However, parenting twins and multiples may put additional strain on the relationship between the parents, depending on the internal and external resources available (Taubman-Ben-Ari et al., 2008).

Assessing parents' history of conception and perception of their stress level is also important. In a metanalysis of research that included 3,000 mothers, there was an association between mothers who had twins or multiples using assistive reproductive technology (ART) for conception and reported stress and depression when compared with mothers of singletons conceived using ART (van den Akker et al., 2016). When considering parents who conceive via ART, some have experienced previous pregnancy loss and may not have intended to have a multiple birth. Understanding the mother's/parents' path to conception, and their perception of life with multiples, can help clinicians provide more effective services.

NON-BIOLOGICAL MOTHERS

Women can take on a mothering role or become mothers without carrying or birthing a child. Non-biological mothers come to their role through foster parenting, step parenting, a partner's pregnancy, or adoption. Non-biological mothers who wanted biological children—and did not or could not have them—who then become mothers through foster parenting, stepparenting, or adoption may share a similar challenge: to grieve what might have been and attach to what is (Waterman, 2001; Robertson, 2006). In the case of adoption, the child experiences the loss of their biological parents. In stepfamilies, stepchildren experience the loss of their family structure and must adjust to a new family. The new adoptive or stepmother shares a similar emotional process of grieving the idealized and hoped-for biological children and embracing their new child/ren and family structure. In this parallel process of grief is an opportunity for attunement, attachment, and bonding between mother and child: "On neither side of the interaction can the attachment process be taken for granted: both mother and child have to work at belonging to one another" (Waterman, 2001, p. 277). Interventions to help mothers and their adoptive child/ren to build strong bonds can be a great way for counselors to support adoptive mothers and their families.

Adoptive Mothers

There are multiple ways to adopt a child; through foster care, a private domestic agency, or through a private international adoption agency. Understanding adoption and the need for adoption is complex and includes babies and children who need homes and prospective families longing to become parents. In the United States, 63,000 children were adopted from foster care in 2018 (US Department of Health and Human Services, 2019). There are 122,000 children in foster care who need adoptive families (Child Welfare Information Gateway, 2022). Long-term, well-documented statistics that include private adoptions are lacking (Sisson, 2022).

The financial cost of adoption varies, with private international adoptions costing a family $70,000 dollars or more (Family Equality, n.d.). However, there is typically no fee to adopt from foster care, and families that adopt children from US foster care agencies receive financial and social/emotional support. Despite the reduced cost to adopt from foster care, there is a potential emotional cost due to the potential trauma children have suffered. Children who experience abuse or neglect and then foster care may struggle with attachment and bonding, which impacts their current relationships with their adoptive family (Roman et al., 2022).

Although their journeys to motherhood are distinct from those of biological mothers or stepmothers, adoptive mothers still experience profound role and identity changes in becoming a mother. All adoptive mothers need support, especially in instances when their adoptive children have experienced neglect, abuse, or trauma. Therefore, it is critical that adoptive mothers have support to help them connect with their adoptive children and to meet their needs for trauma-informed services (Brodzinsky et al., 2022). Becoming a parent changes a person emotionally and in every other dimension, whether the route to parenthood is biological or through adoption, marriage, or surrogacy.

Stepmothers

Becoming a stepparent is a life experience that almost 50 percent of people in the United States and Canada experience (Gosselin & David, 2007). Stepmothers are diverse and have a variety of life stories and circumstances. Women become stepparents after dealing with infertility or not having biological children, after lacking a desire for children, or adding a partner's child to their previously born biological child/ren. As unique as the journey to becoming a stepmother is, the experience of being a stepmother is diverse and varies for each individual and family. Another recent term for stepmother is "bonus mom."

Role salience is about identifying as a mother (Desio, 2008). Being a stepmother usually involves a shared role of mothering with the biological mother still involved, which makes it distinct from adoptive mothering and biological mothering. The rare exception would be when the biological mother is deceased, and the stepmother therefore is the only living mother.

The adjustment to becoming a stepmother is different for each person, and this adjustment is impacted by the person's other life roles and identities, especially if they are already a parent. For a childless woman, becoming a stepmother provides an opportunity to be a parent, to mother a child (or children), and assume a role that might otherwise not be available to them. Desio (2008) discusses two types of stepmothers—stepmothers with children (SWC) and childless stepmothers (CSM). Desio (2008) further suggests there are two distinct groups of childless stepmothers (CSM): those who have wanted to become a mother but have not had the opportunity and those who have intentionally remained child-free.

For stepmothers, finding a balance of making new rules for their home can be challenging and lead to stress and self-doubt. Stepmothers experience increased anxiety as they attempt to balance their new role with the biological mother's role. Stepmothers interviewed in a qualitative study felt left out of important decisions and sought acceptance from the biological mother while also critiquing the biological mother's values (Doodson, 2014). Some stepmothers attempt to make the transition between homes seamless and less disruptive for the child's wellbeing. Others may take a different approach to managing their household and do not accommodate to the rules of the other home. The biological parents' rules, expectations, and way of living may not align with the stepparents' ideal or optimal way of living (Doodson, 2014). We recommend that counselors explore the family's experience of decision-making, rule setting, and differences between the two homes and transitioning the child.

Common Challenges of Stepmother Role

- The stepmother is responsible for mothering but is not *the* mother.
- The stepmother is a caretaker and not a total decision-maker.
- The stepmother may drive their stepchildren to school, but typically does not have an equal say in the school they attend.

- Holidays will forever be shared.
- One household's rules and routines are often incongruent with the other household's rules and routines.
- The stepmother will support their partner in conflicts with the biological mother but cannot fight for them.
- In some cases, a stepmother may be perceived as responsible for the end of the previous relationship between the child(ren)'s parents.

Clinical Responses and Themes to Explore

- Explore what aspects of parenting the stepmother has control over.
- Assess the qualities of the relationship with the stepchild(ren).
- Assess the roles the stepmother plays with her stepchild(ren)—mother, friend, mentor, confidant, etc.
- Assist the stepmother/family in developing holiday traditions and rituals that are meaningful and accommodate the other household/parents.
- Assist the stepmother in redefining motherhood to accommodate the identities and roles they experience.

Stepmother–Child Relationship

There are challenges that stepmothers experience in joint-custody arrangements, especially with the parenting triangle of the biological mother, partner/father, and themselves. Gates (2019) identified a sequential five-phase process that occurs when stepmothers adjust to their new role: "a. the honeymoon phase, b. stepping back, c. searching for voice and clarity, d. acceptance, and e. focusing on the relationship with the stepchildren" (p. 256). Stepmothers benefit by focusing on the relationship between themselves and their stepchildren rather than what they cannot control and working their way towards that realization they may be in different stages of the sequential process described above (Gates, 2019).

My (Carly Paro-Tompkins) stepdaughter was younger when we met, and she was prepared to become a family very quickly. In fact, during one of our first times meeting she crawled into my lap and asked, "Will you be my stepmom?" That was six years ago now and we have journeyed many ups and downs together. There are times she wants to pull me close and others she is not quite sure she would not rather turn back time and have her family of origin intact.

Societal Expectations

Negative stereotypes of stepfamilies and particularly stepmothers have persisted for decades as they continue to be depicted in film as "evil" or "wicked" and originated in classic movies like *Cinderella* (Skeen et al., 1985). These negative stereotypes can also impede stepmothers from seeking support from other stepmothers (Craig & Johnson, 2010). Both families and children are affected by this toxic stereotyping. Stepmothers notice the judgment from others, including bioparents, their stepchildren, and social institutions and may internalize the stigma themselves by comparing themselves to gendered stereotypes about what a mother should be (Miller et al., 2018). On the other hand, a more recent term for stepmother is the term "bonus mom." This might be a useful reframe for a counselor to use in session, particularly with a stepmother struggling with negative societal judgment.

Societal expectations of gender and mothering play a significant role in how a person experiences themselves and their roles and responsibilities as a mother. The mother's role is typically the glue of the family (Lorber, 1996, as cited in Shapiro, 2014). Stepmothers can feel powerless as compared with the biological mother, based on how they view the biological mother as powerful and themselves as not powerful (Gates, 2019). When the stepmother is expected to be the peacekeeper, while also not stepping on the biological mother's toes, this role can be especially challenging.

Stepmothers experience societal stereotyping and challenges being marginalized as a woman and a stepmother (Shapiro, 2014). Stepmothers may have fewer buffers to stress than stepfathers and experience higher levels of stress compared with other high-need parent groups, such as parents whose children have disabilities (Shapiro, 2014). Effective clinical approaches to supporting stepmothers would acknowledge these stressors while also highlighting stepmothers' and families' strengths and relationships.

Lesbian Non-biological Mothers

A specific identity as a non-biological mother is that of the lesbian non-biological partner or wife. In a lesbian parenting relationship, typically one woman carries the child and the other is technically the non-biological mother. Lesbian couples face choices about what egg to use, what sperm to use, and who becomes pregnant to carry the child and give birth (Markus et al., 2010). Some lesbian parents with multiple children might take turns carrying the children to share the experience of biological motherhood. Due to the gender-based constructions of motherhood and parenthood often normed on heterosexual/heteronormative relationships, same-sex lesbian couples co-construct their roles, up to and including the language their child will use, such as mommy, momma, etc.

FAMILY DYNAMICS

Relationships between and among extended family members change profoundly with the birth of a first baby, as the parents' own mothers and fathers become grandparents and the couple become parents (Simkin et al., 2010; Newman & Newman, 2018). This shift is most pronounced when a couple's first baby is also a first grandchild, a first niece/nephew, etc., to be welcomed into an extended family. A family's cultural values shape how parent and grandparent roles are structured (Cox, 2018). For families that align with White European American cultural values, honoring the new roles for everyone involves making room for the parents' parents to become grandparents while respecting the new parents' autonomy as *the parents*. Relinquishing power, responsibility, and control might be a new experience for first-time grandparents who have been used to being head of the household in the parent role. Families who identify with Latino cultural traditions that prioritize interdependence have different expected grandparent roles (Contreras, 2008). Grandmothers often have an active role in parenting decisions, especially in the case of adolescent mothers (Contreras, 2008). Chinese cultural traditions and ideals including the value of "continue the family lineage" mean that grandparents make personal sacrifices to help their children in dual-income couples by providing childcare for their grandchildren (Low & Goh, 2015). In other families when there are issues that prevent a parent from being present to parent their child or children (e.g., incarceration), grandparents step into the mother and father roles (Bachay & Buzzi, 2010).

Cultural values and identities also inform the expected involvement and decision-making power of extended family such as aunts, uncles, and cousins. Extended family may want to help with the baby, but sometimes their well-intentioned comments may not be well-received, increasing the need for assertive communication and effective boundary-setting. With the birth of another baby, an only child becomes a sibling, and this also changes the relationships between the firstborn and their mother and father. The whole family experiences an adjustment process when a baby is born, or a child is welcomed into the family through marriage or adoption. Other extended family members, including the new parents' siblings, experience role shifts too, as they become aunts and uncles (Newman & Newman, 2018). Aunts, uncles, and cousins, in time, are all part of this child's support network and contribute to the family's wellbeing. Moreover, depending on the family dynamics, extended family members are part of a natural support system that clinicians can help families to nurture and/or set boundaries with.

CHANGES IN FRIENDSHIPS

New mothers, fathers, partners, and parents may experience changes in their friendships, as the activities they previously enjoyed becoming impossible or difficult with a baby in tow. Further, subtler changes can create the need for existing friendships to change and develop to allow for this new parenting role and the baby in the friendship. Friends who are experiencing different stages of life may not understand the demands of motherhood because the arrival of a child often marks a major shift in responsibilities. In a qualitative study exploring women's friendships and motherhood, when a woman or their close friend becomes a parent, the friendship patterns, activities, and conversations change, as their identities change to adjust to motherhood and its concomitant responsibilities (Cronin, 2015). Becoming a mother can lead some friendships to dwindle or even end, while creating new friendships or even new types of friendships—mom friends (Cronin, 2015). While some friendships that began prior to motherhood may suffer with this transition to motherhood, other friendship bonds strengthen and grow.

MULTIPLE PERSPECTIVES: FATHER/PARTNER AND EXTENDED FAMILY RELATIONSHIPS

Fathers and other caregivers experience significant role changes when they become parents or welcome a baby into the family. For first-time fathers and partners welcoming a first child, this shift is especially pronounced, as it marks a change in identity from being an adult without a child to being a parent. The transition to fatherhood marks a significant change in a man's life, but men often do not receive support or acknowledgment from their employers about this enormous life shift (Atkinson, 2022).

Fathers bonding with their infants can support dyadic bonding between the parents and can also support each parent's quality of life (Escribano et al., 2022). In addition, the father's involvement in infant care early on has a positive impact on bonding and the mother's wellbeing; when the father's involvement is lacking, there is significant association with a mother's development of PPD (Séjourné et al., 2012). While fathers/partners are not responsible for a mother's wellbeing, there are benefits to fathers/partners providing direct infant care. While we have focused more on stepmothers in this chapter, stepfathers go through role transitions as well. Stepfamilies can be created in several ways: specifically biological father and stepmother relationships, and biological mother and stepfather. Introducing a non-biological stepfather is a common experience in families.

First-time Fathers

Becoming a parent is life-transforming for both mothers and fathers (Kowlessar et al., 2015). There is a need for increased awareness of the needs of expectant first-time fathers for support in their transition into parenthood during their partner's pregnancy and after the birth of their baby. A qualitative study with ten first-time fathers found that fathers feel "undervalued and unsupported," especially during their partner's pregnancy (Kowlessar et al., 2015, p. 4). While overall first-time fathers reported anxiety more than multi-child fathers, only some reported significant anxiety levels in the early postpartum period (Daire et al, 2022). Screening for anxiety could identify fathers/partners who need early intervention services (Daire et al., 2022). Fathers' needs for mental health support often go unmet in the peripartum, and clinicians can work to advocate to address the need for support for fathers, especially first-time fathers (Davenport & Swami, 2022).

Fathers' experiences are impacted by their birthing partner's experiences, moods, and behaviors. Although there is a range of roles for biological fathers, including fathers who do not reside with their child, we focus on those who reside with their partners and are involved in pregnancy, birth, and postpartum care. These fathers may need counseling support for their role transition, especially if their partner is struggling with PPD. Adoptive fathers experience many of the same transitions as other fathers, as they welcome a baby or child into their family.

MULTICULTURAL CONSIDERATIONS

In this section, we explore specific cultural considerations related to counseling peripartum clients. We caution clinicians from assuming that a client's alignment with one cultural identity would make them a good fit for a specific intervention or treatment protocol. As always, your relationship with your client(s) and your clinical judgment are essential to ensuring culturally competent practice. It is important to connect with clients using core counseling skills of rapport building, empathy, and unconditional positive regard.

"Mother" and "motherhood" are gendered terms that communicate sociocultural embedded expectations about accepted mothering behavior (Forbes et al., 2021). "Father" and "fatherhood" are also gendered terms with specific expectations and ideas about who a father is and what a father does. These heteronormative, binary terms for parents can be exclusionary and restrictive (Moreira, 2018). For parents who identify as lesbian, gay, bisexual, transgender, gender non-binary, or have other expansive sexual, affectional or gender identities, these terms may or may not fit with their lived experiences and identities (Moreira, 2018). To be culturally competent, we recommend that counselors apply the *Competencies for Counseling with Lesbian, Gay, Bisexual, Queer, Questioning, Intersex, and Ally Individuals* (ALGBTIC LGBQQIA Competencies Taskforce, Harper et al., 2013) and the *Competencies for Counseling with Transgender Clients* (ALGBTIC, 2010).

A challenge for non-birth parents can be feeling recognized as a parent, so supporting them in their parenting and providing validation can be very powerful. With families that are created through adoption, transracial adoption is common. Clinicians help adoptive families understand the needs of their adoptive child/ren from another racial or ethnic background and supporting their racial/ethnic identity development could be a focus of clinical attention (Malott & Schmidt, 2012). Whatever route to parenthood a family experienced, clinicians need to be aware of the various influences of cultural and familial background on their lived experience.

APPLICATIONS TO COUNSELING

A common counselor consideration when working with first-time parents, adoptive parents, stepparents, and/or parents of multiples, is to allow space for these clients to share a range of emotions they may be feeling. Avoid imposing sociocultural norms that put pressure on new mothers/parents to express happiness while suppressing other feelings they may have. When counseling families, our own family of origin issues can arise. Therefore, a core consideration we recommend is self-reflection about potential countertransference, personal biases, and lived experiences and how those can impact interactions and reactions to clients (Corey et al., 2019). Counselors seeking to demonstrate sensitivity to cultural and familial values should also be aware of avoiding imposing their beliefs about what a family is or should be (Gold & Wilson, 2002). Developing and sustaining an ongoing relationship with a clinical supervisor or colleague you can turn to when issues come up for you is an excellent way to engage in reflective counseling practice (Young, 2021).

Promoting Emotional Wellness

All mothers could benefit from interventions emphasizing and enhancing wellness, especially with the prevalence of social comparison due to online exposure to idealized images of motherhood (Kirkpatrick & Lee, 2022). Feeling worse as a mother than the idealized images promoted on social media can increase envy and state anxiety among mothers (Kirkpatrick & Lee, 2022). Counselors can help clients set social media boundaries—such as adjusting time engaged on social media, and reality-testing of self–other comparison based on social media. Counselors can also encourage realistic expectations about parenthood and normalize both the beautiful and messy moments. To promote positive self-esteem, counselors can help clients develop their own metric for their worth as mothers that is not tied to social media portrayals.

Although social media can negatively impact new mothers, as with the social comparison described above, online interventions can be beneficial for new mothers as complements to therapy. For instance, an online self-compassion program for mothers of infants, which consisted of psychoeducational materials including two videos and a tip sheet derived from compassion-focused therapy, was shown to be beneficial (Mitchell et al., 2018). Results demonstrated that mothers experiencing birth or breastfeeding challenges benefited, with increases in self-compassion, decreases in post-traumatic stress disorder (PTSD) symptoms (e.g., hyperarousal, intrusive thoughts), and increase in satisfaction with breastfeeding (Mitchell et al., 2018).

Addressing Couple and Family Relationships in Counseling

To effect change in a family system, counselors may need to engage in joint family treatment. Another approach is to work with the couple to strengthen their relationship. For first-time parents, whether they are parents through birth, adoption, marriage, or surrogacy, the partners have coexisted without compromising about what values, beliefs, traditions, rituals to teach their child or children. Prospective first-time parents can benefit from discussing these parenting themes and their worldview about parenting. With a baby's arrival, counselors can work with each parent to identify and strengthen their own cultural identity, communicate with each other, and develop a family culture that they feel comfortable with, helping them marry the two systems together to create their new family culture. Family genograms can be used as interventions during the perinatal period to open conversations about family constellations and explore relationship structures and dynamics by representing them visually (White, 2018). Genograms can also be helpful to explore family relationships for mothers who are bisexual (Tasker & Dolvoye, 2018).

Applying a marriage and family counseling lens can be helpful when working with mothers (and parents) because rarely is a presenting problem solely an individual problem, especially in the peripartum. This can give parents a language to use with each other to avoid perpetuating feelings of isolation and resentment that can exist when going through such as significant transition as becoming a parent. Emotionally focused family therapy is a recommended approach to address the complexities of parenting and to improve couples' attachment relationships (Furrow et al., 2019). Furrow et al. (2019) developed a comprehensive manual for implementing this approach entitled: *Emotionally Focused Family Therapy: Restoring Connection and Promoting Resilience*. For further information about working with couples on common peripartum issues including sexuality and parenting, see Chapter 8.

Some families' specific life experiences warrant clinical focus. For families adopting from the foster care system, the whole family may have more extensive clinical needs depending on the child's trauma history. For instance, a child with multiple family placements and a history of childhood trauma may need support services including family counseling. Communicating effectively about the child's family of origin and maintaining their confidence as adoptive parents are two key clinical goals.

Stepfamilies have specific family/couple counseling needs. The needs of blended families should be considered, as children are adjusting to new siblings through marriage. When working with stepfamilies, some clinicians include both families. For instance, marriage and family therapist and researcher Constance Ahrons (2007) treats the bi-nuclear family in family therapy working with all stepparents and family constellations. Bi-nuclear family refers to coparenting after divorce and parental remarriage, such that there are two nuclear families that the children grow up in (Ahrons, 2007).

Individual Counseling: The Journey of Motherhood

The journey of motherhood can be accompanied by a range of emotions, including joy and grief. First-time mothers often grieve the loss of independence and freedom to do things at will as they adjust to taking care of their infant (or infants in the case of multiples). They may experience what has been described as a fracturing of identity, have a sense of self-loss and go through a process of re-configuring their identity (Laney et al., 2015). Counselors can help mothers work toward reconfiguring an identity that includes motherhood. For mothers at risk of developing PPD, short-term process-oriented group psychotherapy is an effective preventative approach with first-time mothers (Pessagno & Hunker, 2013). Treatment approaches such as interpersonal psychotherapy (IPT) and cognitive behavioral therapy (CBT) are discussed in Chapter 11. Counselors can also normalize that bonding takes time, whether for biological, adoptive, or stepmothers.

If infertility is a part of a mother's journey, this should be addressed in counseling. For instance, some adoptive mothers may have struggled with infertility prior to choosing adoption. Similarly, paths to pursuing parenthood in same-sex couples could be a topic for exploration in counseling. Grief counseling could be the initial focus of therapy when working with clients with infertility history. For instance, for some stepmothers who have experienced infertility and have not had a biological child (or children), grief and loss may need to be addressed in treatment. Online support groups may be a good complementary treatment for childless stepmothers (CSMs) in need of social support (Craig & Johnson, 2010).

ETHICAL AND LEGAL CONSIDERATIONS

Working with families requires that the counselor be aware of the need for consent to treatment from parents/caregivers and the minor's assent to treatment (Herlihy & Corey, 2015). When parents are divorced, being aware of the state laws regarding joint decision-making about medical and educational treatment interventions is needed. This will often be detailed in divorce settlement paperwork that parents can provide the counselor with.

Legal permission to provide treatment for stepparents and their children would depend on the custody agreement and divorce settlement. Stepparents can be involved in treatment but cannot give legal consent for a counselor to treat the child unless they are the legal guardian. Providing psychoeducation to stepparents and addressing issues related to parenting would only need to the consent of the stepparent themselves, but any time the child is involved, the parent (or parents) with legal decision-making authority would need to consent to treatment. Counselors should reference laws in their place of practice. Ethically, the counselor must consider what is in the best interests of the child and treatment efficacy while also considering parental rights and the limits of confidentiality when working with minor clients (Herlihy & Corey, 2015). It is also recommended that counselors use a decision-making model about how to address the child's treatment needs and how to move forward in engaging parents and guardians in treatment. With adoption, counselors should be aware of the laws in their state.

Counselors should engage in crisis planning and need to ensure that any clients who are experiencing symptoms of PPD should be advised to see a primary care provider for a full physical evaluation and assessment of their mental state (Stephanie Anderson, Nurse Practitioner (NP), personal communication). Further, depending on the severity of symptoms, referral to a psychiatrist for a psychiatric evaluation may also be needed. Clinicians must always remember to practice with the scope of practice of their licensure.

BARRIERS TO TREATMENT

Individuals and families sometimes do not realize or perceive the need for treatment for themselves, their family, or their children. For instance, sometimes parents do not perceive their child as needing treatment, although their symptoms indicate they would benefit from it (Kim & Kim, 2021). For mothers, the discrepancy between what they thought motherhood would be like and what their experience is actually like can contribute to a sense of being out of step with others. Expecting prospective clients to move beyond this and seek treatment can be daunting, especially in this highly vulnerable stage of life.

Even if a parent or family overcomes the emotional/internal barriers of pursuing treatment, other factors such as family and cultural beliefs, financial constraints, and logistical challenges can be barriers. Structural barriers to accessing mental health services disproportionately impact Black and Latinx people seeking services (Loeb et al., 2022).

Among Asian Americans, cultural belief systems about seeking psychological care and the stigma associated with mental illness impact help-seeking behavior and may be a barrier to treatment (Tung, 2011). Financial costs are also a major barrier for many people in pursuit of treatment. Even those with private health insurance may not have mental health coverage. A great aspect of destigmatizing mental health care is that practices have been filling up with clients, especially during the early years of the COVID-19 pandemic. Logistical barriers to seeking treatment are huge, especially with a mother experiencing depression, and if they have limited family or childcare support. Telehealth options for mental health treatment may increase access to care and can help address some logistical challenges, especially for mothers with newborns and mothers of multiples. Finding a provider with specialized training and/or experience with peripartum, post-adoption, stepparenting, and parent–child attachment issues can be especially challenging.

RESOURCES FOR TREATMENT

> Open Path Collective for low-cost counseling options with quality providers (may be particularly useful for those without mental health insurance coverage or underinsured, who have financial hardship): https://wellness.openpathcollective.org/
>
> Theraplay and directory of providers: https://theraplay.org/directory/
>
> Postpartum Support International provides a variety of services and offers a provider search on their website.
>
> https://www.childwelfare.gov/topics/adoption/adopt-parenting/
>
> https://postpartumhealthalliance.org/postpartum-search-providers/

IMPACT OF THE COVID-19 PANDEMIC

The COVID-19 pandemic resulted in changes and stressors for pregnant women, mothers, parents, and families. For first-time mothers who gave birth early in the pandemic, governmental restrictions and recommendations for social distancing impacted the way they experienced the transition to motherhood (Gray & Barnett, 2021). For instance, mothers in England who welcomed a baby during the British "lockdowns" (periods of behavioral restrictions that included closure of non-essential businesses and restricted social behavior) reported experiencing "an overwhelming sense of responsibility for their baby which was heightened by the pandemic" (Gray & Barnett, 2021, p. 534).

The restrictions due to the COVID-19 pandemic presented challenges to first-time mothers, and they experienced disruptions "to the birthing experience, an inability to connect with close friends and family, and limited healthcare support" (Gray & Barnett, 2021, p. 534). Despite these challenges associated with being a first-time mother in the early days of the pandemic, the reduced social expectations associated with the pandemic coupled with the increased presence of a partner were seen as positive impacts (Gray & Barnett, 2021).

As discussed above, COVID-19 had major impacts, both positive and negative, and mixed, on families. For some families, the flexibility of remote work was beneficial. For instance, in the case study described below, the mother could work from home after her twin sons were released from the NICU. This allowed her to attend to their needs, avoid additional financial hardship of childcare costs, and avoid putting them in out-of-home care for longer.

Case Study: Ceci

Ceci, a Cuban American Catholic, wife, and mother of three. She was raised in South Florida with her mother, father, brother, and sister. Charles is White and was raised in a non-religious family in Northeast Florida. They met in college. She holds a master's degree in Architecture and maintains a passion for building and design. She works in a related profession and finds great satisfaction with her work. Ceci and Charles married at the age of 29 and later at 33 had their first child, William. She had a miscarriage before both her singleton and her twin births.

After years of trying to get pregnant again after the miscarriage, she went to a doctor, who stated she was premenopausal and would need help to get pregnant and carry to term. She said no way and they went on with life assuming she could not get pregnant. Ceci wanted William to have siblings.

At 38, Ceci found herself pregnant again, this time with identical twins. They had mixed emotions surrounding the demands that would come with twins. Ceci and Charles were both midcareer professionals in management positions. Ceci felt great during pregnancy and although she had some morning sickness with the twins felt emotionally well. Their family was supportive and excited. Overall, her pregnancy would be considered healthy, however, a medical condition called cholestasis of pregnancy (which impacts the liver) began when she was 36 weeks pregnant, and she was induced. Her twins were born via a vaginal delivery. She stayed in the hospital because she experienced significant loss of blood during delivery and other complications including pruritic urticarial papules and plaques of pregnancy (PUPPP). The twins were born at five pounds each and were in NICU for six weeks. Albert had issues with lung development, and Gavin was born feet-first and swallowed his meconium during birth. She could not hold both babies at the same time for six days because of their treatments in the NICU and felt out of control and incomplete.

Once the twins came home, Ceci took time off first. She felt very supported by her boss after having the twins. Charles was home for several months, eight weeks of which were paid, to avoid putting the twins in daycare, later transitioning to in-home care. Given his job demands, he worked more during the COVID-19 pandemic's early days.

However, Ceci's dad died a day after the babies came home from the NICU. She was devastated by her father's death—it was sudden, and he did not get to meet the twins.

She experienced depressive symptoms that she called "babies blues" and felt overwhelmed. While the twins were in the NICU, she maintained a tiring schedule, as she would stay until 10 pm, take her son to elementary school the next morning and do it again the next day. Her OB/GYN prescribed antidepressants, and she got support from family and friends but no formal treatment.

Given the stress of caring for the twins and loss of her dad, the social distance of COVID seemed less important in comparison. Then Charles's mother died nine months later, which added stress for the family.

Reflection Questions for Clinicians

- If you were working with this family, what sort of assessment instruments would you use in your initial assessment?

- Are any details of this case personally triggering for you? If so, what sort of consultation or supervision could you use to process the countertransference?

- What cultural considerations need to be accounted for, considering your own cultural identity and the differing cultural identities of both partners and the bicultural identities of their children?

- When you read this, are you automatically drawn to focus on the client's or family's strengths or presenting problems? Whatever you gravitate toward, take a moment to pause and consider the other dimension. For

> instance, if you gravitated toward focusing on the presenting problem, take a moment to consider the various strengths and resilience factors of this mother and family.

APPLYING THE STRENGTHS MODEL—THE CASE OF CECI

Significant Individual, Infant, Family, Societal, and Cultural Factors

- Ceci became pregnant with twins after thinking she couldn't become pregnant again.
- She experienced the medical complication of PUPPP while in the hospital after birth.
- Her twins were in the NICU after birth.

Treatment Barriers

- She disclosed symptoms of OB/GYN and got antidepressants.
- She did not pursue counseling.
- Perceiving treatment as selfish; time away from her family.

Risk Factors

- She experienced medical complications at birth.
- Twins in NICU.
- The sudden death of her father after her twins were discharged from NICU.

Enlisting Support from Family, the Community, and Medical Professionals

- Maintain relationship with OB/GYN and get referral to counselor or therapist.
- Support group for new mothers.
- Joint sessions with both parents to help with family adjustment with twins discharged from NICU and back home.

Noticeable Symptoms, Severity, & DSM-5-TR Diagnosis OR Needs Identified by Family & Treatment Team

- Feeling overwhelmed.
- Frequent crying spells.
- Insomnia.

Goals Identified by Family

- Help Ceci with grief about loss of her father.
- Adjustment to life with the twins at home and make time for fun together.
- Treat Ceci's mood symptoms.

Treatment Recommendations

- Evaluation by a psychiatrist.
- Grief counseling for Ceci and family.
- IPT to enhance relationship functioning, with inclusion of expressive modalities.

Helpful, Protective, and Resilience Factors

- Both parents have strong extended family support.
- Both parents successful in their careers.
- In a committed long-term relationship.

Self-Care & Wellness

- Ceci sought help from her OB/GYN.
- Identifying activities to do when leaving the house is not feasible (due to either COVID-19 and/or twins' medical condition or just having twins and an older child).
- Ask for help from others so that she can implement self-care and positive coping activities.

REFERENCES

Ahrons, C. (2007). Family ties after divorce: Long-term implications for children. *Family Process, 46*(1), 53–65. doi:10.1111/j.1545-5300.2006.00191.x

ALGBTIC LGBQQIA Competencies Taskforce: Harper, A., Finerty, P., Martinez, M., Brace, A., Crethar, H. C., Loos, B., Harper, B., Graham, S., Singh, A., Kocet, M., Travis, L., Lambert, S., Burnes, T., Dickey, L. M., & Hammer, T. (2013). Association for Lesbian, Gay, Bisexual, and Transgender Issues in Counseling Competencies for Counseling with Lesbian, Gay, Bisexual, Queer, Questioning, Intersex, and Ally Individuals. *Journal of LGBT Issues in Counseling, 7*(1), 2–43. doi:10.1080/15538605.2013.755444

Association for Lesbian, Gay, Bisexual, and Transgender Issues in Counseling. (ALGBTIC). (2010). American Counseling Association Competencies for Counseling with Transgender Clients. *Journal of LGBT Issues in Counseling, 4*(3), 135–159.

Atkinson, J. (2022). Involved fatherhood and the workplace context: A new theoretical approach. *Gender, Work and Organization, 29*(3), 845–862. doi:10.1111/gwao.12789

Bachay, J. B., & Buzzi, B. M. (2012). When grandma and grandpa become mom and dad: Engaging grandfamilies in clinical practice. *Kriminologija & Socijalna Integracija, 20*(1), 63–70.

Brodzinsky, D., Gunnar, M., & Palacios, J. (2022). Adoption and trauma: Risks, recovery, and the lived experience of adoption. *Child Abuse and Neglect, 130*(2), 105309. doi:10.1016/j.chiabu.2021.105309

Chavis, L. (2016). Mothering and anxiety: Social support and competence as mitigating factors for first-time mothers. *Social Work in Health Care, 55*(6), 461–480. doi:10.1080/00981389.2016.1170749

Child Welfare Information Gateway (2022). All-In Foster Adoption Challenge. A report from the US Department of Health and Human Services. Retrieved November 1, 2022, from: https://www.childwelfare.gov/topics/adoption/allinadoptionchallenge/

Contreras, J. M. (2004). Parenting behaviors among mainland Puerto Rican adolescent mothers: The role of grandmother and partner involvement. *Journal of Research on Adolescence,14*(3), 341–368. doi:10.1111/j.1532-7795.2004.00078.x

Corey, G., Corey, M., & Corey, C. (2019). *Issues and ethics in the helping professions* (10th ed.). Cengage.

Cox, C. (2018). Cultural diversity among grandparent caregivers: Implications for interventions and policy. *Educational Gerontology, 44*(8), 484–491. doi:10.1080/03601277.2018.1521612

Craig, E., & Johnson, A. (2010). Role strain and online social support for childless stepmothers. *Journal of Social and Personal Relationships, 28*(6), 868–887. doi:10.1177/0265407510393055

Cronin, A. M. (2015). "Domestic friends": Women's friendships, motherhood and inclusive intimacy. *The Sociological Review, 63*(3), 662–679. doi:10.1111/1467-954X.12255

Daire, C., de Tejada, B. M., & Guittier, M. J. (2022). Fathers' anxiety levels during early post-partum: A comparison study between first-time and multi-child fathers. *Journal of Affective Disorders, 312*, 303–309. doi:10.1016/j.jad.2022.06.052

Davenport, C. J., & Swami, V. (2022). Getting help as a depressed dad: A lived experience narrative of paternal postnatal depression, with considerations for healthcare practice. *Journal of Psychiatric and Mental Health Nursing*, 1–7. doi:10.1111/jpm.12854

Desio, A. R. (2008). *A Comparison of Childless Stepmothers and Stepmothers with Children: The Significance of Role Salience and Role Strain in Marital and Psychological Well-Being* (Publication No. 3307639) [Doctoral dissertation, State University of New York at Buffalo]. ProQuest Dissertations and Theses Global.

Doodson, L. J. (2014). Understanding the factors related to stepmother anxiety: A qualitative approach. *The Journal of Divorce and Remarriage, 55*(8), 645–667. doi:10.1080/10502556.2014.959111

Escribano, S., Oliver-Roig, A., Juliá-Sanchis, R., & Richart-Martínez, M. (2022). Relationships between parent–infant bonding, dyadic adjustment and quality of life, in an intra-partner sample. *Health & Social Care in the Community, 30*, e5017–e5026. https://doi-org/10.1111/hsc.13917

Family Equality (n.d.). Average Adoption costs in the United States. Retrieved November 18, 2022 from: https://www.familyequality.org/resources/average-adoption-costs-in-the-united-states/

Feldman, R., & Eidelman, A. I. (2004). Parent-infant synchrony and the social-emotional development of triplets. *Developmental Psychology, 40*(6), 1133–1147. doi:10.1037/0012-1649.40.6.1133

Forbes, L. K., Lamar, M. R., & Bornstein, R. S. (2021). Working mothers' experiences in an intensive mothering culture: A phenomenological qualitative study. *Journal of Feminist Family Therapy: An International Forum, 33*(3), 270–294. doi:10.1080/08952833.2020.1798200

Furrow, J., Palmer, G., Johnson, S., Faller, G., & Palmer-Olsen, P. (2019). *Emotionally focused family therapy: Restoring and promoting resilience.* Routledge.

Gates, A. (2019). Stepmothers coparenting experience with the mother in joint custody stepfamilies. *The Journal of Divorce and Remarriage, 60*(4), 253–269. doi:10.1080/1050.2556.2018.1488124

Gray, A., & Barnett, J. (2021). Welcoming new life under lockdown: Exploring the experiences of first-time mothers who gave birth during the COVID-19 pandemic. *British Journal of Health Psychology, 27*(2), 534–552. doi:10.1111/bjhp.12561

Gold, J. M., & Wilson, J. S. (2002). Legitimizing the child-free family: The role of the family counselor. *The Family Journal, 10*(1), 70–74. doi:10.1177/1066480702101011

Golombok, S., Blake, L., Slutsky, J., Raffanello, E., Roman, G. D., & Ehrhardt, A. (2018). Parenting and the adjustment of children born to gay fathers through surrogacy. *Child Development, 89*(4), 1223–1233. doi:10.1111/cdev.12728

Golombok, S., Readings, J., Blake, L., Casey, P., Marks, A., & Jadva, V. (2011). Families created through surrogacy: Mother–child relationships and children's psychological adjustment at age 7. *Developmental Psychology, 47*(6), 1579–1588. doi:10.1037/a0025292

Gosselin, J., & David, H. (2007). Risk and resilience factors linked with the psychosocial adjustments of adolescents, stepparents, and biological parents. *The Journal of Divorce and Remarriage, 48*(1/2), 29–53. doi:10.1300/J087v48n01_02

Herlihy, B., & Corey, G. (2015). *ACA ethical standards casebook* (7th ed.). American Counseling Association.

Kim, I., & Kim, N. (2021). Parental perceived need for counseling for adolescents' anxiety and depression symptoms: A cross-sectional study. *Counseling Outcome Research and Evaluation, 13*(2), 91--100. doi:10.1080/21501378.2021.1874240

Kirkpatrick, C. E., & Lee, S. (2022). Comparisons to picture-perfect motherhood: How Instagram's idealized portrayals of motherhood affect new mothers' well-being. *Computers in Human Behavior, 137*, 1–13. doi:10.1016/j.chb.2022.107417

Kowlessar, O., Fox, J. R., & Wittkowski, A. (2015). First-time fathers' experiences of parenting during the first year. *Journal of Reproductive and Infant Psychology, 33*(1), 4–14. doi:10.1080/02646838.2014.971404

Laney, E. K., Carruthers, L. L., Hall, M. E. L., & Anderson, T. L. (2013). Expanded the self: Motherhood and identity development in faculty women. *Journal of Family Issues, 35*(9), 1227–1251. doi:10.1177/0192513X13479573

Laney, E. K., Hall, M. E. L., Anderson, T. L., & Willingham, M. M. (2015). Becoming a mother: The influence of motherhood on women's identity development. *Identity, 15*(2), 126–145. doi:10.1080/15283488.2015.1023440

Loeb, T. B., Viducich, I., Smith-Clapham, A., Adkins-Jackson, P., Zhang, M., Cooley-Strickland, M., Davis, T., Pemberton, J. V., & Wyatt, G. E. (2022). Unmet need for mental health services utilization among under-resourced Black and Latinx adults. *Families, Systems, & Health.* doi:10.1037/fsh0000750

Low, S. S. H., & Goh, E. C. L. (2015). Granny as nanny: Positive outcomes for grandparents providing childcare for dual-income families. Fact or myth? *Journal of Intergenerational Relationships, 13*(4), 302–319. doi:10.1080/15350770.2015.1111003

Malott, K. M., & Christopher D. Schmidt, C. D. (2012). Counseling families formed by transracial adoption: Bridging the gap in the multicultural counseling competencies, *The Family Journal, 20*(4), 384–391. doi:10.1177/1066480712451231

Markus, E., Weingarten, A., Duplessi, Y., & Jones, J. (2010). Lesbian couples seeking pregnancy with donor insemination. *Journal of Midwifery & Women's Health, 55*(2), 124–132. doi:10.1016/j.jmwh.2009.09.014

Mezzacappa, E. S., & Endicott, J. (2007). Parity mediates the association between infant feeding method and maternal depressive symptoms in the postpartum. *Archives of Women's Mental Health, 10,* 259–266. doi:10.1007/s00737-007-0207-7

Miller, A., Cartwright, C., & Gibson, K. (2018). Stepmothers' perceptions and experiences of the wicked stepmother stereotype. *Journal of Family Issues, 39*(7), 1984–2006. doi:10.1177/0192513X17739049

Mitchell, A., Wittingham, K., Steindl, S., & Kirby, J. (2018). Feasibility and acceptability of a brief online self-compassion intervention for mothers of infants. *Archives of Women's Mental Health, 21,* 553–561. doi:10.1007/s00737-018-0829-y

Moreira, L. (2018). Queer motherhood: Challenging heteronormative rules beyond the assimilation/radical binary. *Journal of International Women's Studies, 19*(2), article 2. https://vc.bridgew.edu/cgi/viewcontent.cgi?article=2001&context=jiws

Newman, B. M., & Newman, P. R. (2018). *Development through life: A psychosocial approach.* (13th ed.). Cengage Learning.

Parazzini, F., Cipriani, S., Bianchi, S., Bulfoni, C., Bortolus, R., & Somigliana, E. (2016). Risk of monozygotic twins after assisted reproduction: A population-based approach. *Twin Research and Human Genetics, 19*(1), 72–76. doi:10.1017/thg.2015.96

Pessagno, R. A., & Hunker, D. (2013). Using short-term group psychotherapy as an evidence-based intervention for first-time mothers at risk for postpartum depression. *Perspectives in Psychiatric Care, 49*(3), 202–209. doi:10.1111/j.1744-6163.2012.00350.x

Prino, L. E., Rollè, L., Sechi, C., Patteri, L., Ambrosoli, A., Caldarera, A. M., Gerino, E., & Brustia, P. (2016). Parental relationship with twins from pregnancy to 3 months: The relation among parenting stress, infant temperament, and well-being. *Frontiers in Psychology, 21*(7). doi:10.3389/fpsyg.2016.01628

Riva Crugnola, C., Ierardi, E., Prino, L. E., Brustia, P., Cena, L., & Rollè, L. (2020). Early styles of interaction in mother-twin infant dyads and maternal mental health. *Archives of Women's Mental Health, 23*(5), 665–671. doi:10.1007/s00737-020-01037-9

Robertson, (2006). Attachment and caregiving behavioral systems in intercountry adoption: A literature review. *Children and Youth Services Review, 28*(7), 727–740. doi:10.1016/j.childyouth.2005.07.008

Roman, M., Palacios, J., & Minnis, H. (2022). Changes in attachment disorder symptoms in children internationally adopted and in residential care. *Child Abuse and Neglect, 130*(2), 105308. doi:10.1016/j.chiabu.2021.105308

Rubio, B., Vecho, O., Gross, M., van Rijn-van Gelderen, L., Bos, H., Ellis-Davies, K., Winstanley, A., Golombok, S., & Lamb, M. E. (2020). Transition to parenthood and quality of parenting among gay, lesbian and heterosexual couples who conceived through assisted reproduction. *Journal of Family Studies, 26*(3), 422–440. doi:10.1080/13229400.2017.1413005

Séjourné, N., Vaslot, V., Beaumé, M., Goutaudier, N., & Chabrol, H. (2012). The impact of paternity leave and paternal involvement in child care on maternal postpartum depression. *Journal of Reproductive and Infant Psychology, 30*(2), 135–144. doi:10.1080/02646838.2012.693155

Sisson, G. (2022). Estimating the annual domestic adoption rate and lifetime incidence of infant relinquishment in the United States. *Contraception, 105,* 14–18. doi:10.1016/j.contraception.2021.08.008

Shapiro, D. (2014). Stepparents and parenting stress: The roles of gender, marital quality, and views about gender roles. *Family Process, 53*(1), 97–108. doi:10.1111/famp.12062

Simkin, P., Whalley J., Keppler, A. et al. (2010). *Pregnancy, childbirth, and the newborn: The complete guide* (4th ed.). Meadowbrook Press.

Skeen, P., Covi, R., & Robinson, B. (1985). Stepfamilies: A review of the literature with suggestions for practitioners. *Journal of Counseling and Development, 64,* 121–125. doi:10.1002/j.1556-6676.1985.tb01049.x

Sockol, L. E., Epperson, C. N., & Barber, J. P. (2014). The relationship between maternal attitudes and symptoms of depression and anxiety among pregnant and postpartum first-time mothers. *Archive of Women's Mental Health, 17*, 199–212. doi:10.1007/s00737-014-0424-9

Tasker, F., & Delvoye, M. (2018). Maps of family relationships drawn by women engaged in bisexual motherhood: Defining family membership. *Journal of Family Issues, 39*(18), 4248–4274. doi:10.1177/0192513X18810958

Taubman-Ben-Ari, O., Findler, L., Bendet, C., Stanger, V., Ben-Shlomo, S., & Kuint, J. (2008). Mothers' marital adaptation following the birth of twins or singletons: Empirical evidence and practical insights. *Health & Social Work, 33*(3), 189–197. doi:10.1093/hsw/33.3.189

Tung, W. (2011). Cultural barriers to mental health services among Asian Americans. *Home Health Care Management & Practice, 23*(4), 303–305. doi:10.1177/1084822311401857

US Department of Health and Human Services. (2019). The AFCARS report: Preliminary FY 2018 estimates as of August 2019 (26). https://www.acf.hhs.gov/cb/report/afcars-report-26

Van den Akker, O., Postavaru, G.-I., & Purewal, S. (2016). Maternal psychosocial consequences of twins and multiple births following assisted and natural conception: A meta-analysis. *Reproductive Biomedicine Online, 33*(1), 1–14. doi:10.1016/j.rbmo.2016.04.009

Waterman, B. (2001). Mourning the loss builds the bond: Primal communication between foster, adoptive, or stepmother and child. *Journal of Loss and Trauma, 6*(4), 277–301. doi:10.1080/108114401317087806

White, J. (2018). Does a Perinatal Infant Mental Health team hold the family in mind? Opportunities and challenges for working systemically in this specialised field. *Australian and New Zealand Journal of Family Therapy, 39*(2), 144–154. doi:10.1002/anzf.1295

Young, M. E. (2021). *Learning and the art of helping: Building blocks and techniques.* (7th ed.) Pearson.

8

Shift in Couple Dynamics

Vanessa Beatriz Teixeira
with contributor Samantha Fernandez

Personal Narrative

This was my first pregnancy, and I became pregnant much quicker than expected only one month after stopping birth control. My husband and I were ready as we had been together seven years and were just married. I was very fit before pregnancy and continued during. I played soccer and regularly exercised while I was pregnant as well as taught Physical Education to high schoolers. I was planning a natural birth and hired a doula. Labor was intensely fast and I labored at home for 20 hours before going into the hospital. When I got to the hospital I continued to labor with no medical interventions. I had terrible back labor but I was determined to make it through. I was 9.5 cm when I could tell something was wrong. I heard the nurse call and the whole room filled up. They said the baby's heart rate has dropped for too long and there would be an emergency C-section, which I wanted to avoid so badly. The first night I got home I felt the whole rush of anxiety hit. During the day I was okay but at night I would get so much anxiety that something bad was going to happen to the baby and intrusive thoughts that I would never be the same again. I would have crying spells where I couldn't see anything except me not being able to do anything and that my body was messed up and I could never be fit again. I would see all these postpartum women who were skinny and just living life with their babies and it made my thoughts worse. I felt like a failure for having a C-section, especially when everyone told me labor was going to be so easy for me. I struggled for over six weeks with not being able to walk and do things on my own, as I was accustomed to being independent and active. Soccer and fitness were my whole life and not being able to be active brought me down. I would sob out of the blue and thought I would never be able to get back to it. I believe a lot of my thoughts were from my unrealistic expectations of how birth and postpartum would go and how it was the complete opposite for me. My husband was a great support during this difficult time but I felt embarrassed to share my thoughts with anyone. I felt like I wouldn't be seen as the strong independent woman that everyone saw me as. I'm 21 months postpartum now and I can still remember how that felt and the struggle I experienced. Recovering from a C-section was a huge toll physically and mentally, so much so that I fear having any more children because of it.

—Anonymous

This chapter spotlights some of the significant changes many couples experience during the peripartum period, with a sudden shift in the couple's dynamics. In the first section, sexuality is discussed, with a focus on sexual difficulties women and their partners often experience during pregnancy and after birth. Effective screening tools and treatment recommendations for these sexual issues are outlined. In the second section of this chapter, modern-day issues related to the swift changes in roles and responsibilities of becoming new parents are explored. Helpful recommendations for navigating and equally sharing new parenting and household duties are presented. The final section of this chapter outlines the challenges of parenting and the importance of increasing intimacy and positive communication among couples.

SEXUAL DIFFICULTIES AND RISK FACTORS

The perinatal period can bring about both psychological and physical changes that impact a woman's sexuality. While every woman is different, pregnancy and childbirth can either positively or negatively impact a woman's sexual function. Through the processes of pregnancy and giving birth, women have reported feeling sexually empowered, more confident, and relaxed with their partners. Many women, however, report serious negative experiences with sexual functioning during and after pregnancy (Bender et al., 2018; Khajehei & Doherty, 2018).

Risk factors associated with decreased sexuality during the perinatal period are significantly related to the many physical and bodily changes related to pregnancy and birth. While every pregnancy and postpartum period is different, many women experience similar physiological difficulties such as hormonal variability, difficulty breastfeeding, and lack of sleep. These problems can persist during pregnancy and long after birth, with potentially harmful impacts to a woman's sexual functioning (Khajehei & Doherty, 2018). Many women report vast unwanted and unwelcomed changes in their body, such as gaining weight, reduced energy, and constant fatigue during the peripartum period. Dissatisfaction with the pregnant body is a significant predictor of PPD, increasing the chances of developing depression during the peripartum period by almost one and a half (Przybyła-Basista et al., 2020). In fact, one study found that 41 percent of women reported feeling less attractive throughout their pregnancy (Pauleta et al., 2010). A more recent study found similar results, with 36 percent of women reporting they did not accept, or only partly accepted, their pregnant bodies (Przybyła-Basista et al., 2020). Likewise, in a qualitative study, women reported feeling that their breasts were no longer sexual, instead "belonging" to the baby. This new less sexual way of perceiving their bodies, along with unpleasant breastfeeding problems such as leaking breastmilk, greatly reduced a desire for sexual intimacy (Bender et al., 2018). These changes, among others, can negatively impact a woman's sexuality by decreasing the feeling of being sexually attractive, potentially leaving little desire for sexual intercourse. Additionally, many women report experiencing dyspareunia, or pain during sex, as far as six months postpartum (De Judicibus & McCabe, 2002). Consistent with a reduced sexual identity and conation, a woman's need and desire for intercourse can decrease during the perinatal period.

The need for physical and emotional intimacy, however, often increases. One qualitative study found that throughout the peripartum period, women reported substantial intimacy needs and still desired to feel close to their partners without sex (Bender et al., 2018). When physical and emotional needs are met, the relationship becomes better balanced during this vulnerable period. Women benefit from this intimacy by feeling close to their partner through sharing their thoughts and feeling appreciated. Physical intimacy without sexual intercourse can include kissing, hugging, cuddling, and verbal affirmations of love (Bender et al., 2018).

Obstetrical Violence

There are numerous other risk factors counselors should be aware of associated with poor sexual functioning during the perinatal period. A significant one that is often overlooked, and rarely discussed, is the trauma many women experience due to obstetric violence during childbirth. This can be defined as medical professionals neglecting the mother's needs and wishes, verbally humiliating the mother, and/or performing invasive practices and forced medical interventions during childbirth (Khajehei & Doherty, 2018). A recent study of 782 post-birth women found that mothers who experienced obstetric violence were at greater risk for developing PPD (Martinez-Vázquez et al., 2022). Examples of obstetric violence include a violation of privacy during labor, doctors performing an episiotomy without the mother's consent, hospital staff holding down the mother during labor and delivery, and doctors urging the mother to have a caesarean section without effectively communicating the need or risk for major surgery. Women who experience obstetric violence often endure painfully invasive and forced medical interventions during childbirth, leaving them feeling neglected, humiliated, and violated by hospital staff. These violations can lead to a decrease in sexual functioning after childbirth (Khajehei & Doherty, 2018). Furthermore, women who experience vaginal injury during childbirth, either related or unrelated to obstetric violence, report more sexual problems than women without vaginal injuries up to 16 months postpartum. Postpartum sexual problems can include decreased sexual interest, arousal, orgasm, lubrication, and satisfaction (Asselmann et al., 2016). Clearly, physical and/or psychological trauma related to childbirth can lead to significant sexual concerns for women postpartum.

Another important risk factor related to lower sexual functioning during the perinatal period is lack of support, intimacy, and communication from a romantic partner. When working with couples, counselors should note that in order to feel a greater sexual connection, many women express a significant need for feeling love and appreciation within the relationship by connecting to their partners on an emotional, mental, and intellectual level (Khajehei & Doherty, 2018; Bender et al., 2018). Moreover, pregnant and postpartum women who are more satisfied with their current romantic partner report feeling higher sexual satisfaction (De Judicibus & McCabe, 2002). In addition to this, it is important for partners to understand that once a newborn joins the family, they quickly become the center of attention in the mother's life, leaving little time and attention for sexual intimacy.

Hence, it is crucial for fathers to become active participants in the parenting role (Bender et al., 2018).

A final important risk factor to consider is PPD, which has been linked to poor sexual functioning in women during the perinatal period, and sometimes long after. Compared with women who have never experienced PPD, women with symptoms of depression before and after birth experience greater decline in sexual desire and report being less satisfied in their sexual relationship up to two years after giving birth (Moel et al., 2010). It is widely known that depression and related symptoms such as shame, guilt, low self-esteem, and worry significantly reduce a person's sexual desire, leaving pregnant and postpartum women at higher risk for developing and maintaining a sexual dysfunction. Women who take medications for depression could be at even higher risk for sexual dysfunctions, as there is evidence that prescription drugs such as SSRIs impair sexual functioning in women. Research shows alarmingly high rates of sexual dysfunction in women taking SSRIs for major depressive disorder, with sexual dysfunction rates as high as 33 percent (Masiran et al., 2014). While counselors should always encourage clients to follow medication recommendations from primary care doctors and psychiatrists, it is essential to recognize the physical and emotional impact depression and prescription medications can have on women during a vulnerable time in their lives.

Assessment of Sexual Difficulties

Recognizing the high prevalence of sexual difficulties women can experience during the perinatal period, clinicians should take note how the severity, frequency, and significance of these sexual issues are impacting the client's mental health. Assessing these issues for potential short-term or long-term sexual dysfunctions can help in the treatment planning process. The DSM-5-TR outlines three different types of sexual dysfunctions women may experience in the course of their lives (APA, 2022). Female orgasmic disorder (F52.31) is characterized by a reduced intensity, delay, infrequency, or absence of orgasms during sexual activity (APA, 2022). Female sexual interest/arousal disorder (F52.22) is diagnosed when women have a significantly reduced interest in sexual thoughts and activity or reduced arousal in excitement and sexual response (APA, 2022). Genito-Pelvic pain/penetration disorder (F52.6) involves persistent fear and/or pain involving sexual intercourse (dyspareunia) or tensing of the pelvic floor muscles when attempting vaginal penetration (vaginismus) (APA, 2022). These sexual dysfunctions can seriously hinder a woman's healthy sexual functioning during pregnancy and after childbirth.

Clinicians can use a variety of assessment instruments to diagnose or rule out a potential sexual dysfunction diagnosis during the peripartum period. The Brief Sexual Function Index for Women (BSFI-W; Taylor et al., 1994) is a no-cost, comprehensive and widely used assessment for sexual dysfunctions in women. This brief self-report measure screens a woman's sexual desire, arousal, frequency, receptivity, orgasm, and sexual problems. The Female Sexual Function Index (FSFI; Rosen et al., 2000) is also a no-cost, brief inventory focused on assessing a woman's sexual desire, arousal, lubrication, orgasm, satisfaction, and pain. The Golombok Rust Inventory of Sexual Satisfaction (GRISS; Rust & Golombok, 1986) assesses numerous sexual problems in women, including anorgasmia, nonsensuality, satisfaction, sexual avoidance, sexual communication, sexual frequency, and vaginismus. Lastly, the Sexual Function Questionnaire (SFQ; Quirk et al., 2002) screens a woman's sexual desire, arousal, lubrication, enjoyment, orgasm, pain, and partner satisfaction.

When using the inventories outlined in Table 8.1, clinicians should not solely focus on diagnosing a sexual dysfunction. These screening tools can also be used to begin a healthy and honest conversation about a woman's sexual life, and any sexual problem she may have encountered during the perinatal experience. Once a clinician discovers and understands the significant sexual challenges their client is currently experiencing, the next step is evaluating treatment options.

Table 8.1
Sexual Dysfunction Screening Tools

Screening Tool	Number of Items	Time to Complete	Sexual Dimensions Assessed	Cost
Brief Sexual Function Index for Women (BSFI-W)	22	15–20 minutes	Sexual desire, arousal, frequency, receptivity, orgasm, satisfaction and sexual problems	No
Female Sexual Function Index (FSFI)	19	15–20 minutes	Sexual desire, arousal, lubrication, orgasm, satisfaction, and pain	No
Golombok Rust Inventory of Sexual Satisfaction (GRISS)	28	15–20 minutes	Anorgasmia, nonsensuality, satisfaction, sexual avoidance, sexual communication, sexual frequency, and vaginismus	Yes
Sexual Function Questionnaire (SFQ)	31	20–30 minutes	Sexual desire, arousal, lubrication, enjoyment, orgasm, pain and partner satisfaction	Yes

PARENTAL ROLES AND RESPONSIBILITIES

It is expected that the birth of a child will bring along a variety of changes and transitions for parents. What may be surprising for some new parents and families is that parenthood will likely cause a shift toward more traditional gender roles, especially for parents engaged in opposite-sex relationships (Perales et al., 2018). While it's important to consider roles and responsibilities amongst diverse families, this section will primarily focus on more traditional male and female relationships. A section on multicultural considerations for LGBTQ+ families can be found later in this chapter.

Despite a major societal shift toward egalitarian gender roles, women in today's society are still spending more time with childcare tasks and doing more housework than their male partners (Baxter et al., 2008; Negraia et al., 2018; Perales et al., 2015). In fact, research shows that new mothers spend an average of six extra hours per week doing household chores such as cleaning, cooking, and organizing (Baxter et al., 2008). When additional children are born, there continues to be an increase in those hours doing housework for women, while men typically reduce the hours they spend helping around the house (Baxter et al., 2008). When it comes to spending quality time with children, mothers are also spending more time doing one-on-one parenting activities such as showing affection with hugs and kisses, providing for physical needs such as feeding and giving baths, helping with homework or attending teacher–parent conferences, attending school plays or sporting events, taking kids out for fun or educational outings such as a museum, and eating together (Negraia et al., 2018). In essence, mothers spend more time parenting their children compared with fathers.

PARENTING

Having a baby can be a time of excitement and bonding, but it is also a very fragile time in the relationship for new parents. Roughly 25 percent of cohabiting parents break up after having a baby, and married parents have significantly lower marital satisfaction than non-parents (Lichter et al., 2016; O'Reilly Treter et al., 2020; Twenge et al., 2003). There are several reasons why couples may experience dissatisfaction after having their first child, including a decline in intimacy, spending less time together, and an increase in negative communication, resulting in poor conflict management (Belsky & Kelly, 1994; Cowan & Cowan, 2000; Dew & Wilcox, 2011; Doss et al., 2009; O'Reilly Treter et al., 2020; Twenge et al., 2003). Counselors can be a source of support and encouragement during this challenging time if couples find themselves struggling in their relationship after having a baby.

Decreased intimacy is often caused by couples spending less time together as well as a sudden decline in emotional, sensual, and sexual emotions (Ahlborg & Strandmark, 2006). After having a baby, it becomes more challenging for couples to facilitate communication and foster emotional intimacy (Dew & Wilcox, 2011). Many new parents no longer have time to engage in valued activities they shared before the baby was born. Free time now belongs to the newborn, and bonding activities between the couple are no longer the top priority. Meeting with the lactation consultant, washing bottles, preparing formula, washing cloth diapers, or sneaking in a quick nap is the new priority for many new parents, leaving little to no time for anything else.

Partners can increase feelings of intimacy and closeness by prioritizing spending quality time together, even during the hectic time of having a newborn. The Gottman Institute proposes the novel idea to "never stop dating your partner." Counselors can encourage couples to plan date nights or quality time alone for the purpose of staying connected through increased intimacy and tackling life as a team (Eldemire, 2016). Since common interests strengthen relationships, it is imperative to help couples find and engage in interests that they may share to improve relationship satisfaction (Ahlborg & Strandmark, 2006). While attending therapy, counselors can also encourage and guide couples through healthy conversations, allowing partners to openly share their feelings in a safe space. Through the openness that often occurs in therapy, emotional intimacy can increase between partners.

While we have established that intimacy is important, it is not the only factor related to dissatisfaction among new parents. Regardless of marital status, couples are likely to experience an increase in negative communication after having a baby (O'Reilly Treter et al., 2020). Healthy communication among couples is vital because it brings awareness to the relationship, leading to increased satisfaction in women transitioning to parenthood (Shapiro et al., 2000). Due to the many demands of pregnancy, some couples start experiencing communication difficulties well before the baby is born. More frequent conflicts during pregnancy lead to lower relationship satisfaction between couples (Kluwer & Johnson, 2007). Not only is it imperative for couples to learn to communicate positively when there is conflict during the peripartum period, but it is also important to decrease the amount of conflict that arises between new parents. Couples will inevitably have disagreements, however, using positive communication to decrease conflict can increase relationship satisfaction (Kluwer & Johnson, 2007; Shapiro et al., 2000).

Improving communication and increasing positive conflict resolution has obvious benefits for the couple's relationship. It is also important to note that poor communication and conflict can have a negative effect on children. Gottman and Gottman (2007) assert that babies are profoundly affected by witnessing arguments between parents. Thus, couples should avoid allowing children to witness arguments until the age of four. When children do witness arguments between their parents, couples should strive to resolve the problem and explain conflict and resolution to the child in terms they understand. Here is an example of this healthy conversation: "Mary, mom and dad got angry with each other, but we talked about it and listened to each other so that we could understand our feelings. Then we worked it out and hugged each other." It is important for parents to understand how relationship conflict can negatively affect their children. For a parent who is resistant to therapy, it may help to encourage that partner to learn how to improve communication and conflict resolution for the wellbeing of their child (Gottman & Gottman, 2007).

MULTIPLE PERSPECTIVES: FATHER/PARTNER

A 2007 Pew Research Center study reported that 62 percent of men and women agree that sharing household chores is very important to marital success. Nevertheless, it's clear that mothers are doing more than their fair share of work related to caring for the needs of their children. When fathers fall short of helping with housework and childcare, mothers are more likely to feel stressed and unhappy in their marriage (Khawaja & Habib, 2007). While fathers are often aware of their lack of involvement in childcare duties and the expectation that mothers should not be doing the bulk of the work, they are still falling short of stepping up to help with their children's needs (Borgkvist et al., 2020). It should be noted that fathers do spend time with their children, perhaps just not in the way mothers want or need them to. Fathers play with their children just as much as mothers do and watch television more with their children than mothers do. Also, when couples are no longer together and "single" parents, tasks associated with the children become more equal (Negraia et al., 2018). While there are exceptions to every rule, a majority of women report feeling disrespected and unsupported when their male partners do not fulfill their parenting role (Gottman & Silver, 2015).

MULTICULTURAL CONSIDERATIONS

A significant multicultural consideration related to parenting roles and sexuality is how parenthood impacts LGBTQ+ couples and parents, as counselors serve diverse parents, including those who are LGBTQ+. A comprehensive research report on LGB-Parent Families by the Williams Institute's UCLA School of Law addresses important research findings on LGB parenting. According to this report, few differences have been found in regard to mental health, parenting stress, and parenting competence among same-sex and heterosexual parents. Similar to heterosexual parents, same-sex parents report a decline in the quality of their mental health and relationship satisfaction during their transition to becoming parents. While support from friends, family, and work can help buffer some challenges of new parenthood, it is important to note that many LGBT parents report receiving less support from their families (Goldberg et al., 2014).

In addition, LGBTQ+ couples and prospective parents face more discrimination than heterosexual couples when attempting to adopt children, as many adoption agencies and birth parents prohibit children from being adopted by same-sex couples (Goldberg et al., 2014). Studies comparing children raised by LGBT parents and heterosexual parents have found few differences related to children's self-esteem, quality of life, psychological adjustment, and social functioning. When it comes to roles and responsibilities, same-sex parents have more egalitarian relationships than heterosexual couples, sharing parenting duties such as childcare, housework, and employment more equally (Goldberg et al., 2014). Increased awareness of the strengths and challenges faced by LGBTQ+ families can be helpful in delivering effective multicultural treatment of PPD.

TREATMENT OF SEXUAL DIFFICULTIES

Whether or not a woman is diagnosed with a sexual dysfunction, sexual problems during the peripartum period can become burdensome. Crooks and Baur (2017) recommend general treatment guidelines for clinicians looking to help clients resolve sexual problems, regardless of where they originate. The guidelines outlined in the following paragraphs, based in research and evidence-based practices, can be a good starting point for counselors working with women and couples presenting with a variety of sexual issues. Adapting these general guidelines to pregnant and postpartum women will also be outlined.

The first treatment guideline for counselors to consider when working with women presenting with sexual issues involves encouraging self-stimulation and arousing fantasies to elicit sensual and erotic responses (Crooks & Baur, 2017). For pregnant and postpartum women, self-stimulation might feel strange because their bodies often look and feel very different from before they became pregnant. Specifically, a woman's breasts, stomach, and genitals can look and feel completely different during pregnancy and after birth. While these new physical changes can be a challenge to accept, clinicians can encourage women and their partners to embrace the way their body looks and feels in the present moment. In addition, a woman's body may respond differently to arousing fantasies due to hormonal fluctuations. Hormones from pregnancy and birth may cause vaginal dryness, potentially hindering a woman's typical vaginal lubrication prior to pregnancy.

The second treatment guideline outlined by Crooks and Baur (2017) entails reducing anxiety related to sex by using psychoeducation and sensate focus techniques. Clinicians can provide helpful resources and education about sexual health during the perinatal period to help women and their partners better understand the normal changes and struggles they may be experiencing with their sexuality. Psychoeducation about sensate focus techniques that couples can try at home can also be useful. Sensate focus is a valuable and effective sex therapy technique created in the 1970s by Masters and Johnson to help couples struggling with sexual issues. The five stages of sensate focus include: 1) body exploration without touching sexual body parts, 2) body exploration with touching sexual body parts, 3) mutual touching, 4) mutual touching with genital-to-genital contact, and 5) mutual touching, genital-to-genital contact, and insertion. One important element to remember about sensate focus exercises is that they ought to be done at home, with privacy, and with the goal of exploration, relaxation and mindfulness (Weiner et al., 2014). In pregnant and postpartum women, sensate focus exercises can be helpful in maintaining and reinforcing partner intimacy without the pressure of sexual intercourse.

The third treatment guideline suggested to resolve sexual dysfunctions includes improved communication and skill in initiating and refusing sexual activity (Crooks & Baur, 2017). Counselors can help couples communicate in a healthy way with their partner when they desire or do not desire sexual contact. During therapy sessions, counselors can encourage clients to openly communicate about how they can approach future sexual advances. Here is an example of both negative and positive communication about sexual contact:

> Husband touches wife's shoulder and begins to run his hands down her body, touching her breasts and buttocks.

Wife negative response: rolls her eyes, shoves husband's hand away and walks out of the room.

Wife positive response: "I appreciate when you touch me and try to initiate intimacy, but sometimes I'm not in the mood for getting touched in a sexual way. Also, my breasts are tender and sore from breastfeeding. Right now, could you give me a shoulder massage instead?"

This type of healthy and productive conversation can lead to more positive sexual experiences for both partners in the future. In the above example, the husband may or may not be satisfied with just giving his wife a massage instead of having sexual intercourse. However, her refusal did not push him away. Instead, she invited him to increase their intimacy without sexual contact. The husband was also reminded that his wife does not always want to be touched in a sexual way, and that him touching her breasts might bring pain instead of pleasure. While this particular style may not work for every couple, counselors can help partners understand and communicate what works or doesn't work in their relationship.

The final treatment recommendation suggested by Crooks and Baur (2017) to resolve sexual issues includes expanding the couple's range of intimacy and sexual activities. Many couples believe sex consists of one definition and purpose; sexual intercourse with orgasm. This is quite a limited and narrow goal of sex, leading to various sexual and intimacy challenges for couples. Wincze and Carey (2001) proposed a menu analogy to reduce performance pressure by accepting a broader definition of sex. With the menu analogy, sex is conceptualized as a meal, allowing clients to pick and choose from a menu based on their particular appetite and taste at the current moment. In this cognitive reframing technique, counselors can help couples shift the focus away from sexual intercourse and identify various types of intimacy and sexual activities. Table 8.2 provides some ideas and examples of ways clients can increase intimacy through both sexual and non-sexual activities. These activities should be done in privacy with no distractions such as children, cell phones, and pets.

Table 8.2

Intimacy Activities

Non-sexual Intimacy Activities	Sexual Intimacy Activities
Giving and receiving massages	Passionate kissing, touching, and grinding
Kissing and cuddling while watching a movie	Sensual naked massages with oil
Writing a love letter or text message	Sharing erotic fantasies in detail
Being silly and laughing together	Masturbating with partner watching
Mindful cooking and eating together	Watching pornography together
Taking a shower together and washing each other's hair	Using sex toys
Verbalizing what each partner is grateful for	Foreplay without penetration

SOLUTIONS FOR SHARING PARENTING ROLES AND RESPONSIBILITIES

Counselors should be aware of the largely inequitable division of labor in parenthood when evaluating and treating heterosexual couples with children. This gender gap can become detrimental to the experience of motherhood, creating long-lasting challenges in the couple's relationship. It would be helpful to openly discuss how this apparent gender gap impacts the mother, children, and the romantic relationship. Counselors can also help couples think about a more pragmatic and realistic plan to equally share parenting tasks. The following section focuses on practical solutions recommended by experts in the field that couples can use to successfully share the many roles and responsibilities of parenthood.

Relationship counselor and expert John Gottman suggests that parents create a *Who Does What List* to help pinpoint and visually see all necessary household and childcare tasks. This list should be comprehensive, including long-term financial planning, grocery shopping, home repairs, planning birthday parties, making doctor appointments for the kids, watering houseplants, etc. When everything is written out on paper, couples can better grasp how one partner does more than the other and can better plan how to share tasks more equally. The main goal is to ensure that the person who feels they are doing all the work, usually the female partner, gets help from the person who does less work, usually the male partner. More importantly, with this approach, members of the couple avoid nagging or asking that the partner complete their task; rather, each partner is entrusted to complete their tasks in a timely manner. As a motivating factor for male partners, Gottman asserts that "women find a man's willingness to do housework extremely erotic" (Gottman & Silver, 1999, p. 214).

Creating a list of all parenting roles and responsibilities can seem daunting for couples. In her best-selling book that takes a business approach to domestic duties, Eve Rodsky (2019) took this intimidating task and made it into a useful and practical card game called *100 Cards of Fair Play*. Rodsky designed this Fair Play system to sensibly organize the domestic ecosystem into five main categories: *the home suit, the out suit, the caregiver suit, the magic suit,* and *the wild suit*. Various domestic tasks such as doing laundry, taking the kids to soccer games, and enrolling the family in health insurance are divided into these five main categories. Whoever holds a particular card has the responsibility of conceiving, planning, and executing that task, without nudges or reminders from their partner. The Fair Play system allows couples to establish mutually agreed-upon expectations that cater to individual strengths and abilities. By playing this game, couples take a vow to let go of past resentments and play their cards consistently, while letting go of control over their partner's cards. The goal of this innovative system is to rebalance the domestic workload and "begin to play fair" (Rodsky, 2019, p. 230).

Another expert in the field, Farnoosh Torabi (2014), is a finance guru who takes a no-nonsense approach for domestic drudgery in her ground-breaking book for women who are the breadwinner in the relationship. She advises women to completely remove the "household chore tug-of-war from our relationships" (p. 123) with a straightforward idea—hiring outside help. Outsourcing housework and childcare duties simplifies many of the complexities busy working couples face on a daily basis. While it may be difficult for hard-working couples to justify hiring a nanny, house cleaner, or mommy's helper, Torabi suggests doing the math and deciding how much the couple's time is worth. For example, if it takes three hours per week to do yardwork that can be done by someone else for $200 per month, is the couple's time worth $16 per hour? If busy and active couples can buy time while simultaneously bringing peace and happiness into their home, then outsourcing timely parenting tasks and dreaded domestic chores is certainly worth it. As Torabi eloquently puts it, "stop complaining, start hiring, and automate your life" (2014, p. 130).

While outsourcing domestic work can make things easier, some couples do not want to spend money paying someone else to complete parenting obligations, and some parents simply do not have the financial privilege to choose that option. Also, creating chore lists and allocating certain tasks might not work for every couple, especially if one partner is unwilling to fulfill their parental duties. When some of the more practical solutions such as the ones offered above are not working, counselors can shift gears and teach couples how to communicate with their partner to get what they want when pragmatic ideas for sharing parenting tasks have not worked.

Imago Therapy Approaches for Addressing Parenting Responsibilities

Imago therapists Harville Hendrix and Helen Hunt (2013) take a different approach to working with couples struggling with equal sharing of parenting responsibilities. Imago therapy centers on teaching couples that their feelings, thoughts, and behaviors related to issues like household chores and childcare obligations are ways in which they are replaying the same unsatisfactory experiences with their partners that they had with childhood caregivers. Subconsciously, the goal is to resolve unmet needs and heal childhood wounds through meaningful interactions with romantic partners. In fact, imago therapy suggests that most arguments or problems in a relationship are superficial in nature and have nothing to do with whose turn it is to wash baby bottles or change diapers. When couples can dig deeper and look past superficial relationship concerns, they find these commonplace issues are actually related to their unmet childhood needs. Consequently, each partner is routinely seeking to satisfy their own emotional needs that were consistently unmet by their childhood caregivers (Hendrix & Hunt, 2013).

How exactly can couples resolve unmet childhood needs while also ensuring that the needs of their children and the home environment are not neglected? One of the first steps is to be aware of what they are trying to get from their partner that they were unable to get from childhood caregivers. It's essential to acknowledge how parents are instinctively using their relationship to heal painful wounds from childhood. After this awareness is gained, the next step involves utilizing and practicing the *Imago Dialogue Process* on a regular basis, which includes mirroring, validating, and empathizing during partner interactions. Table 8.3 provides an example of this key active listening process.

Table 8.3

Imago Dialogue Process

Wife: I'm feeling really frustrated with all the cooking and cleaning I do with little help from you or the kids. I'm exhausted.
Husband: You're saying that you're really exhausted and frustrated, especially because you do so much around the house with little help from us. Did I get it right? **(Mirroring)**
Wife: Yes … that's right, and I don't know how long I can do this by myself.
Husband: You make sense. **(Validating)**
Wife: I've asked so many times for help and I just feel so hopeless.
Husband: Since you do so much around the house for me and the kids, you're hitting a point where you can't do it alone anymore and need help so you're not feeling so hopeless, frustrated and tired. **(Empathizing)**

Note: Copyright Imago Relationships North America. Reprinted with permission (https://www.imagorelationshipswork.com).

As couples are learning to use this type of healthy dialogue, they are also feeling less defensive, better understood, and more acknowledged by their partners. The more couples can calmly discuss their struggles with parenting tasks, the easier they will find solutions that work for everyone. Imago therapy emphasizes the importance of forming a more stable and healthy relationship. Frequently using humor, communicating wants and needs in a straightforward way rather than expecting partners to be mind-readers, and frequently sharing positive affirmations will create a more positive relationship dynamic, with less resentment and defensiveness when dealing with parenting duties (Hendrix & Hunt, 2013). The more couples communicate effectively, the more they can learn to share and balance the oftentimes overwhelming roles and responsibilities of parenthood.

APPLICATION TO COUPLES COUNSELING

When looking to help new parents decrease conflict and increase positive communication, counselors can focus on well-researched and evidence-based theories and interventions. The next section focuses on two widely used theories; Gottman Method and Emotionally Focused Therapy (EFT). These two counseling modalities have been widely researched and used with diverse couples to achieve positive communication and relationship satisfaction.

Relationship expert and founder of the Gottman Institute, John Gottman, began researching the intricacies, behaviors, and patterns of happy and unhappy couples in the early 1970s. With nearly 50 years of scientific research with couples and families, the Gottman Institute is recognized as a valuable resource for counselors in search of effective and successful methods for helping diverse families. Counselors can improve communication between parents by changing the way they manage conflict. To start, couples should *soften* how they start a discussion, recognizing that there are two valid viewpoints to each argument. Next, each partner can learn to use physiological self-soothing to calm down and hit the pause button when dealing with conflict. Once both partners have cooled down, a calmer conversation can eventually lead to a compromised resolution (Gottman & Gottman, 2007).

Some couples may think that happy couples never argue, but the truth is that disagreements within a relationship are inevitable. What helps reduce negative conflict is the way that couples choose to handle their disagreements. One important way for couples to decrease negative conflict is to be direct when confronting a problem, and how partners handle their directness. Gottman (1999) suggests approaching discussions with sympathy and understanding instead of accusations. Below are some examples of soft start-ups compared with harsh start-ups.

Soft vs. Harsh Start-ups

Harsh start-up: "You never help me with the baby."

Soft start-up: "I appreciate it when you help me feed the baby so that I can have a moment to relax while taking a shower. Would you be able to feed the baby when you get home?"

Harsh start-up: "All you do when you get home is watch TV."

Soft start-up: "I appreciate when you help me clean-up around the house while I cook dinner. Would you be able to help me pick up for a few minutes?"

This simple technique is an effective way for partners to be honest and direct, without causing defensiveness. Even if couples struggle with their start-up, it is still better for them to be direct about an issue they are facing, which can motivate change in each other. When partners confront problems indirectly, ambiguous information is given on how to fix problems, leading to an ineffective resolution (McNulty & Russell, 2010). In addition to this, the most important part of the conflict resolution process is to make attempts at repairing and de-escalating. This means doing things to stop an argument from getting out of control. A repair attempt can include apologizing, taking actions to calm down, sharing feelings, sharing appreciation, or stopping a discussion when it feels as though it is getting out of control (Gottman, 1999).

Attachment style is also an important consideration when looking at positive or negative communication among couples. To improve communication and healthy attachment among their relationship, couples should *turn towards* each other and *accept bids* for connection. These two terms were coined by John Gottman and refer to making positive verbal statements or actions to connect with a partner. It should be noted that no matter what attachment style a couple has, romantic relationships are more likely to endure if one partner can transition an argument into a positive conversation. To improve communication, partners must feel that the other is accessible, by giving their attention and emotional availability. They must also feel responsiveness from their partners, in which each partner accepts the other's needs and comforts them. Lastly, they must feel engagement from their partner in the form of emotional presence and involvement (Johnson, 2014). A good exercise to try in or out of a therapy session is to practice 20-minute conversations a few times a week with no interruptions. This means not looking at phones, watching TV, or playing with the kids. This type of exercise increases emotional availability, responsiveness, and emotional presence, leading to better communication and attachment among couples.

While the Gottman method can be successful and effective with new parents, Emotionally Focused Therapy (EFT) can also be beneficial for couples struggling with communication. This type of therapy focuses on changing the couple's interaction patterns to develop new solutions. EFT has been widely researched and is effective across diverse couples as it focuses on emotions and the attachment style of each partner, and how it may be affecting the communication patterns within their relationship. One major benefit of using this therapeutic orientation is that the counselor can help create a plan for continued success when therapy has been terminated (Gehart, 2014). This is especially important for couples with a newborn since they may not have time to commit to weekly sessions for a prolonged period.

EFT consists of three stages: *De-Escalation of Negative Cycles, Change Interactional Patterns and Creating Engagement,* and *Consolidation and Integration*. In the first stage, the goal of treatment is to establish a therapeutic alliance with the couple so that they are comfortable exploring difficult emotions and to develop a case conceptualization that is based on attachment theory. The therapist helps the couple reframe their negative interactions so that instead of seeing the issue as a problem with each other, they see their negative interaction cycle as the enemy (Gehart, 2014).

Stage 2 of EFT begins by focusing on the more emotionally withdrawn partner to help them identify and express their attachment needs. This is important because it allows the withdrawer to reconnect and makes it easier for their partner (the pursuer) to be vulnerable and ask for needs in a way that does not seem like complaining or nagging. Once the therapist helps the withdrawer identify and express their attachment needs, they will do the same for the pursuer. During this phase, both partners will learn to respond to *bids for connection*, which are attempts that partners make to connect. Below are some examples of ineffective and effective responses to bids for connection.

Bids for Connection Examples

Bid for connection: "Can you believe how much it rained today?"

Ineffective response: (In a dry tone, while continuing to read the paper) "We live in Florida, it rains every day."

Effective response: (Puts newspaper down to look at their partner) "I know! I thought there was going to be a swimming pool in the back yard!"

> **Bid for connection:** (While watching TV, one partner sighs loudly)
>
> *Ineffective response*: "Great. What's wrong now?"
>
> *Effective response*: "What's on your mind, honey?"

Showing couples how to effectively respond to bids allows more opportunities for turning towards each other and feeling acknowledged by their partner, creating a secure attachment in the relationship. In the third and final stage of EFT, couples use their newly learned techniques and patterns to work through new and old relationship issues. The therapist helps the couple identify when they are using old unhealthy patterns and reconnect to their new, more helpful patterns. This process helps couples develop a sense of safety and love, so they are able to work through issues outside of therapy (Gehart, 2014).

The process of becoming new parents brings about an additional set of challenges for couples. By becoming aware of what may cause a decline in relationship satisfaction for first-time parents, counselors are better equipped to help couples navigate this new transition. Counselors should focus on increasing intimacy, increasing quality time spent together, and increasing positive communication and conflict resolution through evidenced-based practices like EFT and the Gottman Method. The more open couples are to the changing roles they are facing as parents, the smoother the transition to parenthood will be.

ETHICAL AND LEGAL CONSIDERATIONS

The *ACA Code of Ethics* (2014) encourages counselors to "practice only within the boundaries of their competence, based on their education, training, supervised experience, state and national professional credentials, and appropriate professional experience" (ACA, 2014, C.2.a, pg. 8). When it comes to the treatment of certain sexual problems and dysfunctions, counselors can refer clients to more appropriate professionals if they are unable to provide clients with safe, ethical, and effective counseling treatments. A combination of counseling with medical treatment can sometimes be the best approach for clients struggling with certain sexual problems during the perinatal period. For example, if a client is suffering from pelvic dysfunction after childbirth, a referral to a medical doctor or physical therapist who specializes in pelvic health would be appropriate.

It is also important to note that mental health counselors and other mental health professionals are not sex therapists, unless they have obtained a certification to ethically provide sex therapy techniques and interventions. The American Association of Sexuality Educators, Counselors, and Therapists (AASECT) have established specific requirements related to education and experiential activities for Sex Therapist Certification. While counselors can provide therapy and education related to sexual issues, certain sex therapy interventions should only be conducted by trained and certified sex therapists. This helpful description of the some of the intricacies related to sex therapy training has been provided by AASECT:

Sex therapy training must involve the learning of specific sex therapy techniques and interventions, not just theory. The training may be achieved through attending a specific sex therapy training program, taking graduate level academic courses that are specific to sex therapy techniques or by attending AASECT workshops which outline specific sex therapy techniques and how those may be applied to working with individuals and couples. As an example: you might attend a workshop on Sensate Focus and learn the theory of this particular therapeutic technique. An additional workshop would be required on how to present this technique, what kind of language to use, how to time and pace the specific assignments, and in which order the assignments are given. Additionally, you would learn how to deal with clients who resist doing the assignments, how to help them deal with being blocked and how to deal with couples where one wants to do the assignments and the other partner does not.

(n.d., Section VI. Sex Therapy Training)

BARRIERS TO TREATMENT

When it comes to the help-seeking and treatment of sexual difficulties, women face various internal and external barriers and challenges. A large research study found that 40 percent of women experiencing sexual problems did not seek help from professionals, while 54 percent reported that they would like to (Berman et al., 2003). Reasons for not seeking help included: embarrassment, believing they could not be helped, and not thinking about seeking help for their sexual issues. For women who did seek treatment for their sexual functioning problems, less than 50 percent experienced positive feelings of validation, hope, relief, assurance, optimism, confidence, and satisfaction related to getting help. Perhaps more concerning, 25 percent of women experienced disgust, 33 percent experienced shame and devaluation, and more than 50 percent experienced frustration and anxiety when seeking help or treatment for sexual issues (Berman et al., 2003).

External barriers to treatment of sexual issues among women also exist, especially among health professionals. These include: a significant lack of research and medical treatments for women's sexual problems, lack of up-to-date knowledge and education among health professionals related to women's sexual dysfunctions, and failure to promptly address sexual issues with women (Feldhaus-Dahir, 2009). Understanding the many internal and external barriers women face when seeking treatment for sexual issues, it is crucial for counselors and other healthcare professionals to be educated, competent, and compassionate in the treatment of women's sexual functioning.

IMPACT OF THE COVID-19 PANDEMIC

The COVID-19 pandemic introduced new challenges for parents navigating the pregnancy and postpartum period. Emerging research shows that the pandemic has been more harmful to parents than non-parents, as parents report a higher rate of psychological and economic toll on their families due to the pandemic (Elder & Greene, 2021). In a recent study, parents and pregnant mothers reported increased levels of anxiety, feelings of uncertainty, loneliness, isolation, and not knowing where to get help. Consequently, these new challenges negatively impacted their parenting, mental health, and wellbeing (Moltrecht et al., 2022). In terms of sharing parenting duties, the gendered childcare gap between dual-earner households was slightly narrowed by fathers spending more time with children during pandemic lockdowns. However, unpaid work increased for mothers, leaving women more dissatisfied with how much household work they did in comparison with their male partners (Craig & Churchill, 2020). On a final note about parenthood stress during the pandemic, one study cautioned the use of alcohol to manage the challenges and stressors parents face during the pandemic, as alcohol use has been found to increase the risk of punitive parenting in times of stress (Wolf et al., 2021). Counselors should be aware that a potential increase in substance use, along with all other stressors parents faced during the COVID-19 pandemic, could potentially disrupt the important bonding process between mother and baby.

The COVID-19 pandemic also had a negative impact on couples' sexuality, as many parents and couples reported greater difficulties and conflicts in their relationship during the pandemic (Luetke et al., 2020). These escalations in conflict often led to a significant decrease in intimacy and sexuality, including a marked decrease in the frequency of "hugging, kissing, cuddling, or holding hands with their partner; decreased solo masturbation; decreased partnered masturbation or touching of each other's genitals; decreased giving or receiving oral sex; and decreased engaging in penile-vaginal intercourse" (Luetke et al., 2020, p. 755). This marked increase in couples' conflict and decrease in sexuality during the pandemic could be attributed to navigating new roles and responsibilities, including working virtually from home and managing childcare and schooling for children unable to attend school or daycare. In order to promptly address the many challenges parents faced during the pandemic, clinicians are encouraged to promote positive stress management and conflict resolution techniques with parents to increase emotional support, intimacy, and healthy sexuality (Luetke et al., 2020).

CONCLUSION

This chapter showcased how the shift in couple dynamics during the peripartum period is multifaceted and ever-changing. Counselors can be a source of support and assistance for women and/or couples who struggle with sexual difficulties during this time. Effectively screening for sexual dysfunctions and providing helpful and appropriate treatment recommendations and resources for clients is vital to restore healthy sexual functioning. Counselors can also help couples who may struggle with the many new and challenging roles and responsibilities of having a newborn. Assisting couples with balancing and sharing parenting obligations can alleviate one partner from becoming overwhelmed by taking on the bulk of household tasks. Lastly, the challenges experienced in parenthood can have a lasting negative impact on relationship satisfaction. Counselors can be proactive and teach couples how to maintain their intimacy and build positive communication when tackling their journey into parenthood.

Case Study: Roberta

Roberta is seeking therapy ten months after having her first baby. She recently found out that she is pregnant with her second child, which was a "happy surprise." Roberta is married, works full time, and reported feeling both excited and overwhelmed about growing her family. After the birth of her daughter, Roberta experienced symptoms of peripartum depression for about seven months, some of which might still be lingering. She reports feeling worried about this pregnancy and potentially going through similar PPD symptoms after the birth of the second baby. One major issue she and her husband are struggling with is a lack of sexual intimacy in their marriage. Roberta worries that, with a second child, this intimacy will become even more distant. She is constantly feeling overwhelmed about her role as a full-time working mother, and her sexuality has taken a back seat in the priorities list. Roberta sometimes feels resentful of how much extra she does for the baby, such as planning the first birthday party, keeping up with the baby book, remembering doctor appointments, daycare schedules, and pumping breastmilk. Sometimes, she feels like there's "way too much on my plate." While her husband does help with some chores around the house, many of the "baby tasks" fall to her. She's worried about how a second child would add to an already full schedule. Additionally, Roberta and her husband have been disagreeing on many parenting decisions, such as co-sleeping, discipline, hiring a babysitter, and taking parenting advice from extended family members. These issues, among others, are further exacerbating their lack of intimacy and sexual desire. Before the new baby arrives, Roberta would like to improve the couple's intimate life, get more help from her husband with baby tasks and make decisions together about parenting.

Reflection Questions for Clinicians

- What are some of your personal values and beliefs related to traditional gender roles and parenting that may come up when working with this client?
- What would be your top priority or topic of higher concern to address with this client based on her presenting issues?
- What is your level of comfort and confidence in appropriately addressing intimate sexual issues and concerns related to this client's sexuality?

APPLYING THE STRENGTHS MODEL—THE CASE OF ROBERTA

Significant Individual, Infant, Family, Societal, and Cultural Factors

- Second pregnancy was unplanned shortly after giving birth ten months ago.
- Working full time and feeling overwhelmed with juggling work and motherhood tasks.
- History of PPD with first child this past year.
- Relationship conflicts, intimacy, and sexual issues after childbirth.

Treatment Barriers

- Feeling a lack of support and understanding from spouse.
- Full-time job may pose as a barrier to prioritizing treatment.

Risk Factors

- History of PPD, with some symptoms still lingering after childbirth.
- Maternal life stressors, including marital problems, perceived lack of support from spouse, working full time and feeling overwhelmed with balancing work and motherhood duties.

Enlisting Support from Family, the Community, and Medical Professionals

- Practical support from spouse with household and childcare tasks.
- Emotional and physical intimacy from spouse.
- Primary care doctor, counselor, or sex therapist to address sexual issues.
- Time off from work to prioritize treatment and self-care.

Noticeable Symptoms, Severity, & DSM-5-TR Diagnosis OR Needs Identified by Family & Treatment Team

- Lingering symptoms of PPD from first pregnancy ten months ago.
- Worrying about developing PPD with current second pregnancy.
- Sexual intimacy and relationship conflicts with spouse.
- Difficulties balancing work and motherhood duties.
- Disagreements with spouse on parenting choices.

Goals Identified by Family

- Improve couple's intimate life.
- Receive more help from spouse with baby tasks.
- Make decisions together about parenting.

Treatment Recommendations

- Interpersonal psychotherapy (IPT) interventions to improve interpersonal relationship functioning and increasing social support.
- Cognitive behavioral therapy (CBT) to develop assertiveness skills to learn how to communicate needs more effectively with spouse and work.
- Couple's therapy to address sexual intimacy issues.

Helpful, Protective, and Resilience Factors

- Positive feelings about second pregnancy.
- Willingly seeking therapy for current personal and relationship issues.
- Dual-income family.

Self-Care & Wellness

- Share parenting` duties with spouse by frequently asking for help or delegating tasks.
- Set firm boundaries at work and take time off (sick or vacation leave) to balance work/home tasks.
- Prioritize more frequent intimacy with spouse.

REFERENCES

Ahlborg, T., & Strandmark, M. (2006). Factors influencing the quality of intimate relationships six months after delivery—First-time parent's own views and coping strategies. *Journal of Psychosomatic Obstetrics & Gynecology, 27*(3), 163–172. doi:10.1080/01674820500463389

American Association of Sexuality Educators, Counselors, and Therapists. (AASECT). (n.d.). AASECT requirements for sex therapist certification, section VI. sex therapy training. https://www.aasect.org/aasect-requirements-sex-therapist-certification

American Counseling Association (ACA). (2014). *ACA code of ethics*. ACA.

American Psychiatric Association (APA). (2022). *Diagnostic and statistical manual of mental disorders* (5th ed., text rev.). doi:10.1176/appi.books.9780890425787

Asselmann, E., Hoyer, J., Wittchen, H.-U., & Martini, J. (2016). Sexual problems during pregnancy and after delivery among women with and without anxiety and depressive disorders prior to pregnancy: A prospective-longitudinal study. *Journal of Sexual Medicine, 13*(1), 95–104. https://10.1016/j.jsxm.2015.12.005

Baxter, J., Hewitt, B., & Haynes, M. (2008). Life course transitions and housework: Marriage, parenthood, and time on housework. *Journal of Marriage and Family, 70*(2), 259.

Belsky, J., & Kelly, J. (1994). *The transition to parenthood: How a first child changes a marriage. Why some couples grow closer and others apart*. Dell.

Bender, S. S., Sveinsdóttir, E., & Fridfinnsdóttir, H. (2018). "You stop thinking about yourself as a woman". An interpretive phenomenological study of the meaning of sexuality for Icelandic women during pregnancy and after birth. *Midwifery, 62*, 14–19.

Berman, L., Berman, J., Felder, S., Pollets, D., Chhabra, S., Miles, M., & Powell, J. (2003). Seeking help for sexual function complaints: What gynecologists need to know about the female patient's experience. *Fertility and Sterility, 79*(3), 572–576. doi:10.1016/S0015-0282(02)04695-2

Borgkvist, A., Eliott, J., Crabb, S., & Moore, V. (2020). "Unfortunately I'm a massively heavy sleeper": An analysis of fathers' constructions of parenting. *Men & Masculinities, 23*(3/4), 680–701. doi:10.1177/1097184X18809206

Cowan, C. P., & Cowan, P. A. (2000). *When partners become parents: The big life change for couples*. Erlbaum.

Craig, L., & Churchill, B. (2020). Dual-earner parent couples' work and care during COVID-19. *Gender, Work and Organization*. doi:10.1111/gwao.12497

Crooks, R., & Baur, K. (2017). *Our sexuality* (13th ed.). Wadsworth Cengage Learning.

De Judicibus M. A., McCabe, M. P. (2002) Psychological factors and the sexuality of pregnant and postpartum women. *Journal of Sex Research, 39*, 94–103.

Dew, J., & Wilcox, B. W. (2011). If momma ain't happy: Explaining declines in marital satisfaction among new mothers. *Journal of Marriage and Family, 73*(1), 1–12.

Doss, B. D., Rhoades, G. K., Stanley, S. M., & Markman, H. J. (2009). The effect of the transition to parenthood on relationship quality: An 8-year prospective study. *Journal of Personality and Social Psychology, 96*(3), 601–619. doi:10.1037/a0013969

Eldemire, A. (2016). The "golden rule" for exhausted new parents that keeps the romance alive. Retrieved from https://www.gottman.com/blog/golden-rule-for-new-parents-that-keeps-romance-alive/

Elder, L., & Greene, S. (2021). A recipe for madness: Parenthood in the era of Covid-19. *Social Science Quarterly, 102*(5), 2296. doi:10.1111/ssqu.12959

Feldhaus-Dahir M. (2009). Female sexual dysfunction: Barriers to treatment. *Urologic Nursing, 29*(2), 81–86.

Gehart, D. R. (2014). *Mastering competencies in family therapy: A practical approach to theory and clinical case documentation* (2nd ed.). Brooks/Cole Pub.

Goldberg, A. E., Gartrell, N. K., & Gates, J. G. (2014). Research Report on LGB-Parent Families. Los Angeles, CA: Williams Institute, UCLA School of Law. http://williamsinstitute.law.ucla.edu/wp-content/uploads/lgb-parent-families-july-2014.pdf.

Gottman, J., & Gottman, J. S. (2007). *And baby makes three: The six-step plan for preserving marital intimacy and rekindling romance after baby arrives*. Three Rivers Press.

Gottman, J. M. (1999). *The marriage clinic: A scientifically-based marital therapy*. W.W. Norton.

Gottman, J. M., & Silver, N. (1999). *The seven principles for making marriage work*. Harmony Books.

Hendrix, H., & Hunt, H. L. (2013). *Making marriage simple: 10 truths for changing the relationship you have into the one you want*. Harmony Books.

Johnson, S. (2014). *Love sense: The revolutionary new science of romantic relationships*. Piatkus.

Khajehei, M., & Doherty, M. (2018). Women's experience of their sexual function during pregnancy and after childbirth: A qualitative survey. *British Journal of Midwifery, 26*(5), 318–328. doi:10.12968/bjom.2018.26.5.318

Khawaja, M., & Habib, R. R. (2007). Husbands' involvement in housework and women's psychosocial health: Findings from a population-based study in Lebanon. *American Journal of Public Health, 97*(5), 860–866. doi:10.2105/AJPH.2005.080374

Kluwer, E. S., & Johnson, M. D. (2007). Conflict frequency and relationship quality across the transition to parenthood. *Journal of Marriage and Family, 69*(5), 1089–1106. doi:10.1111/j.1741-3737.2007.00434.x

Lichter, D. T., Michelmore, K., Turner, R. N., & Sassler, S. (2016). Pathways to a stable union? Pregnancy and childbearing among cohabiting and married couples. *Population Research and Policy Review, 35*(3), 377–399. doi:10.1007/s11113-016-9392-2

Luetke, M., Hensel, D., Herbenick, D., & Rosenberg, M. (2020). Romantic relationship conflict due to the COVID-19 pandemic and changes in intimate and sexual behaviors in a nationally representative sample of American adults. *Journal of Sex & Marital Therapy, 46*(8), 747–762. doi:10.1080/0092623X.2020.1810185

Martinez-Vázquez, S., Hernández-Martínez, A., Rodríguez-Almagro, J., Delgado-Rodríguez, M., & Martínez-Galiano, J. M. (2022). Relationship between perceived obstetric violence and the risk of postpartum depression: An observational study. *Midwifery, 108*. doi:10.1016/j.midw.2022.103297

Masiran, R., Sidi, H., Mohamed, Z., Mohd. Nazree, N. E., Nik Jaafar, N. R., Midin, M., Das, S., & Mohamed Saini, S. (2014). Female sexual dysfunction in patients with major depressive disorder (MDD) treated with selective serotonin reuptake inhibitor (SSRI) and its association with serotonin 2 A-1438 G/A single nucleotide polymorphisms. *Journal of Sexual Medicine, 11*(4), 1047–1055. doi:10.1111/jsm.12452

McNulty, J. K., & Russell, V. M. (2010). When "negative" behaviors are positive: A contextual analysis of the long-term effects of problem-solving behaviors on changes in relationship satisfaction. *Journal of Personality and Social Psychology, 98*(4), 587–604. doi:10.1037/a0017479

Moel, J. E., Buttner, M. M., O'Hara, M. W., Stuart, S., & Gorman, L. (2010). Sexual function in the postpartum period: Effects of maternal depression and interpersonal psychotherapy treatment. *Archives of Women's Mental Health, 13*(6), 495–504. doi:10.1007/s00737-010-0168-0

Moltrecht, B., Dalton, L. J., Hanna, J. R., Law, C., & Rapa, E. (2022). Young parents' experiences of pregnancy and parenting during the COVID-19 pandemic: A qualitative study in the United Kingdom. *BMC Public Health, 22*(1), 523. doi:10.1186/s12889-022-12892-9

Negraia, D. V., Augustine, J. M., & Prickett, K. C. (2018). Gender disparities in parenting time across activities, child ages, and educational groups. *Journal of Family Issues, 39*(11), 3006–3028. doi:10.1177/0192513X18770232

O'Reilly Treter, M., Rhoades, G. K., Scott, S. B., Markman, H. J., & Stanley, S. M. (2020). Having a baby: Impact on married and cohabiting parents' relationships. *Family Process*. doi:10.1111/famp.12567

Pauleta, J. R., Pereira, N. M., & Graça, L. M. (2010). Sexuality during pregnancy. *Journal of Sexual Medicine, 7*(1), 136–142. doi:10.1111/j.1743-6109.2009.01538.x

Perales, F., Baxter, J., & Tai, T. (2015). Gender, justice and work: A distributive approach to perceptions of housework fairness. *Social Science Research, 51*, 51–63.

Perales, F., Jarallah, Y., & Baxter, J. (2018). Men's and women's gender-role attitudes across the transition to parenthood: Accounting for child's gender. *Social Forces, 97*(1), 251–276. doi:10.1093/sf/soy015

Pew Research Center. (2007, July 18). Modern marriage: "I like hugs. I like kisses. but what I really love is help with the dishes." [Report]. https://www.pewsocialtrends.org/2007/07/18/modern-marriage/

Przybyła-Basista, H., Kwiecińska, E., & Ilska, M. (2020). Body acceptance by pregnant women and their attitudes toward pregnancy and maternity as predictors of prenatal depression. *International Journal of Environmental Research and Public Health, 17*(24), 9436. doi:10.3390/ijerph17249436

Quirk, F. H., Heiman, J. R., Rosen, R. C., Laan, E., Smith, M. D., & Boolell, M. (2002). Development of a sexual function questionnaire for clinical trials of female sexual dysfunction. *Journal of Women's Health & Gender-Based Medicine, 11*(3), 277–289. doi:10.1089/152460902753668475

Rodsky, E. (2019). *Fair play: A game-changing solution for when you have too much to do (and more life to live)*. G.P. Putnam's Sons.

Rosen, R., Brown, C., Heiman, J., Leiblum, S., Meston, C., Shabsigh, R., Ferguson, D., & D'Agostino, R., Jr. (2000). Female Sexual Function Index (FSFI) [Database record]. APA PsycTests.

Rust, J., & Golombok, S. (1986). The GRISS: A psychometric instrument for the assessment of sexual dysfunction. *Archives of Sexual Behavior, 15*(2), 157–165. doi:10.1007/BF01542223

Shapiro, A. F., Gottman, J. M., & Carrère, S. (2000). The baby and the marriage: Identifying factors that buffer against decline in marital satisfaction after the first baby arrives. *Journal of Family Psychology, 14*(1), 59–70. doi:10.1037/0893-3200.14.1.59

Taylor, J. F., Rosen, R. C. & Leiblum, S. R. (1994). Self-report assessment of female sexual function: Psychometric evaluation of the brief index of sexual functioning for women. *Archives of Sexual Behavior, 23*, 627–643 (1994). doi:10.1007/BF01541816

Torabi, F. (2014). *When she makes more: 10 rules for breadwinning women*. Hudson Street Press.

Twenge, J. M., Campbell, W. K., & Foster, C. A. (2003). Parenthood and marital satisfaction: A meta-analytic review. *Journal of Marriage and Family, 65*, 574–583.

Weiner, L., Cannon N., & Avery-Clark, C. (2014). Reclaiming the lost art of sensate focus: A clinician's guide. *Family Therapy Magazine, 13*(5), 46–48.

Wincze, J. P., & Carey, M. P. (2001). *Sexual dysfunction: A guide for assessment and treatment* (2nd ed.). The Guilford Press.

Wolf, J. P., Freisthler, B., & Chadwick, C. (2021). Stress, alcohol use, and punitive parenting during the COVID-19 pandemic. *Child Abuse & Neglect, 117*. doi:10.1016/j.chiabu.2021.105090

9

Finding a Rhythm as a Mother and Connecting with Baby

Vanessa Beatriz Teixeira
with contributor Dawn Hoffman

Personal Narrative

As a first-time mom, I had a plan for childbirth, and that plan went down the toilet. What I wanted was a birth with no medical interventions, no hospital, no formula and back home in four hours after delivery to settle in as a family. What I got was a birth at the hospital, a C-section, and a baby drinking formula instead of my breastmilk. My water broke and I never progressed past 2 cm dilated. After 30 hours of labor her heart rate was dropping, and we had to go with a C-section. I was heartbroken, tired, and overwhelmed. I was crying, my husband was crying, it was a hard thing for both of us to experience. But we got our baby earth side healthy, beautiful, and perfect. She was good, and I should have been too right? No. I hate asking people for help. I find it a source of weakness. And all of a sudden, I had to ask for help to even stand up. Talk about my own personal hell. My mom and husband were so helpful, to the point that I held my daughter for maybe 30 minutes the first three days. I didn't change my daughter's first diaper until a week old. Everyone was trying so hard to help me that I didn't have to engage with her. So I didn't. I was told to sit, heal, focus on pumping, etc., my husband or mom would take care of it. While I am forever grateful for their love and support, I disconnected. I tried to breastfeed but it was painful, so I started pumping. I wasn't producing so we had to use formula. That made me feel like a failure. Failure to breastfeed. Failure at giving birth. Failure all around. Through sheer determination, I ended up exclusively pumping. It was so easy for everyone else, why wasn't it for me? When my mom left after a week, I started holding her and changing her. I love my daughter. But, for the first three months I had a really hard time connecting with her. I knew she was my child, I love her, I don't want anything bad to happen to her. But that connection everyone talks about? That magical take your breath away instant head over heels in love feeling didn't happen. I think the birth was very traumatic for me, and didn't let me connect. No one knows I have felt this way. No one. I still treat it as my dirty secret. Thankfully, given enough time and some space to deal with what happened, I can now say I have connected with my daughter.

—*Anonymous*

This chapter explores different ways that mothers, partners, and families can find their rhythm when a new baby joins the family unit. It also examines the negative effects of untreated PPD on mother–infant bonding, helping counselors recognize concerning developmental challenges or delays presented in the baby's early development. Additional resources for women, such as lactation consultants and breastfeeding support groups are also outlined as a way to help mothers and babies bond and connect during the peripartum period.

ENHANCING THE MOTHER–BABY BOND

A woman's journey to find her rhythm as a mother is unique, as she is tasked with understanding the needs of her infant while also navigating how to enhance the mother–baby bond. This rhythm can be interrupted if she is faced with overwhelming struggles related to motherhood and/or PPD. Various activities enhance maternal–infant bonding and foster secure attachment between infant and caregiver, namely warm and responsive reactions to the infant's needs, cooperative and stimulating interaction and play between mother and infant, and frequent breastfeeding (Crucianelli et al., 2019; Paulson et al., 2006; Slomian et al., 2019). It is vital for counselors to help women foster a secure bond with their infants through some of the evidence-based techniques discussed in the following section.

Bonding inspires a feeling of intense emotional connection that motivates a new mother to provide her infant with unconditional love and protection (Bowlby, 1969). Mother–baby bonding is important for both infant survival and healthy cognitive development. As a mother provides affection and care to her unique new infant, she is building a firm foundation for a healthy and secure relationship while simultaneously enhancing her infant's cognitive, social, and emotional development (Bowlby, 1969). As the process of mother–infant bonding is vitally important for child development, many mothers and professionals express concern when bonding with an infant is impaired.

Changes occurring in a pregnant or new mother's brain may produce alterations in a woman's mood (O'Connor et al., 2019). These chemical changes in the brain can potentially affect a mother's ability to bond and care for her infant by producing typical symptoms of a depressive disorder including sadness, hopelessness, loss of interest in familiar activities, and withdrawal from family and friends, in addition to persistent self-doubt that may, in extreme cases, include thoughts of harming herself or her infant (O'Connor et al., 2019). Mothers who experience PPD experience a spectrum of emotions, including intense guilt, shame, fear, and stigma. They often neglect their own care based on their childcare needs, concerns about the cost of treatment, and for fear of having their children removed from them (O'Connor et al., 2019). When treating women for PPD, counselors should incorporate a focus on developing skills to enhance the mother–baby bond. Counselors can promote healthy mother–baby bonding by encouraging warm and responsive care, opportunities for cooperative and stimulating interaction and play, and frequent breastfeeding within the context of a welcoming and safe therapeutic relationship (Table 9.1).

Table 8.1
Mother–Baby Bonding

Warm and Responsive Care	Interaction and Play	Frequent Breastfeeding
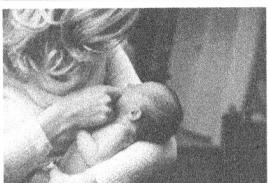	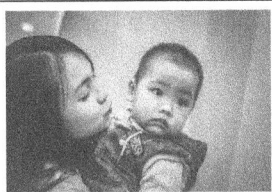	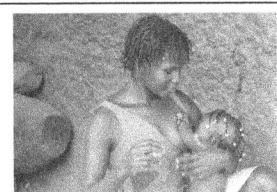
Skin-to-skin contact. Frequent holding, rocking, kissing, gently stroking. Baby wearing. Infant massage and bathing. Singing, reading, baby sign language. Including baby in visits with friends and family, support groups, and daily exercise routines.	Reading books. Playing games. Making silly faces, laughing, tickling, telling funny stories, singing funny songs. Making time for playgroups and community groups that emphasize learning and play.	Frequent nursing. Healthy diet and hydration. Rest. Incorporating the help of a lactation consultant. Social support from community groups.

Note: All images downloaded from Pixabay.com.

Warm and Responsive Reactions to Infant Needs

A new mother develops an intimate knowledge of her unique infant by spending a great deal of time with her new baby. As a mother bonds with her infant and develops a history of providing warm and responsive care, a deep emotional connection emerges that is commonly referred to as attachment (Bowlby, 1969). All babies express evidence of their unique personalities at birth. A mother's task involves learning how her baby communicates and how to meet the basic needs of her infant with loving care. When PPD unexpectedly emerges and becomes a part of a new mother's journey, some women are unable to connect and form a secure bond with their new baby (Bowlby, 1969). Unsurprisingly, many women begin to feel a deep sense of inadequacy rather than a deep emotional connection to their baby. This lack of connection can produce feelings of guilt, fear, hopelessness, and shame, often resulting in isolation and withdrawal.

As counselors, encouraging new mothers with PPD to develop a new way of coping with these challenges involves motivating women to engage in new experiences that challenge temporary limitations and expectations of themselves. The symptoms of PPD act on a new mother's brain by challenging her abilities to recognize her infant's efforts to communicate, hindering a nurturing response (Crucianelli et al., 2019). In addition to changes in social functioning, women who experience PPD also experience changes in brain structure and function that limit bonding by producing changes in oxytocin and dopamine (Gholampour et al., 2020; Piallini et al., 2015). Knowing that change does not happen quickly, it would be unreasonable for a counselor or mother to expect new behaviors to produce immediate relationship changes. Instead, a counselor can help mothers develop a sequence of consistent behaviors that expand on the foundational conditions of attachment theory, encouraging warm and responsive reactions by focusing on physical proximity and shared emotional connection (Crucianelli et al., 2019).

Research shows that early intervention in PPD is essential (O'Connor et al., 2019). Hence, counselors can help women build a healthy and close bond with their infants starting as early as pregnancy. False assumptions often lead mothers and professionals to believe that bonding does not begin until the child is born. However, activities involving physical touch and positive engagement should include developing a mother's sensitivity and involvement with her growing baby during the pregnancy period (Bernard et al., 2018). Counselors can use practical strategies to encourage pregnant mothers to interact with their growing belly as their pregnancy progresses. New mothers can spend time stroking their abdomen, providing light pressure as the baby kicks, integrating self-massage, and involving their partners in belly massages. These bonding activities can be done anytime throughout the day, including during daily walks, a warm bath, or even as part of an exercise routine.

Bonding activities should continue throughout the peripartum experience, especially right after birth. After the infant is born it is important to include plenty of opportunities for maternal touch with the baby outside of mealtime (Bowlby, 1969). A new mother should be encouraged to spend time interacting with her infant by providing skin-to-skin contact, holding, rocking, kissing, gently stroking, bathing, baby wearing, and massaging her new baby several times a day (Bowlby, 1969). These special experiences using touch can be enhanced by integrating scented soaps and lotions, soft baby blankets, toys, special lighting, heat, music, and other creative ideas to improve the sensory experience. A counselor can also encourage a new mother to integrate behaviors that communicate positive engagement with their infants. During the infant stage, a mother might devote time to holding her infant while gazing into her baby's eyes or following her baby's gazes and speaking softly about their shared experiences (Crucianelli et al., 2019). A new mother can also sing to her infant, read to her infant, take her baby for daily walks, teach her baby sign language, visit a friend with her infant, take her baby to support groups, or attend mother baby exercise classes. Focusing on skills that rely on maternal touch and opportunities for positive engagement can improve bonding and attachment as well as the physical and mental health of mother and baby.

Cooperative and Stimulating Interaction and Play between Mother and Infant

Play is an important part of the bonding experience for both mothers and infants. Counselors can continue to build on the tenets of attachment theory by encouraging new mothers to spend time having fun and playing with their infant. Outside influences can diminish creative ways for new mother to play with their baby. In some cases, this means buying expensive baby equipment and toys that capture a baby's interest for a brief amount of time. While these purchases can at times be useful, a baby wants nothing more than to have close contact with their affectionate mother. As a result, opportunities for play can be fun and economical. Practical strategies for encouraging bonding and attachment through play include reading playful books, playing games like peek-a-boo, making funny faces, laughing, tickling, telling funny stories, and singing fun songs (Paulson et al., 2006). The internet is a valuable resource for learning creative ways to play with an infant. Also, many local libraries and community centers host weekly groups that encourage play and social interaction. Shared play experiences not only soothe and reduce stress, but can also increase an infant's language abilities and teach them valuable social skills (Allen & Oliver, 1982; Frodi & Smetana, 1984). Some women may find it useful and enjoyable to document their daily interactions and playful experiences using a baby book, a personal journal, pictures, or videos. Counselors can encourage mother–baby bonding by encouraging mothers who are experiencing PPD to engage in playful opportunities that encourage learning and social development.

Frequent Breastfeeding

Nursing is another beneficial way for a mother and baby to bond (Kendall-Tackett & Mohrbacher, 2010). However, a mother's decision to breastfeed is personal and often complex, as some women who want to breastfeed may encounter difficulties doing so. In the context of the attachment relationship, breastfeeding represents the earliest opportunity to enhance the mother–baby bond. In addition to inspiring early bonding, breastfeeding can positively affect the mother–baby relationship by reducing stress and inspiring relaxation (Gribble, 2006). In contrast, many women who experience PPD find themselves facing significant breastfeeding problems that affect their bonding experience in an undesirable way (Slomian et al., 2019). Many women feel intense guilt when they find themselves unable to begin, or continue, breastfeeding. As a result, some women develop negative beliefs about themselves and a sense of inadequacy when they compare their plans for breastfeeding their infant with their current reality. Counselors can best help mothers who are struggling with breastfeeding by building confidence, knowledge, and access to resources that support their goals for feeding their new baby. This may include providing contact information for local lactation specialists, reading material, and information about online breastfeeding communities. Counselors can empower women to seek solutions and adapt to challenges by emphasizing the importance of sensitive interactions over specific feeding methods (Britton et al., 2006). This means that breastfeeding is not always the only or best feeding option for mothers and infants. When treating mothers for PPD, counselors can educate women about how mother–baby bonding is best inspired by sensitive interactions including alternative feeding techniques that promote infant and maternal health (Jansen et al., 2008).

On a final note, counselors may experience a lack of confidence in their abilities to inspire the conditions of attachment theory when working with families. PPD symptoms may sharply contrast evidence that parents are able to function as emotionally sensitive primary caregivers for babies (Bowlby, 1969). Therefore, counselors can focus on conveying a safe and welcoming therapeutic relationship and allowing space for a hurting mother to see herself as worthy of love and trust. Counselors who are committed to approaching their clients with unconditional positive regard help by validating and normalizing a new mother's journey with PPD. Approaching opportunities for teaching new skills or reflecting on life experiences using a warm and responsive counselor orientation is the first step in this process. A counselor who is dedicated to modeling sensitive caretaking skills with their clients can improve maternal and infant consequences of PPD by encouraging relationship conditions that improve mother–baby bonding and attachment (Erickson et al., 1989; Stern, 1985).

IMPLICATIONS OF UNTREATED PPD FOR BABY'S DEVELOPMENT

Finding a rhythm and connecting with the baby during pregnancy and postpartum is an important part of a baby's development. Research literature on child development affirms that during all developmental stages, babies need a caregiver who consistently provides a safe, loving, and nurturing environment to foster and advance their cognitive and social-emotional growth. Being emotionally available by consistently responding to a baby's cues and cries is essential to healthy development during all stages and milestones (Halfon et al., 2014).

Providing an infant with the responses they need can be especially difficult for mothers experiencing depression. For mothers who experience varying symptoms of PPD, bonding with their infant can be disrupted due to the challenging affective and cognitive symptoms associated with depression. Mothers experiencing PPD might experience more difficulty in responding to their infant's needs, especially during challenging developmental periods that may make their baby fussy, such as teething, changes in sleep patterns, or growth spurts. Hence, PPD symptoms can lead to more hostile parenting approaches and negative parent–child interactions, such as mother feeling angry or shouting at an infant when they are crying or when the infant is not soothed easily (Hentges et al., 2021).

A major concern related to a lack of connection between mother and baby is the potential short- and long-term consequences to the infant. Research indicates that PPD, especially when it is severe and untreated, and other mental health issues experienced by the mother during pregnancy and postpartum, can have a lasting negative impact on a baby's development (Elitok et al., 2020; Tuovinen et al., 2018). It is important for counselors to recognize a variety of implications related to the baby's development and meeting specific milestones if a mother is presenting with mental health symptoms during the peripartum period.

Research has found that a mother's experience with PPD is associated with her child's lower developmental milestones, including *fine and gross motor, communication, problem-solving, and personal/social skills* (Tuovinen et al., 2018). *Gross motor skills* include central body movements such as the child's ability to sit, stand, crawl, walk, jump, climb, and run. In contrast, fine motor skills include the child's hand dexterity such as grasping a toy, holding a crayon, using utensils to eat, opening and closing a zipper, turning the pages of a book, and brushing their teeth. It's important for counselors to know when babies are expected to meet standard motor skill milestones. For example, infants should typically be able to roll over from front to back and vice versa by the time they are five months old and should be throwing a ball before their first birthday. Counselors can encourage mothers to develop and/or improve their baby's physical development through playing games, experiential learning activities and, if necessary, occupational therapy.

Communication skills are sometimes harder to assess than physical development and can include a variety of communication abilities such as making eye contact, using gestures, pointing to objects, babbling, comprehending and following directions, and saying words. During PPD treatment, counselors can ask mothers about their baby's communication skills, or lack thereof. For example, 9-month-old babies should follow simple commands like "give it to me" without the mother's use of gestures, while an 18-month-old should follow more complex commands like "go get your blanket in your room" (Squires & Bricker, 2009). Counselors can help mothers find creative ways to stimulate their child's communication skills through interactive play, reading books, rhyming words, and singing songs. If a child is showing signs of communication delays, recommending early intervention with a speech therapist can be greatly beneficial (Kaplan et al., 2014).

Problem-solving skills involve how a child plays with different toys and solves problems through play. This skill helps the child explore their world while learning and understanding how things work. Problem solving can look like a baby trying to find a toy that was just hidden under a pillow or turning a cup upside down to dump out a cheerio (Squires & Bricker, 2009). As the baby grows, their understanding of problem solving also develops. For example, a 6-month-old baby should be able to pick up a toy from the floor after it's dropped, while a 12-month-old baby should be able to imitate their mother's actions. The best way to stimulate a child's problem-solving skills is through interactive play, being silly, and having fun with different toys and games (Twombly & Fink, 2004). Counselors can encourage mothers to participate in these fun activities with their babies daily to foster their learning, growth, and development.

Finally, *personal/social skills* include the child's self-help skills as well as their interactions with others. A baby might show personal self-help skills by eating a snack on their own or washing their body with a washcloth during a bath. Social skills and interacting with others can include asking or gesturing for help with a toy, waving "bye-bye" to a friend, or hugging a doll. As with other developmental skills and milestones, personal/social skills continue to improve as the baby grows and gains more independence. For example, an 18-month-old baby should be able to feed themselves with a spoon, even though they might make a big mess (Squires &

Bricker, 2009). Counselors can encourage mothers to foster their child's independence by allowing different independent activities like self-feeding with a spoon or drinking milk from a cup.

While there is some evidence related to the negative impacts of PPD on a child's developmental stages, research literature does appear to show conflicting and mixed results when it comes to the implications of untreated PPD for a baby's development (Śliwerski et al., 2020). Most studies do show a connection between a mother's current depression symptoms and a disruption in the mother–child bonding process, especially if the depressive or mental health symptoms are severe (Closa-Monasterolo et al., 2017; Śliwerski et al., 2020). In fact, if a mother's mental health symptoms are left untreated and persist for years, elementary school age children can also be negatively impacted and potentially develop their own mental health problems such as anxiety, depression, somatic complaints, social problems, thought problems, attention problems, rule-breaking behavior, and aggressive behaviors (Closa-Monasterolo et al., 2017). Therefore, effective treatment is essential to help both mother and child.

Recognizing that infants, toddlers, and older children can be negatively impacted by a mother's persistent and untreated mental health issues, counselors can learn to recognize early signs of developmental delays or mental health problems in children. Using developmental milestones evaluations, such as the Ages and Stages Questionnaire (ASQ; Squires & Bricker, 2009) or charts recommended by the American Pediatrics Society can be helpful for counselors. Helping mothers be emotionally available, consistently respond to their infant's cues and cries, and increase positive parent–child interactions can be greatly beneficial in the treatment of PPD.

COPING WITH THE CHALLENGES OF MOTHERHOOD AND PPD

Finding a personalized rhythm as a mother and connecting with a new baby are not something mothers should be expected to do entirely alone. In fact, social support is widely known as a strong protective factor against developing PPD (Beck, 1996). There are numerous social connections and resources to help mothers achieve a healthy rhythm after having a baby. In this section, a variety of resources and support networks will be discussed that can offer positive coping for mothers struggling with the many challenges of motherhood. It is important for counselors to be well informed of the difficult challenges faced by parents with infants, as well as the range of social support available to help these families.

New mothers may not be aware of the strong social bond that is created with other mothers after childbirth. This type of fusion of identity, which is the strong connection mothers feel with other mothers, can be an unexpected, yet empowering experience for women who recently gave birth. This instant and deep bond can help new mothers feel a sense of unity and camaraderie with other mothers who have also experienced the often isolating, painful, as well as physically and emotionally draining and challenging, experience of childbirth (Tasuji et al., 2020). Support groups specifically tailored for mothers can make great use of this new bond and shared meaning amongst women. These groups provide women with a unique and positive experience during the peripartum period.

MULTIPLE PERSPECTIVES

While encouraging maternal bonding is essential, counselors can also shift the focus and explore bonding between babies and other family members, such as the father or other parent who did not physically give birth to the child. Research suggests that paternal care of infants assists in the successful transition to fatherhood, and better parental outcomes positively impact paternal infant bonding, especially in the infant's first few days of life (Bieleninik et al., 2021). Although research on paternal bonding is sorely lacking, several studies have found that paternal bonding has benefits to both fathers and infants (Shorey et al., 2016). An integrative literature review concluded that fathers who spend extra time providing their infants with skin-to-skin contact report a smoother transition to their paternal roles, healthier interactions with their infants, better infant responses to the father, and a decrease in stress and anxiety (Shorey et al., 2016). Another study related to new fathers' brain chemicals asserted that assuming the parenting role and actively engaging in the physical care of infants can produce and increase brain chemicals related to parent–child bonding (Abraham et al., 2014). Understanding the benefits of paternal bonding can help counselors encourage both mothers and fathers to find a rhythm and connect with their babies during the peripartum period, with tailored interventions aimed at promoting early paternal bonding.

MULTICULTURAL CONSIDERATIONS

While it is important for counselors to consider how culture impacts parental bonding with infants, very limited research exists on examining bonding relationships among ethnic minority populations (Zhang et al., 2020). One important issue for counselors to consider is that Black mothers are less likely to breastfeed than White mothers and other ethnic minorities (Li et al., 2019). Experiencing institutionalized racism, such as racism at work or by police, negatively impacted breastfeeding initiation and duration among 2,017 Black mothers in the United States (Griswold et al., 2018). While not breastfeeding could potentially have a negative impact on the process of maternal bonding, counselors should be sensitive to the systemic factors that can negatively impact breastfeeding and also support mothers with other ways to enhance maternal bonding. By understanding the importance of maternal bonding, and the significant impact it can have on infants, counselors can prioritize educating and helping mothers form positive and healthy interactions with their babies during the peripartum period, whether or not they are breastfeeding. Furthermore, counselors who are inspired to work toward systemic-level change can pursue advocacy efforts to address the societal inequities such as poverty and racism that impact parenting behavior.

Another important multicultural perspective for counselors to consider is the similarities and differences in parental bonding among LGBTQ+ parents. One study comparing heterosexual parents with same-sex parents found no differences in child adjustment related to the parent's sexuality. Instead, supportive coparenting was associated with better child adjustment, regardless of a family's structure (Farr & Patterson, 2013). Regarding attachment, research also yields positive results for LGBTQ+ parents. A recent study found that attachment security for children born to gay fathers and lesbian mothers did not differ from that of children born to heterosexual parents (Carone et al., 2020). Developing and nurturing affectionate and positive bonds with infants is associated with parental behaviors, not their sexual identity.

While many of the recommendations to develop a caregiver–infant bond discussed throughout the chapter can apply to same-sex parents, it is important for counselors to be aware of the unique needs of same-sex couples. For instance, among non-birth mothers in lesbian relationships who participated in a qualitative study, researchers reported themes of an insecure connection and seeking legitimacy as a parent, as these non-biological mothers navigated their role in a cultural context that prioritizes heteronormative family structures and biological mothers (McInerney et al., 2021). Understanding the unique struggles LGBTQ+ parents with infants may face, counselors can provide extra supports so that parents can form healthy early bonds and attachments.

APPLICATIONS TO COUNSELING

Counselors can encourage women to attend support groups that are specific to their personal struggles with motherhood. Group therapy has been found to be effective in reducing PPD symptoms (Goodman & Santangelo, 2011). Support groups that are designed specifically for mothers struggling with PPD may be most helpful for women struggling with symptoms of resentment, fear, inadequacy, and guilt related to PPD. These groups can provide mothers with a safe space in which to feel heard and accepted, and share the physically and emotionally painful feelings associated with PPD. During group meetings, mothers can experience a sense of community, encouraging healthy relationships among members and an increase in overall health, self-esteem, and self-worth. Being in a room with other women who have a shared meaning of PDD can be powerful in alleviating the pervasive symptoms of this disorder (Anderson, 2013; Cook et al., 2019). While PPD support groups can be helpful, mothers can also benefit from other types of support groups based on their personal difficulties and challenges related to motherhood. Counselors can help mothers find a support network that works best for their individualized needs as well as the needs of their baby.

While community support groups can be valuable, mothers can also seek a support network much closer to home. Family and spousal support can be a tremendous source of encouragement for women struggling with motherhood. While mothers often seek help and support from in-laws, their own parents, or other members of the family, many women rely heavily on their spouse as a primary source for physical, emotional, and social support during the perinatal period. Research suggests that spousal and other family support can directly lower the risk of mothers developing PPD (Kızılırmak et al., 2020; Xie et al., 2010). Counselors can provide practical guidance for couples and key family members to regularly seek, request, and provide one another with physical, emotional, and social supports during and after pregnancy. Physical support can include helping with childcare tasks such as giving the baby a bath, washing baby bottles or breast pumping parts, as well as helping the mother with personal needs such as showering after a C-section, preparing and cooking healthy meals, driving to doctors' appointments, or simply being physically present and willing to help with any immediate needs or requests. Physical support can give mothers a much-needed break from childcare tasks so they can focus on their own physical, emotional, and social needs.

Conversely, emotional support is less tangible than physical support but can be just as helpful to mothers. Emotional support for new mothers can include showing physical affection such as holding hands or giving a massage, as well as providing empathic listening, validation, reassurance, and shared problem solving related to the motherhood experience. When a mother receives emotional support, she feels less lonely and isolated knowing that someone else is sharing this sometimes challenging and demanding experience with her. Counselors can guide family members to give less advice and provide more active listening during the peripartum time. This can be difficult for some family members who have become accustomed to giving mothers oftentimes unsolicited, incorrect, or unhelpful advice. Giving mothers the space to openly discuss their doubts, fears, joys, and wonders can be liberating. Furthermore, it is important to allow mothers the space to find their own answers and solutions to the challenges of parenting and encourage them to communicate with their spouses or partners about ways to manage these challenges.

The third type of support counselors should encourage for mothers is social support. This type of support can help mothers feel less isolated and more connected to others during the peripartum period. Connecting with social supports can be done in various ways, including meeting with friends, neighbors, extended family, and healthcare providers in the community or virtually through social media, video calls, or written communication. Attending church, joining a mother's group, or enrolling in a baby yoga class are all examples of healthy social supports for mothers. For family members, ensuring these social supports are consistently accessible to mothers is key. Engaging in social supports can also be a good opportunity for family members to either join the mother in the community or take care of the baby to give the mother some independent time. Knowing that this is a vulnerable time for mothers, counselors can urge family members and spouses to regularly provide mothers with positive and healthy physical, emotional, and social supports during and after pregnancy. Figure 9.1 illustrates this complex support system for new mothers.

Figure 9.1
Support for New Mothers

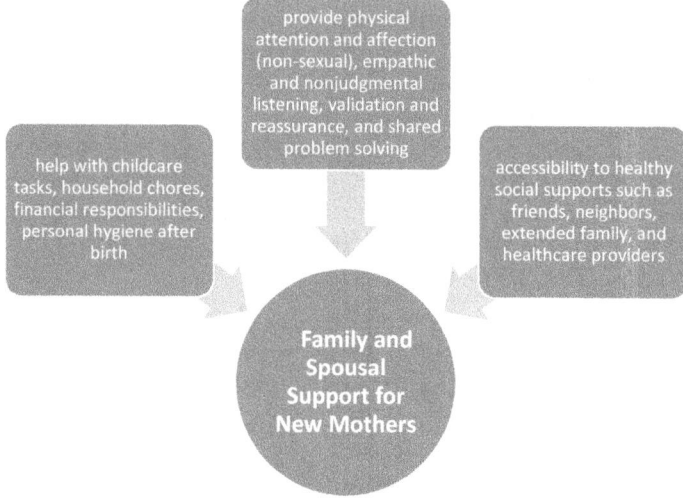

When community and family supports are not sufficient, counselors can educate families regarding other treatment options for PPD. The research consensus is that the first line of treatment for PPD is psychotherapy and/or medications for depression, depending on the severity of the woman's symptoms (Freeman et al., 2012). As counselors strive to provide ethical and individualized treatment for mothers and their families, all treatment modalities, including pharmacologic options, should be considered and discussed with the family. While it is important for women and their families to be aware of treatment options that may effectively treat PPD symptoms during and after pregnancy, they should also be made aware of any potential risks or side effects related to these treatments.

Many women are hesitant and worried about taking medications for PPD symptoms during pregnancy or while breastfeeding their infant for the fear that their baby will be exposed to those medications (Freeman et al., 2012). Counselors can educate themselves on psychopharmacology and breastfeeding and provide resources to breastfeeding mothers such as the Drugs and Lactation Database (LactMed) available online via the National Library of Medicine—National Center for Biotechnology Information, which includes information about medications and breastfeeding infants (National Library of Medicine, 2006), while being careful not to step outside of their scope of practice. For example, counselors should not give medical advice and should not suggest that women start or stop specific medications for their PPD symptoms as this is outside the scope of practice and competence for counselors. Instead, counselors can refer clients to a psychiatrist or healthcare provider and work closely with that provider to provide support and monitor clients for medication adherence and side effects. Providing women and their families with psychoeducation about their PPD diagnosis, medication compliance, and consulting with the client's healthcare provider are exceptionally beneficial for treatment success and relapse prevention.

In one study, mothers who chose to take medications for PPD while pregnant or breastfeeding noted that it was particularly encouraging and valuable to attend support groups with facilitators who normalized the use of antidepressant medications during the peripartum period (Cook et al., 2019). Being part of a group that not only accepts, but openly encourages medication compliance and adherence during this vulnerable and stressful time, was rarely found among healthcare professionals and was highly valued and appreciated by mothers experiencing PPD (Cook et al., 2019). Acknowledging this as a significant area of need for women, counselors can become a source of nonjudgmental support, openly advocating for a woman's right to be educated about and choose the treatment options she believes are best for her and her child. More information about counseling treatment interventions for PPD as well as psychopharmacology treatment resources can be found in Chapter 11 of this book.

ETHICAL AND LEGAL CONSIDERATIONS

The American Counseling Association *Code of Ethics* (2014) encourages counseling professionals to only practice within the boundaries of their competence. This competence is based on proficient training, education, supervised experience, and professional credentials (ACA, 2014, Section C.2.a). Although most mental health counseling graduate programs do not have a specific course focused on maternal mental health, counselors are expected to recognize their limitations and seek continuing education training to increase their competence on important and current mental health concerns (ACA, 2014, Section C.2.f). Remaining informed regarding best practices for working with diverse populations and clinical issues is essential to maintaining professional competence (ACA, 2014, Section C.2.f).

Clinicians are becoming increasingly aware that perinatal women are an at-risk, vulnerable population whose unique mental health needs must be prioritized (McCloskey & Ragudaran, 2019). Counselors who feel unprepared, uncomfortable, or lack in knowledge and training related to mother–infant bonding, breastfeeding, infant development, and other topics covered in this chapter can seek out appropriate education, credible training, and professional experience to improve their level of competence to address and effectively treat these presenting problems in counseling.

BARRIERS TO TREATMENT

In order to expand on existing treatments for PPD, clinicians are called to develop an awareness of barriers that frequently influence treatment outcomes for women at the individual, local, and macrosystem level (Coffman et al., 2020). At the individual level, many new mothers are familiar with the physical and emotional exhaustion that emerges during the first few months of their new baby's life. This exhaustion often detracts mothers from self-care practices that contribute to their physical and emotional health. New mothers who do not recognize symptoms of PPD may minimize their tiredness and low levels of energy rather than discuss them with a healthcare professional (Canty et al., 2019). Similarly, attitudinal barriers including stigma and underlying feelings of guilt and shame may prevent women from seeking professional help for concerning PPD symptoms (Fonseca et al., 2015). Additionally, women often fear being labeled as a bad mother, experiencing disapproval from loved ones, and being labeled as mentally ill (Fonseca et al., 2015). Women seeking treatment for PPD must also overcome additional challenges such as finding childcare, organizing transportation, and securing time off from work (Coffman et al., 2020). For many women, these stressors are intensified by socioeconomic factors that further serve as barriers. Even when new mothers are able to identify PPD symptoms, find a provider, and organize schedules and resources to prioritize their own care, they often fear that honest disclosure of their symptoms may result in child protective services involvement and someone taking their baby (Coffman et al., 2020).

Following an individual's recognition or awareness of PPD symptoms, social support networks become increasingly important. The burden of barriers experienced at the individual level can be drastically reduced by the presence of a strong social support network within the community (Canty et al., 2019). New mothers often turn to friends, relatives, and family members to share their symptoms and need for support (Fonseca et al., 2015). Family and community are vital emotional support systems that can help women cope with symptoms of PPD and other competing priorities associated with taking care of their families (Canty et al., 2019). The recent use of telehealth improves access to care and support for women by providing opportunities to supplement or expand on existing support networks (Lackie et al., 2021).

At the local level, barriers continue to exist in the community and healthcare systems for women seeking PPD treatment. Most women first report their symptoms to an OB/GYN or a pediatrician rather than a mental health professional (Prevatt et al., 2018), while other mothers completely overlook their child's pediatrician as a resource due to labeling the doctor as the child's provider (Canty et al., 2019). Pediatricians can support women experiencing PPD by learning to identify symptomology, devoting adequate time during pediatric appointments to assessing mothers who present with anxiety and depression, and by helping women find mental healthcare providers in their area (Coffman et al., 2020). Improving public health practices associated with PPD requires collaboration among providers in order to screen, diagnose, treat, and offer helpful resources (Coffman et al., 2020).

Further, barriers at the macrosystem level can be significantly reduced by ensuring that uninsured or underinsured women have access to affordable mental health services (Canty et al., 2019). The field of eHealth has become instrumental in making information, education, and resources both accessible and cost effective (Lackie et al., 2021). That said, providers still experience barriers related to a lack of funding, training, and systematic screening across agencies (Canty et al., 2019). Reducing barriers at the macrosystem level requires passionate political advocates that support screening and additional funding to support women who experience PPD.

COVID-19 AND ONLINE SUPPORT

Keeping up with current trends which became especially relevant and prominent during the COVID-19 pandemic, online resources for mothers and babies can be a tremendous help for women who want access to quick and up-to-date information about their perinatal experience. Online platforms have become the new way to gain information, ask questions, and create a social support network for mothers. Worried parents can get answers to their questions from experts as well as other parents at any time of day or night, from the comfort of their own home, through websites and social media platforms. Pregnant and postpartum women are frequently using websites and social media for parenting information, social support, and increased connection with others. The internet provides parents with opportunities to blog, communicate with other parents on message boards, and watch videos about how to install car seats, soothe sore nipples from breastfeeding, and change baby diapers. It is becoming a normalized and ubiquitous part of parenting to use social media and the internet for practical and useful answers to questions related to pregnancy, childbirth, and newborn growth and development (Archer & Kao, 2018; Baker & Yang, 2018; Price et al., 2018). Counselors are encouraged to jump on board the internet bandwagon, if they haven't done so already, and familiarize themselves with the myriad of online resources available to parents. Counselors should also advise their clients to look for reliable sources of information online, such as government websites and trusted organizations, and be critical consumers of online content.

It's evident that a majority of women are using social media to not only seek information about the peripartum experience, but to also build a social network that may combat loneliness and isolation that can occur during the peripartum period, which could serve as a protective factor against developing PPD. Counselors have an additional responsibility to be aware of reliable sources as well as helping parents vet the information they are finding to ensure that it is accurate and credible (Baker & Yang, 2018). For example, counselors can guide mothers who struggle with breastfeeding to find assistance through La Leche League International, an entirely free, trustworthy, and highly regarded resource for women who are able and choose to breastfeed their baby. This international organization focuses on helping families succeed in their breastfeeding goals by providing a plethora of online resources as well as local support groups with trained parent volunteers. If internet and social media platforms are not enough, counselors should also be aware of and help parents find local community resources that fit their needs. For instance, for mothers who want or require further help with breastfeeding, a lactation consultant may be more helpful. While there may be a charge for trained lactation consultants such as a Board-Certified Lactation Consultant (IBCLC), many insurance companies will pay for this healthcare service. Counselors can guide families to their local hospital, birth center, pediatrician, or insurance company for help with finding a lactation consultant to help prevent and manage common breastfeeding problems and concerns. More credible and reputable resources that may be helpful for counselors can be found in Table 9.2.

Table 9.2
Online Resources

Motherhood Challenge	Credible Resource
Breastfeeding	La Leche League International (https://www.llli.org/) International Lactation Consultant Association (https://ilca.org/)
Depression, anxiety, substance abuse, suicidal ideation & other PPD symptoms	National Alliance on Mental Illness (nami.org) Substance Abuse and Mental Health Services Administration (samhsa.gov) Health Resources and Services Administration Maternal & Child Health (mchb.hrsa.gov/national-maternal-mental-health-hotline) Postpartum Support International (postpartum.net) U.S. Department of Health & Human Services- Office on Women's Health (womenshealth.gov) 988 Suicide and Crisis Lifeline (988lifeline.org/) National Institute of Mental Health (nimh.nih.gov)
Parenting, development, and attachment	Zero to Three—Early Connections Last a Lifetime (zerotothree.org) Healthychildren.org Circle of Security Parenting (circleofsecurityinternational.com) Kids Health from Nemours (kidshealth.org) Attachment Parenting International (attachmentparenting.org)

CONCLUSION

This chapter highlighted the significance of providing mothers with the necessary support and resources to develop a healthy bond with their babies. Symptoms of PPD or other mental health problems can significantly impact parental bonds, subsequent attachment, and an infant's developmental milestones. Counselors are encouraged to help mothers enhance their connection with their babies through various forms of physical contact while also bolstering their own wellbeing through various means of support, including family, social, and community supports. Exploring various types of supports, resources, and levels of treatment is essential when a mother's PPD symptoms interfere with her ability to bond with her baby to prevent infant attachment and developmental problems.

Case Study: Kennedy

Kennedy, a 35-year-old Korean American mother of two older children currently in college, found out she was pregnant shortly before the COVID-19 pandemic. Kennedy and her family felt delighted about the pregnancy, as she was newly remarried and had been trying to conceive for six months with her new husband. This pregnancy was not as easy as her first two, especially with all the inflexible Covid restrictions set by her prenatal care and hospital, such as not allowing any family members to sit in during pregnancy ultrasounds, only allowing her husband for support during labor and delivery and being required to wear a mask during and after labor. Kennedy did not want any family members or friends to visit her newborn, for the fear that she would possibly catch Covid. While she attempted to breastfeed, she couldn't get the baby to latch and was too afraid to meet with lactation specialists for help. Her husband was not allowed to attend any of her doctor's visits due to Covid restrictions, and they both felt very isolated at home, with no help or support from family or medical professionals. Kennedy became increasingly afraid of getting Covid and refused to leave the house for the first three months after giving birth. When the baby was six months old, her husband finally convinced her to see a therapist virtually so she could gain some emotional support about her fears. During the first virtual therapy appointment, Kennedy revealed that she feels anxious most of the time, doesn't feel like she is bonding with her baby like she did with her first two children, and feels guilt about not being able to breastfeed. Most days, she lacks motivation to be productive, tries her best not to leave the house or meet up with people, and watches a lot of television with her baby. She did report feeling concern and guilt about her baby's development, noting that he is still not sitting up or attempting to crawl. On the rare occasion she does take him to the playground, he doesn't seem interested in other children and doesn't make much eye contact with other adults. Kennedy feels like she has failed as a parent but doesn't know how to move past her fears and anxiety of Covid.

APPLYING THE STRENGTHS MODEL—THE CASE OF KENNEDY

Significant Individual, Infant, Family, Societal, and Cultural Factors

- Limited family and medical supports due to isolation and Covid restrictions.
- Infant delayed in motor and communication skills, potentially due to isolation and mother's mental health symptoms.
- COVID-19 restrictions in the community.

Treatment Barriers

- Social isolation of mother and baby

- Fear and anxiety about seeking help.
- Not recognizing red flags or signs of PPD or other mental health concerns.

Risk Factors
- Significant life stressors due to Covid restrictions.
- Limited social supports for mother and child.
- Community restrictions of medical supports due to COVID-19.

Enlisting Support from Family, the Community, and Medical Professionals
- |Family members and friends for social support.
- Lactation specialist for breastfeeding support.
- Pediatrician for infant development support.

Noticeable Symptoms, Severity, & DSM-5-TR Diagnosis OR Needs Identified by Family & Treatment Team
- Severe fear and anxiety related to leaving the house.
- Severe social and medical isolation.
- DSM-5-TR diagnosis: 300.02 Generalized Anxiety Disorder.

Goals Identified by Family
- Increase social supports.
- Decrease fear and anxiety related to COVID-19 pandemic.
- Increase number of times mother and child leave the home.
- Increase healthy bonding activities between mother and child.

Treatment Recommendations
- "Baby and me" sessions to help mother form healthier interactions with baby.
- CBT interventions to reduce level of fear and anxiety.
- Pediatric referral to evaluate baby's development.
- Pharmacological referral to psychiatrist or primary care doctor for evaluation for anxiety medications.

Helpful, Protective, and Resilience Factors

- Spousal support for seeking and attending treatment.
- Willingness to attend mental health counseling.
- Availability of virtual treatment options due to Covid restrictions.

Self-Care & Wellness

- Psychological self-care by attending weekly mental health counseling sessions.
- Emotional self-care by enjoying new or old hobbies.
- Personal self-care by fostering social interactions with friends, family members, and community supports.

REFERENCES

Abraham, E., Hendler, T., Shapira-Lichter, I., Kanat-Maymon, Y., Zagoory-Sharon, O., & Feldman, R. (2014). Father's brain is sensitive to childcare experiences. *Proceedings of the National Academy of Sciences of the United States of America, 111*(27), 9792–9797. doi:10.1073/pnas.1402569111

Allen, R. E., & Oliver, J. M. (1982). The effects of child maltreatment on language development. *Child Abuse & Neglect, 6*(3), 299–305. doi:10.1016/0145-2134(82)90033-3

American Counseling Association. (ACA). (2014). *2014 ACA code of ethics.* https://www.counseling.org/docs/default-source/default-document-library/2014-code-of-ethics-finaladdress.pdf

American Psychiatric Association. (APA). (2013). *Diagnostic and statistical manual of mental disorders* (5th ed.). American Psychiatric Association.

Anderson, L. N. (2013). Functions of support group communication for women with postpartum depression: How support groups silence and encourage voices of motherhood. *Journal of Community Psychology, 41*(6), 709–724. doi:10.1002/jcop.21566

Archer, C., & Kao, K.-T. (2018). Mother, baby and Facebook makes three: Does social media provide social support for new mothers? *Media International Australia, Incorporating Culture and Policy, 168*(1), 122–139. doi:10.1177/1329878X18783016

Baker, B., & Yang, I. (2018). Social media as social support in pregnancy and the postpartum. *Sexual & Reproductive Healthcare, 17*, 31–34. doi:10.1016/j.srhc.2018.05.003

Beck, C. T. (1996). A meta-analysis of predictors of postpartum depression. *Nursing Research, 45*(5), 297–303. doi:10.1097/00006199-199609000-00008

Bernard, K., Nissim, G., Vaccaro, S., Harris, J. L., & Lindhiem, O. (2018). Association between maternal depression and maternal sensitivity from birth to 12 months: A meta-analysis. *Attachment & Human Development, 20*(6), 578–599. doi:10.1080/14616734.2018.1430839

Bieleninik, L., Geretsegger, M., Mössler, K., Assmus, J., Thompson, G., Gattino, G., Elefant, C., Gottfried, T., Igliozzi, R., Muratori, F., Suvini, F., Kim, J., Crawford, M. J., Odell-Miller, H., Oldfield, A., Casey, Ó., Finnemann, J., Carpente, J., Park, A. L., Grossi, E., … TIME-A Study Team (2017). Effects of improvisational music therapy vs enhanced standard care on symptom severity among children with autism spectrum disorder: The TIME-A randomized clinical trial. *JAMA, 318*(6), 525–535. doi:10.1001/jama.2017.9478

Bowlby J. ([1969]1982). *Attachment and loss* (2nd ed., vol. 1). Basic Books.
Britton, J. R., Britton, H. L., & Gronwaldt, V. (2006). Breastfeeding, sensitivity, and attachment. *Pediatrics, 118*(5), e1436–e1443. doi:10.1542/peds.2005-2916
Canty, H. R., Sauter, A., Zuckerman, K., Cobian, M., & Grigsby, T. (2019). Mothers' perspectives on follow-up for postpartum depression screening in primary care. *Journal of Developmental and Behavioral Pediatrics: JDBP, 40*(2), 139–143. doi:10.1097/DBP.0000000000000628
Carone, N., Baiocco, R., Lingiardi, V., & Kerns, K. (2020). Child attachment security in gay father surrogacy families: Parents as safe havens and secure bases during middle childhood. *Attachment & Human Development, 22*(3), 269–289. doi:10.1080/14616734.2019.1588906
Closa-Monasterolo, R., Gispert-Llaurado, M., Canals, J., Luque, V., Zaragoza-Jordana, M., Koletzko, B., Grote, V., Weber, M., Gruszfeld, D., Szott, K., Verduci, E., ReDionigi, A., Hoyos, J., Brasselle, G., & Escribano Subías, J. (2017). The effect of postpartum depression and current mental health problems of the mother on child behaviour at eight years. *Maternal & Child Health Journal, 21*(7), 1563–1572. doi:10.1007/s10995-017-2288-x
Coffman, M. J., Scott, V. C., Schuch, C., Mele, C., Mayfield, C., Balasubramanian, V., Stevens, A., & Dulin, M. (2020). Postpartum depression screening and referrals in special supplemental nutrition program for women, infants, and children clinics. *Journal of Obstetric, Gynecologic & Neonatal Nursing, 49*(1), 27–40. doi:10.1016/j.jogn.2019.10.007
Cook, C., Goyal, D., & Allen, M. (2019). Experiences of women with postpartum depression participating in a support group led by mental health providers. *MCN: The American Journal of Maternal/Child Nursing, 44*(4), 228–223. doi:10.1097/NMC.0000000000000533
Crucianelli, L., Wheatley, L., Filippetti, M. L., Jenkinson, P. M., Kirk, E., & Fotopoulou, A. K. (2019). The mindedness of maternal touch: An investigation of maternal mind-mindedness and mother-infant touch interactions. *Developmental Cognitive Neuroscience, 35*, 47–56. doi:10.1016/j.dcn.2018.01.010
Elitok, G. K., Bülbül, L., Erden, S. Ç., Beşirli, A., & Bülbül, A. (2020). Effect of postpartum depression and anxiety on infant development at 12 months: A one-year follow-up study. *Istanbul Medical Journal, 21*(6), 423–429. doi:10.4274/imj.galenos.2020.58265
Erickson, M. F., Egeland, B., & Pianta, R. (1989). The effects of maltreatment on the development of young children. In D. Cicchetti, & V. Carlson (Eds.), *Child maltreatment: Theory and research on the causes and consequences of child abuse and neglect* (pp. 647–684). Cambridge University Press. doi:10.1017/CBO9780511665707.021
Farr, R. H., & Patterson, C. J. (2013). Coparenting among Lesbian, Gay, and Heterosexual Couples: Associations with adopted children's outcomes. *Child Development, 84*(4), 1226–1240. doi:10.1111/cdev.12046
Fonseca, A., Gorayeb, R., & Canavarro, M. C. (2015). Women's help-seeking behaviours for depressive symptoms during the perinatal period: Socio-demographic and clinical correlates and perceived barriers to seeking professional help. *Midwifery, 31*(12), 1177–1185. doi:10.1016/j.midw.2015.09.002
Freeman, M. P., Joffe, H., & Cohen, L. S. (2012). Postpartum depression: Help patients find the right treatment: Accessibility of treatment, patient preference, breast-feeding help guide decisions. *Current Psychiatry, 11*(11), 14–21. https://cdn.mdedge.com/files/s3fs-public/Document/September-2017/1111CP_Freeman1.pdf
Frodi, A. M., & Smetana, J. (1984). Abused, neglected, and nonmaltreated preschoolers' ability to discriminate emotions in others: The effects of IQ. *Child Abuse & Neglect, 8*(4), 459–465. doi:10.1016/0145-2134(84)90027-9
Gholampour, F., Riem, M., & van den Heuvel, M. I. (2020). Maternal brain in the process of maternal-infant bonding: Review of the literature. *Social Neuroscience, 15*(4), 380–384. doi:10.1080/17470919.2020.1764093

Goodman, J. H., & Santangelo, G. (2011). Group treatment for postpartum depression: A systematic review. *Archives of Women's Mental Health*, 12(4), 277. doi:10.1007/s00737-011-0225-3

Gribble, K. D. (2006). Mental health, attachment and breastfeeding: Implications for adopted children and their mothers. *International Breastfeeding Journal*, 1(1), 5. doi:10.1186/1746-4358-1-5

Griswold, M. K., Crawford, S. L., Perry, D. J., Person, S. D., Rosenberg, L., Cozier, Y. C., & Palmer, J. R. (2018). Experiences of racism and breastfeeding initiation and duration among first-time mothers of the Black Women's Health Study (2018). *Journal of Racial Ethnic Health Disparities*, 5(6), 1180–1191. doi:10.1007/s40615-018-0465-2

Halfon, N., Larson, K., Lu, M., Tullis, E., & Russ, S. (2014). Lifecourse health development: Past, present and future. *Maternal and Child Health Journal*, 18(2), 344–365. doi:10.1007/s10995-013-1346-2

Hentges, R. F., Graham, S. A., Plamondon, A., Tough, S., & Madigan, S. (2021). Bidirectional associations between maternal depression, hostile parenting, and early child emotional problems: Findings from the all our families cohort. *Journal of Affective Disorders*, 287, 397–404. doi:10.1016/j.jad.2021.03.056

Jansen, J., de Weerth, C., & Riksen-Walraven, J. (2008). Breastfeeding and the mother–infant relationship—A review. *Developmental Review*, 28(4), 503–521. doi:10.1016/j.dr.2008.07.001

Kaplan, P. S., Danko, C. M., Everhart, K. D., Diaz, A., Asherin, R. M., Vogeli, J. M., & Fekri, S. M. (2014). Maternal depression and expressive communication in one-year-old infants. *Infant Behavior & Development*, 37(3), 398–405. doi:10.1016/j.infbeh.2014.05.008

Kendall-Tackett, K., & Mohrbacher, N. (2010). *Breastfeeding made simple: Seven natural laws for nursing mothers*. New Harbinger Publications.

Kızılırmak, A., Calpbinici, P., Tabakan, G., & Kartal, B. (2020). Correlation between postpartum depression and spousal support and factors affecting postpartum depression. *Health Care for Women International*, 42(12) 1325–1339. doi:10.1080/07399332.2020.1764562

Lackie, M. E., Parrilla, J. S., Lavery, B. M., Kennedy, A. L., Ryan, D., Shulman, B., & Brotto, L. A. (2021). Digital health needs of women with postpartum depression: Focus group study. *Journal of Medical Internet Research*, 23(1), e18934. doi:10.2196/18934

Li, R., Perrine, C. G., Anstey, E. H., Chen, J., MacGowan, C. A., & Elam-Evans, L. D. (2019). Breastfeeding trends by race/ethnicity among US children born from 2009 to 2015. *JAMA Pediatrics*, 173(12), e193319. doi:10.1001/jamapediatrics.2019.3319

McCloskey, R. J., & Ragudaran, S. (2019). Creation and evaluation of a maternal mental health course. *Social Work Education*, 38(2), 227–240. doi:10.1080/02615479.2018.1509952

McInerney, A., Creaner, M., & Nixon, E. (2021). The motherhood experiences of non-birth mothers in same-sex parent families. *Psychology of Women Quarterly*, 45(3), 279–293. doi:10.1177/03616843211003072

National Library of Medicine (2006). Drugs and Lactation Database (LactMed). https://www.ncbi.nlm.nih.gov/books/NBK501922/

O'Connor, E., Senger, C. A., Henninger, M. L., Coppola, E., & Gaynes, B. N. (2019). Interventions to Prevent Perinatal Depression: Evidence Report and Systematic Review for the US Preventive Services Task Force. *JAMA*, 321(6), 588–601. doi:10.1001/jama.2018.20865

Paulson, J. F., Dauber, S., & Leiferman, J. A. (2006). Individual and combined effects of postpartum depression in mothers and fathers on parenting behavior. *Pediatrics*, 118(2), 659–668. doi:10.1542/peds.2005-2948

Piallini, G., De Palo, F., & Simonelli, A. (2015). Parental brain: Cerebral areas activated by infant cries and faces. A comparison between different populations of parents and not. *Frontiers in Psychology*, 6, Article 1625. doi:10.3389/fpsyg.2015.01625

Prevatt, B. S., Lowder, E. M., & Desmarais, S. L. (2018). Peer-support intervention for postpartum depression: Participant satisfaction and program effectiveness. *Midwifery, 64*, 38–47. doi:10.1016/j.midw.2018.05.009

Price, S. L., Aston, M., Monaghan, J., Sim, M., Murphy, G. T., Etowa, J., Pickles, M., Hunter, A., & Little, V. (2018). Maternal knowing and social networks: Understanding first-time mothers' search for information and support through online and offline social networks. *Qualitative Health Research, 28*(10), 1552–1563. doi:10.1177/1049732317748314

Shorey, S., He, H.-G., & Morelius, E. (2016). Skin-to-skin contact by fathers and the impact on infant and paternal outcomes: an integrative review. *Midwifery, 40*, 207–217. doi:10.1016/j.midw.2016.07.007

Śliwerski, A., Kossakowska, K., Jarecka, K., Świtalska, J., & Bielawska-Batorowicz, E. (2020). The effect of maternal depression on infant attachment: A systematic review. *International Journal of Environmental Research and Public Health, 17*(8), 2675. doi:10.3390/ijerph17082675

Slomian, J., Honvo, G., Emonts, P., Reginster, J. Y., & Bruyère, O. (2019). Consequences of maternal postpartum depression: A systematic review of maternal and infant outcomes. *Women's Health, 15*, 1745506519844044. doi:10.1177/1745506519844044

Squires, J., & Bricker, D. (2009). *Ages & Stages Questionnaires®, Third Edition (ASQ®-3): A Parent-Completed Child Monitoring System*. Paul H. Brookes Publishing Co.

Stern, D. N. (1985). *The interpersonal world of the infant: A view from psychoanalysis and developmental psychology*. Basic Books.

Tasuji, T., Reese, E., van Mulukom, V., & Whitehouse, H. (2020). Band of mothers: Childbirth as a female bonding experience. *PLoS ONE, 15*(10), 1–24. doi:10.1371/journal.pone.0240175

Tuovinen, S., Lahti-Pulkkinen, M., Girchenko, P., Lipsanen, J., Lahti, J., Heinonen, K., Reynolds, R. M., Hämäläinen, E., Kajantie, E., Laivuori, H., Pesonen, A.-K., Villa, P. M., & Räikkönen, K. (2018). Maternal depressive symptoms during and after pregnancy and child developmental milestones. *Depression and Anxiety, 35*(8), 732–741. doi:10.1002/da.22756

Twombly, E. & Fink, G. (2004). *Ages & Stages learning activities*. Paul H. Brookes Publishing Co.

Xie, R., Yang, J., Liao, S., Xie, H., Walker, M., & Wen, S. (2010). Prenatal family support, postnatal family support and postpartum depression. *Australian & New Zealand Journal of Obstetrics & Gynaecology, 50*(4), 340–345. doi:10.1111/j.1479-828X.2010.01185.x

Zhang, Y., Edwards, R. C., & Hans, S. L. (2020). Parenting profiles of young low-income African American and Latina mothers and infant socioemotional development. *Parenting: Science & Practice, 20*(1), 28–52. doi:10.1080/15295192.2019.1642088

10

Career and Identity in the Peripartum

Isabel A. Thompson

Personal Narrative

I have wanted to be a mom all my life. I got a head start when I married a man with a child and became a bonus mama to a beautiful 3-year-old. When my time came to carry my own baby, I was surprised at my immediate worry about if I could do it. I have taken care of kids my whole life and I had been a teacher for almost ten years. I am a constant worrier, so I wasn't THAT surprised. Anxiety and depression had been a part of my life since I was a teen and worrying about stuff was an unwelcome past time. I had a worrisome pregnancy in the beginning due to having three Subchorionic hemorrhages. They resolved themselves around 12 weeks, but I worried the rest of the pregnancy. My sweet baby was born October of 2019 and I loved being home with him until January of 2020 when I had to return to my job as a Pre-K teacher. Going back was tough in more ways than one. I worried constantly about him being with someone who wasn't me. I was grateful to be friends with his nanny, but he did not take kindly to bottles and he spent months not eating for her and then keeping me up all night. I worried every day about him eating for her only to be disappointed at each pick up. Postpartum anxiety and depression snuck up then, teaming up with my everyday anxiety and depression. I began thinking how I wasn't enough for my baby and my family and how they would be better off without me. Thankfully I caught myself in some harmful intrusive thoughts one day and immediately took the day off and went to the doctor. I also called my husband and told him what was going on. I felt so much support from my husband, who did everything he could and still does to help me protect my mental health so I can be the best mama I can be. I learned one thing from my friends and the reading I did throughout my pregnancy and that was to ask for help. I needed help—from my doctor. From my husband. From my family. And I needed it immediately. I am thankful for an amazing support system. And I am prepared to lean on them again should I need them again as I prepare for the arrival of our third child. I have since become a stay at home due to the uncertainty of things with COVID-19 as well as my desire to be home and raise my children. I have found it even more important to keep an eye on my mental health as now I never leave the house and spend my whole

DOI: 10.4324/9780429440892-10

day with children 2 and under. I wouldn't change my life for the world though. I am where and who I am meant to be. And being a mama is my favorite.

—*Anonymous*

In this chapter, we examine parenthood and identity, especially the impact of gender role socialization on mothers as they navigate their roles, identities, and responsibilities at home, at work, and in society. Since gender role expectations impact parents and replicate gender-based inequities in society (Roskam & Mikolajczak, 2020), we focus on how gender role socialization and expectations impact mothers and their careers. For instance, mothers are expected to spend more time caring for their infants than fathers and to serve as primary caregivers (Lamar et al., 2019), which results in time away from paid employment. In addition, we address how mothers face discrimination in the workplace (Crowley, 2013).

We also explore specific role and identity challenges of stay-at-home mothers and explore the impact of the lack of guaranteed paid maternity leave and other forms of parental leave on mothers and families. While we primarily focus on mothers, we explore the challenges fathers and partners face navigating work and parenting roles. We discuss multicultural considerations specific to work-related issues, ethical and legal considerations, barriers to treatment, and the impact of the COVID-19 pandemic on the landscape of work.

WOMEN, IDENTITY, AND CAREER

Women experience complicated interrelationships between career, identity, and family roles and responsibilities, which can manifest as dual identities and role conflicts. Motherhood heightens these complications and the likelihood of identity conflicts, but work can also contribute to a mother's wellbeing by enhancing life satisfaction and self-esteem when they perceive work and mothering identities as compatible (Zagefka et al., 2021). However, when there is identity conflict, working mothers' wellbeing may be negatively impacted (Zagefka et al., 2021).

Mothers can experience identity and/or role conflict in all seasons of motherhood, but it is especially challenging to manage these roles during pregnancy, birth, and the early postpartum. Mothers of newborns are often sleep deprived and face sleep disruptions, while caring for their infant and trying to meet their own needs. For working mothers, learning how to reintegrate into work roles after an often too-brief period of leave from work adds to the stresses of life with a new baby.

An ethnographic exploration of work and motherhood suggests that motherhood (in North American society) is constructed as a private responsibility, in which women are responsible for providing care to their child(ren) (Vair, 2009). The responsibilities of motherhood are often understood as the mother's sole realm. Working mothers who have recently had a baby experience additional stress as they navigate this huge role shift and making childcare arrangements in the private sphere of family life.

The cultural view of motherhood and parenthood as private responsibilities is reflected in the lack of support for childcare in the United States, as the government does not provide subsidized or free childcare for all families. The American Rescue Plan provided a brief period (during the COVID-19 pandemic) in 2021 when eligible families received advanced child tax credit payments monthly (Internal Revenue Service [IRS], 2022). This program had a tremendous positive benefit in reducing family stress and assisting parents with caring for their children's basic needs. This program (as of this writing) has not been extended, although efforts were made to make the credits permanent.

Societal and cultural expectations about motherhood impact how working mothers navigate career and family demands (Forbes et al., 2021). The prevalence of intensive mothering culture increases stress, with intensive mothering defined as a gender role that is "normative and desirable" and involves mothers prioritizing others' needs above their own, at times to the detriment of their own mental and physical health and wellbeing (Forbes et al., 2021). Intensive mothering culture negatively impacts mothers as well as women who are not mothers, who fall outside this gender-based cultural norm (Forbes et al., 2021). For working mothers, the expectations of intensive mothering culture coupled with a lack of universal childcare means managing the stresses of arranging and paying for childcare along with professional demands.

NAVIGATING WORK AND MOTHERHOOD WHILE EXPERIENCING PPD

Mothers with symptoms of PPD, or other mood disorders, experience additional stress and complexity as they navigate motherhood and career roles. For example, consider a first-time mother of a six-week-old infant who is having crying spells frequently, feeling a loss of pleasure, and simultaneously dealing with painful mastitis, sleep disruption, and feeling isolated at home as her partner has returned to work. Then imagine this mother, now with a 12-week-old infant, returning to work, arranging childcare, managing her emotions, feeding and caring for her infant, and handling her professional role. Discerning what is typical stress of having a newborn, what are symptoms, and whether to seek treatment takes time, energy, and effort, all of which are in short supply for new mothers.

Due to societal stigma regarding mental illness, working mothers experiencing PPD or other mood disorders may face additional discrimination or be fearful of potential discrimination and may be reluctant or cautious about sharing their symptoms, especially with their employer or work colleagues. When we consider the context of lack of paid parental leave in the United States and resulting pressure to return to work soon after childbirth, mothers with PPD can experience challenges in work performance due to caring for a newborn, the impact of PPD, and returning to paid employment quickly after childbirth.

WORKING MOTHERS

Given the myriad of considerations—personal, financial, and familial—many women and families struggle with the decision about whether and/or when a mother will return to the paid workforce. Furthermore, in a qualitative study, working mothers shared feelings of guilt and pressure about both work and family roles (Forbes et al., 2021). New working mothers may struggle to care for their infants as they would like to and feel guilty about missing special moments, while simultaneously trying to sustain a high level of work performance like before they had a baby. American society can be viewed as particularly unforgiving for new working mothers, as there is not guaranteed paid leave of sufficient duration for a slow return to work.

For working mothers, juggling the demands of career and motherhood often takes precedence in their lives and they "still have primary responsibility for their children and homes" (Dugan & Barnes-Farrell, 2020, p. 63). This has been described as a second shift—the unpaid labor of childcare and housework that takes up a lot of time outside of paid employment and still falls primarily on the mother (Dugan & Barnes-Farrell, 2020). Therefore, working mothers often experience time pressure and overload attempting to meet career and family demands (Dugan & Barnes-Farrell, 2020).

Working mothers experience a gender-based double-bind pressure to function at work "as if they are not mothers" and "mother as if they are not workers." This double-bind pressure may create a scenario in which a mother feels like she is failing in the two most important roles of her life. Furthermore, a lack of competence and self-efficacy as a mother or experiencing challenges with childcare and/or the transition back to paid employment can increase maternal life stress, which can be a risk factor in the development of PPD (Julian et al., 2021).

Working mothers also experience discrimination in the workplace. For instance, in a qualitative study with 54 interviews of mostly middle-class heterosexual women, researchers reported that "as mothers, they are seen as not meeting the ideal worker standard of performance nor as capable as non-mothers by their employers" (Crowley, 2013, p. 192). These types of concerns increase the pressure on working mothers to demonstrate their efficacy.

Maternity Leave (or Lack Thereof)

The United States of America is the only large democratic country worldwide that lacks federal laws that guarantee paid maternity leave (Addati et al., 2014). The pressure to return to work before a mother (let alone a partner/father!) feels ready creates stress and tensions for mothers and families, who are trying to live up to ideals of motherhood and family life, while facing a lack of social, cultural, and instrumental support without guaranteed paid leave or universally available, affordable, and accessible childcare.

In the United States, leave time from work is often short, sometimes six weeks or less. It takes time for infants to settle into a sleep pattern with fewer night awakenings. At 12 weeks postpartum most mothers have stopped bleeding and may have a better handle on their routines with a new baby but may not be emotionally ready to leave their new baby. However, FMLA only guarantees 12 weeks of unpaid leave in specific types of employment settings and many mothers get less time (Andres et al., 2016).

Researchers studying mothers' perceptions of maternity leave developed the Quality of Maternity Leave Scales (QMLS), to assess "time off, flexibility, coworker support, discrimination, microaggressions, and benefits (e.g., pay, health care, disability insurance)" (Sterling & Allan, 2020, p. 337). They reported an association between positive perceptions of maternity leave and overall work conditions, including greater job satisfaction and less reported discrimination (Sterling & Allan, 2020). Counselors can help validate mothers' experiences and provide space for them to share positive and negative aspects of their leave experience and adjustment to life with a baby. Dispelling the myth of maternity leave as a "vacation" is needed, as this could not be farther from the lived reality of caring for a newborn.

Returning to Work after Maternity Leave

What factors might contribute to a woman not feeling ready to return to work six, eight, or twelve weeks after giving birth? In the case of natural birth scenarios, a woman gives birth to a baby, births the placenta, loses blood, and her body adjusts to the hormonal changes. In surgical births, a mother has had surgery and is healing from that, in addition to the hormonal changes of giving birth. For a mother with a newborn, self-care tasks such as taking a shower or eating are difficult to prioritize and they have little time to recover from childbirth (Lambermon et al., 2020). Returning to work, with expectations for professional appearance and functioning, can be daunting, especially when a postpartum mother is frequently still bleeding for weeks after giving birth and focused on caring for her baby.

The reality of returning to work can vary, depending on how long a woman was able to be home with her baby (or babies), how she feels about her infant in someone else's care, her childcare options, and how her sleep and self-care have been impacted. If a mother returns to work before she has had enough time to bond with her newborn, this can impact her interactions with her baby. In a study of 3,850 working mothers and their children, Plotka reported that "early return to work and early separation might make it harder for a mother to develop higher levels of attunement to her child's needs or higher levels of sensitivity towards her child's cues" (2012, p. 110). Since sensitivity towards a child's cues has been associated with the development of positive parent–child interactions (Plotka, 2012), an early return to work may have negative impacts for the mother and baby. A shorter maternity leave can negatively impact mothers' personal and marital distress levels, thereby increasing her risk factors for developing depression (Hyde et al., 2001). Working mothers face numerous stressors and demands on their time, attention, and energy and counselors can invite them to explore these stressors and resources for support.

Breastfeeding Working Mothers

Returning to work (or school for mothers pursuing educational goals) poses unique challenges for mothers who are breastfeeding (Bell et al., 2022). The *Breaktime for Nursing Mothers* federal law is intended protect nursing mothers by giving them time, privacy, and a space (that is not a bathroom) to express milk (DOL, 2010). However, this law only provides for unpaid breaks, does not specify the length of breaks, and does not apply to salaried workers and students, who may need its protection (Johnson & Salpini, 2017). Even mothers working in female-dominated fields including midwifery and teaching experience breastfeeding barriers, like not wanting to take too many breaks or not having sufficient time during the day to pump (Burns et al., 2022).

Breastfeeding mothers who are working and want to maintain breastfeeding take time to either directly breastfeed their infants (if their childcare/work arrangements allow) and/or express milk via pumping. Pumping involves multiple steps and considerations, including the privacy, cleaning, and storing of the pump, and ensuring safe storage of the expressed milk. Switching between professional activities and nursing and/or pumping has been described as a form of interspersed labor called a "simultaneous second shift" (Avishai, 2004 as cited in Johnson & Salpini, 2017). This interspersed labor is stressful, with mothers switching modes, roles, and activities to meet professional demands and their nursing/pumping schedule.

Breastfeeding working mothers also need to maintain their professionalism while attending to the tasks of pumping or nursing. I (Isabel Thompson) have personally experienced the stresses of this form of interspersed labor while nursing both my children, such as needing to take breaks to pump or nurse my infant between meetings, which required time and energy to regroup and resume professional activities. These stresses were manageable due to the flexibility I had with a private office and working from home sometimes. Mothers who return to work or educational settings and want to breastfeed may experience structural/institutional challenges (such as lack of suitable place to pump or breastfeed or lack of sufficient break time to do so) that make continuing to breastfeed hard despite their desire to do so (Bell et al., 2022).

Benefits of Paid Employment for Working Mothers

Despite the challenges associated with mothers returning to paid work, paid employment can have many benefits for mothers, especially those who are in a meaningful career path that contributes to their sense of self-worth and/or are a way that they contribute their talent to society. For many women, work is a huge part of their identity and can contribute to wellbeing (Zagefka et al., 2021). Some working mothers may feel socially disconnected during maternity leave and miss the positive reinforcement they receive at work, which may less common caring for a newborn who does not yet smile or speak. These personal factors are only part of the picture when exploring a mother's return to work, as financial factors and a lack of affordable childcare play a role in the decisions about when and whether to return to paid work (Dagher et al., 2014).

STAY-AT-HOME MOTHERS

We view being a stay-at-home mother (SAHM) as a family and career choice, as it impacts a woman's identity and defines her responsibilities. Furthermore, SAHMs are completing domestic labor and childcare (Aslam & Adams, 2022). Many women take some sort of leave from work after the birth of a child and therefore experience a temporary period as stay-at-home mother. This can often be a welcome opportunity to focus on motherhood. For others, even a brief period away from a meaningful career can bring a sense of loss of identity or grief. For women who choose or need to remain at home longer term after the birth, counselors should learn how they perceive this circumstance. For example, a woman who identified herself with her career prior to becoming a stay-at-home mother may experience loss and conflicting emotions when choosing to be a stay-at-home mother (Rubin & Wooten, 2007). For other women, being a stay-at-home mother may have been a life-long goal to provide their children with the love and caring attention in the home setting.

For a SAHM, there is no separation between the work context and the home, as the home is the labor setting for SAHMs completing domestic labor and caregiving for their child (or children) (Aslam & Adams, 2022). Furthermore, working hours for a SAHM lack a clearly defined end (Aslam & Adams, 2022). The expectations of mothers and the work of motherhood, especially the intensive mothering standards that many mothers face, are demanding for both working mothers and SAHMs (Crowley, 2014).

Babies and children require constant monitoring and attention to be safe and to thrive and grow in their environment. Providing that constant care and attention means that stay-at-home mothers have not had a break for the entire day by the time a working spouse or partner (if applicable) comes home. Stay-at-home mothers benefit from strong support systems, including family and friends who are also stay-at-home mothers. Finding ways to meet their own needs while simultaneously meeting the needs of their baby and/or children is helpful, such as taking outings to parks or other settings.

Working mothers with paid employment are responsible for many of the same tasks in the domestic sphere as SAHMs and they experience what has been called a second shift consisting of housework and childcare in addition to completing their paid employment, which is distinct from the experience of working fathers (Dugan & Barnes-Farrell, 2020). For heterosexual couples, persistent gender inequities in the domestic sphere mean that working mothers experience more labor demands in terms of housework and care of children than working fathers (Dugan & Barnes-Farrell, 2020). Social support, including support from employers and family and childcare, can enhance working mothers' perceptions of work and family role balance and job satisfaction (Wiens et al., 2022).

WORK FROM HOME MOTHERS

Work from home mothers (WFHMs) describes mothers who complete paid work while also caring for their child (or children) at home. The COVID-19 pandemic and switch to remote work for many professionals resulted in many mothers who had previously worked outside the home becoming de facto work from home mothers. For mothers working from home during the initial period of the COVID-19 pandemic, simultaneously trying to fulfill caregiving roles while also meeting paid employment responsibilities resulted in added stress (Brannon & Wiant Cummins, 2022). Work from home mothering offers flexibility, but often includes interspersed labor and shifts of attention between mothering and work-related activities. The lack of work–life balance/separation and the potential impact on burnout can be a clinical focus with this population.

NAVIGATING MATERNAL ROLES WITH PROFESSIONAL ROLES AND PRIORITIES

Navigating maternal roles with professional roles and priorities can sometimes feel like a no-win scenario, especially pronounced when women first become mothers or with the birth of another baby. While factors such as a flexible workplace and working at home may reduce the tension between work and family roles for mothers (Schott, 2011), the demands of family caregiving and professional responsibilities leave little time or energy for self-care or reflection. Working mothers also experience more cumulative work with responsibilities to home and family constituting what has been called "the second shift": "The persistently gendered nature of the home/family work role results in heavy cumulative workload (i.e., paid work plus home/family work) for working mothers that can excessively drain time and energy resources, resulting in stress" (Dugan & Barnes-Farrell, 2020, p. 64). National data indicate that working mothers complete twice as much housework as working fathers (Dugan & Barnes-Farrell, 2020).

Women who work in less flexible settings with rigid demands struggle when challenges like a sick child or baby needing to be home conflict with required in-person attendance. Women in academia and other professional fields that require advanced education experience a conflict of timing and the pressure to meet maternal and career demands simultaneously, as the reproductive years are concurrent with when they are expected to be the most productive professionally. Sharing her personal experience as an academic mother, Karen Miller writes: "Like many academic moms, my attention was constantly divided between children's needs, the mundane tasks of keeping a household fed, clean, and orderly, learning the explicit and implicit rules of my new institution, and the work of teaching, research, and service" (2021, p. 262). While Dr. Miller acknowledges the privileges that come with a faculty position, including flexibility and typically a private office that allows for pumping breast milk (2021), the demands of both roles can leave a person feeling overwhelmed and unsuccessful.

As discussed above, issues for women in academia include the potential conflict between the tenure clock and the biological clock, as many women who are faculty members delayed having children until after the completion of their PhD and getting settled in an academic position (Miller, 2021). When I (Isabel Thompson) was a junior faculty member, I had my first baby approximately two years after getting my first faculty position. Waiting longer to have children could have jeopardized my fertility; however, giving birth when I did was not optimal when viewed from the lens of advancing an academic career, as I took FMLA after my first son's birth. After my second son's birth approximately four years later, I took FMLA again, pressing pause on professional and career-related pursuits to recover from giving birth, fulfill my mothering role, and connect with my second son.

For women in many careers, taking time away beyond FMLA would be forfeiting years of higher education without a guarantee of being able to find the same level of position in their field. Therefore, many women, including myself, return to work prior to feeling ready, because they do not want to risk putting their career advancement into jeopardy or give up their career. Mothers often successfully juggle the demands of motherhood and career, but the burdens can be fearsome and societal lack of empathy does not help.

Women experience numerous employment disadvantages that are rooted in gender-related discrimination, with increased discrimination against mothers (Peterson Gloor et al., 2021). Working mothers may be perceived as less committed or less engaged than women without children. The combination of discrimination and childcare demands puts working mothers in often challenging situations of juggling childcare needs while meeting professional demands. The individualistic approach to childcare was highlighted by the COVID-19 pandemic, as employers expected mothers and parents to continue working as before, even as the entire childcare and schooling infrastructure of in-person learning dissolved almost overnight. The tenuous nature of working parents' ability to be successful in the paid workforce was starkly noticeable, with a differential impact on mothers.

Even prior to the pandemic and its accompanying differential gendered impact on women and working mothers especially, inequities in the load that working mothers often bear were substantial: "mothers with a child under the age of 6 spend an average of 2.68 hours per day caring for household children; fathers spend 1.58 hours" (US Bureau of Labor Statistics, 2017, as cited in Linde Leonard & Stanley, 2020, p. 1534). Further, married women who become mothers experience an increase in household labor while fathers contribute less to household labor (Linde Leonard & Stanley, 2020). After the birth of a child, gender roles among opposite-sex couples become more traditional (even among couples who had thought of themselves as egalitarian), resulting in married women with children carrying more of the burden of both childcare and household labor (Katz-Wise et al., 2010). While there are exceptions to these general statistics and trends, with some fathers and partners providing more household labor and caring for their children in equitable ways, it is important to validate mothers' lived experiences of inequity. Invalidating a mother's lived experience of inequity, whether in the home or at work, or both, constitutes a sexist and gender-based microaggression. To be culturally competent, counselors must be attuned to the impact of those gender roles and expectations on their client's stress level and mental wellbeing.

But what, might you ask, does childcare and household work have to do with paid employment? For a working mothers (and partners/fathers), childcare is essential in allowing them to perform their best at work while also being able to spare a few moments for self-care. When working mothers spend more time on household labor and childcare than their partners, they are more stressed and overwhelmed. These gender-specific patterns of women being burdened by "second shift" (Dugan & Barnes-Farell, 2020) and/or "interspersed second shift" labor reflects gender-based inequity that impacts domestic division of labor and is also present in the paid work environment. Thus, mothers often experience discrimination and increased labor in home and paid work environments, with decreases in recognition and wages, respectively. What has traditionally been viewed as "women's work" in the home, such as childcare, cooking, and cleaning, is often undervalued both within the home environment and by society at large.

FEMINISM AND SEXISM IN THE WORKPLACE AND GENDER ROLE SOCIALIZATION

Women's life stages, role changes, and caregiving responsibilities sometimes conflict with workplace expectations and demands. These sorts of conflicts are heightened during pregnancy and in the immediate postpartum. For instance, employers might be displeased when a person becomes pregnant and be concerned about their job performance and/or the impact of upcoming leave time, though they are not legally allowed to discriminate against a pregnant person due to the *Pregnancy Discrimination Act of 1978*, which was enacted to protect pregnant people in employment settings. Discrimination also impacts women who do not have children but are perceived to be of childbearing age and therefore may become pregnant after being hired, as explored in a study of hiring managers' attitudes (Peterson Gloor et al., 2021).

Applying a feminist framework, one of the primary principles of which is that "the personal is political," can be helpful when counseling working mothers (Gladding & Newsome, 2018, p. 319). For example, while a working mother who chooses to breastfeed and returns to her paid employment has made a personal choice for their baby, this choice can have broader implications. Depending on the nature of the work setting, her personal choice to breastfeed may be perceived as political as she strives to pump and sustain her breastfeeding goals while also meeting her work requirements.

The feminist approach, which emphasizes empowerment and an egalitarian relationship between the client and the counselor (Gladding & Newsome, 2018), can be especially effective when addressing work-related issues in which gender and/or motherhood has been a source of discrimination or inequity. Counselors employing a feminist therapy framework can help their clients explore gender role socialization and analyze messages they receive around being a woman and mother and how these may impact their self-efficacy in work settings.

The gender role expectations of women as caregivers impacts how they relate to their work roles and their domestic roles as mothers. For example, in her memoir

Becoming, Michelle Obama wrote about tempering her work ambitions so that she could support her two daughters when her husband, former President Barack Obama, was serving as state senator and commuting between their home in Chicago and his apartment at the Illinois state capital (Obama, 2018). She also describes the juggling of roles and mental load that working mothers experience, such as using a lunch hour to pick up a quick birthday present for her daughter's friend's upcoming party while also trying to grab a quick bite to eat (Obama, 2018).

Employees who are mothers may be perceived as less committed to their work than other women. Researchers conducting a meta-regression analysis of 49 studies found that the United States drove the motherhood wage penalty and that the penalty was approximately 4 percent per child (Linde Leonard & Stanley, 2020). This result could reflect both the added household labor working mothers are doing as compared with working fathers, as well as the cost to career advancement of birthing and caring for young children and the resulting increase in accompanying household labor that primarily falls to women (Linde Leonard & Stanley, 2020). Validating working mothers' experiences and helping working mothers have a place to share their load and find resources to support them is essential in effective clinical work.

MULTIPLE PERSPECTIVES: FATHERS/PARTNERS

While this chapter primarily focuses on the challenges that mothers face when trying to navigate their career and motherhood, fathers and partners also face work-related challenges with their parenting roles. For instance, the lack of guaranteed paid family leave in the United States often negatively impacts new fathers and partners. This negative impact is especially salient for families who are living in poverty or working in industries that do not protect workers' rights.

Fathers or same-sex partners sometimes return to work before they feel ready, often a few days or less than a week after their baby is born, due to financial stressors and needing to keep their employment. This can negatively impact their bonding with their baby and their capacity to provide support for the mother (or parent) providing primary childcare. Some couples are forced to ration unpaid leave time between them, while other workers with gig employment may not have any guaranteed unpaid leave.

Working fathers are under pressure to demonstrate that their commitment to their employer remains strong, while taking time to care for their children and adjust to the demands of fatherhood. Working fathers may face penalties in the workplace if they adjust their working hours or responsibilities to take on more caregiving of their children (Kelland et al., 2022).

Stay-at-home fathers (SAHFs) may experience societal discrimination from other adults due to taking on a role that is inconsistent with gendered norms around parenting (Holmes et al., 2020). In a study of SAHFs, they report increased stress and reduced happiness with interacting with adults as compared with spending time with their children (Holmes et al., 2020).

MULTICULTURAL CONSIDERATIONS

Mothers who are members of other marginalized groups or marginalized identities experience discrimination based on their intersectional identities, including their role as a mother. From an intersectional perspective, a Black cisgender working mother who is a lesbian has a differential experience from a White cisgender heterosexual working mother. While both may experience discrimination based on their identities as women and working mothers, the White working mother simultaneously experiences privileges due to her White cisgender identity whereas the Black working mother who is also a lesbian may experience discrimination based on her race and sexual orientation. Transgender working mothers may face discrimination based on their gender identity, perceived gender, and being a working mother.

Being aware of the pervasive impact of gender role expectations, including the unrealistic standards of intensive mothering culture, is essential, as these expectations negatively impact all mothers, regardless of employment status (Forbes et al., 2021). Counselors and other mental health professionals need to apply this awareness to avoid imposing their own beliefs and/or perpetuating micro-aggressions:

> Without such knowledge and awareness, mental health professionals may inadvertently engage in harmful micro-aggressions or potentially perpetuate the intensive mothering expectations with the clients and families they treat (e.g., suggesting a mother stay-at-home with her children if being a working mother is too stressful).
>
> (Forbes et al., 2021, p. 272)

When working with clients facing career-related concerns, it is often helpful to turn to career-specific resources such as the Minimum Competencies for Multicultural Career Counseling and Development, which address the need for counselors to "practice in ways that promote the career development and functioning of individuals of all backgrounds" (National Career Development Association [NCDA], 2009, p. 1). While these competencies do not directly address pregnancy and motherhood, counselors can apply these principles to the needs of pregnant and working mothers. Understanding that career issues and mental health concerns are often intertwined is also essential to effectively working with career-related issues (Niles & Harris-Bowlsbey, 2017), especially with working mothers navigating the unique demands of melding career and motherhood.

APPLICATIONS TO COUNSELING

Motherhood is a sea change in a person's life. There are different challenges associated with being a working mother or a stay-at-home mother. Whatever path a mother chooses, she may feel judged for her choice. Counselors and other mental health professionals working with mothers need to avoid intentionally or unintentionally communicating judgment about a mother's choice and can help a mother consider options, while being cautious not to impose their own values. If a mother is considering stepping away from paid employment for longer than FMLA, some career paths offer more flexibility for extended leave, but in others a mother is "punished" for taking time off to care for children and may struggle to regain the career trajectory she would have had with a shorter leave. Given the potential career impacts of taking longer leave, career-related considerations such as advancement may be a high priority, even if the financial renumeration for a mother working is equivalent or just slightly more than the cost of paid childcare (in the short-term).

We also recommend exploring if a new mother misses her paid employment and longs to reconnect to her career identity. For mothers who feel torn between their career and role as a mother, exploring possibilities in the non-judgmental, objective setting of a counselor's office can be welcome. Bringing the spouse/partner/baby's father into the conversation and/or encouraging the mother to discuss options can facilitate a family conversation about the benefits and downsides of the mother's return to paid employment or staying at home.

Mothers returning to their paid work roles may feel pressured to perform as they did before, regardless of the new demands on their time and energy as mothers. Given the challenges inherent in the individualistic cultural construction of motherhood, mothers can be left feeling like they are failing or underperforming both as mothers and in their paid employment. Demonstrating empathy about how the stresses of an intensive mothering culture impacts working mothers is a crucial way that counselors can demonstrate attunement to their lived experiences (Lamar et al., 2019).

ETHICAL AND LEGAL CONSIDERATIONS

There are legal protections related to pregnancy, childbirth, and breastfeeding, especially in employment and educational contexts. According to the U.S. Department of Health and Human Services, students in any education setting or activity that receives federal funding have legal protection against discrimination under Title IX (1972), which prohibits sex discrimination, including discrimination based on pregnancy status, a person's sexual orientation, and a person's gender identity (HHS, n.d.). Counselors working in college and university settings and those working with women in educational programs can help clients get needed protections (if applicable).

Sex discrimination due to pregnancy is legally prohibited by the Pregnancy Discrimination Act of 1978, an amendment to Title VII of the Civil Rights Act of 1964, which protects people who are pregnant, those who have recently given birth, and those with related medical conditions (Pregnancy Discrimination Act, 1978). Nursing women who are working have legal protection under the *Breaktime for Nursing Mothers* law, which mandates that employers offer reasonable breaktime for nursing mothers to express milk in a private location that is not a bathroom (DOL, 2010). While these laws are in place to protect pregnant women and mothers who are working, employment settings vary in their level of attentiveness to the needs of pregnant women and working mothers. Counselors can help working pregnant women and mothers to advocate for their needs to be met in compliance with these laws.

BARRIERS TO TREATMENT

Barriers to treatment and early intervention of PPD and other maternal mood disorders include individual factors, such as women not realizing they need treatment or being afraid of the stigma associated with having a mental illness, and systemic factors, such as the lack of guaranteed paid parental leave in the United States (Addati et al., 2014). This leaves many families in the lurch and increases the pressure on mothers as well as fathers/partners to return to paid employment quickly after a child's birth. The duration of maternity leave matters for the health and wellbeing of both mother and baby; maternal mental and physical health and child development are negatively impacted by shorter leave, with increased rates of infant mortality also associated with shorter maternity leave (U.S. Department of Health and Human Services, Maternal and Child Health Bureau, 2011).

While some parents' employers offer paid family leave, this varies by employer and may depend on whether the mother/parent can use paid sick time or vacation time as part of FMLA leave, which leaves many families with unpaid or reduced pay during leave. Returning to work can be a barrier to treatment because a mother may feel too busy and overwhelmed by both her work and parenting responsibilities to find a way to seek treatment and identify a provider they can trust.

Women's experiencing PPD or other mood disorders face compounded challenges of how to manage their mental health symptoms, when and how to seek treatment, and may feel shame as well as an imperative to hide this health concern due to societal stigma around mental health and fear of discrimination or concerns about how employers will perceive their professional competence. This occurs within a society in which misogyny and societal inequities increase the pressure and stress that women feel overall, especially with regards to career development. Gender role expectations and the competing demands of motherhood and career can leave many women feeling overwhelmed and burned out, whether they have a diagnosable or diagnosed mood disorder. Having PPD or another postpartum mood disorder adds another layer of stress for new mothers about to return to the paid workforce. Below are some of the types of questions women with PPD or other peripartum mood disorders may be asking themselves:

Will my symptoms be manageable by the time I am supposed to return to work?

How will I cope with the additional stressors and demands of paid employment?

Will the benefits I derive personally and financially from paid employment be worth the risks of returning to work and spending time apart from my baby?

IMPACT OF THE COVID-19 PANDEMIC

The COVID-19 pandemic shed light on the challenges that many working mothers, fathers/partners, and families faced prior to the pandemic and exacerbated existing challenges. During the early years of the COVID-19 pandemic, many professional women who transitioned to remote work also served as the primary parent responsible for caring for their infants or toddlers (often while overseeing their older children's remote learning). Some women left the workforce to care for their babies, toddlers, or young children and/or facilitate remote schooling for their school-aged children. The gendered impact of the COVID-19 pandemic highlighted the ongoing struggle many women were already facing to meet both caregiving and work responsibilities (Miller, 2021).

Securing childcare is essential to working mothers/parents and their families. Mothers of school-aged children who were "working from home often went back and forth between work and school in what we refer to as a simultaneous shift. Essential workers were engaged in a sequential shift, engaging with children's schoolwork after work and trading off with partners" (Lutz et al., 2022, p. 1). In both cases, working mothers experienced the added stress of directly managing children's schooling.

Even with the greater return to normalcy in the later years of the pandemic, some daycare centers closed permanently, further exacerbating the scarcity of high-quality affordable childcare. The pandemic left working mothers and their families in the lurch, trying to meet childcare demands without previous resources such as in-person schooling and daycare. In the face of these challenges and new demands that primarily fell on mothers, many mothers left the workforce.

The implicit (or sometimes even explicit) message to working mothers during the start of the COVID-19 pandemic with its ensuing disruptions seemed to be "take care of your families and keep them safe while continuing to function professionally as if things are normal, but also upend your whole life and juggle your responsibilities without all the structures you had in place to perform your job and take care of yourself too." The added stress of a global pandemic and childcare resources pulled out from underneath made this a recipe for exhaustion and burnout for many working mothers. In various parts of the world, and in the United States, these direct stressors continued for years, with school and childcare disruptions as new surges required safety measures that precluded in-person schooling or childcare.

CONCLUSION

Mothers work in all sorts of ways. As well as doing unpaid work in the home and caring for their child (or children), the majority also have paid work either at home, by telecommuting, or in an employment setting outside the home. Helping mothers identify their strengths as well as their needs can be a powerful way to leverage their skills to aid in finding a way to navigate various aspects of their identity and get the support they need for their own wellbeing. While there are numerous challenges associated with being a working mother, working mothers demonstrate flexibility and adaptability to manage the numerous demands they encounter at home and at work. Counselors can explore ways for working mothers to increase their social support and access resources.

> **Case Study: Paisley**
>
> Paisley is a White stay-at-home mother (SAHM) who worked for seven years as a special education teacher and worked throughout her pregnancy. Her husband Carl is a police officer. She became pregnant during the first few months of the COVID-19 pandemic. They made the decision for Paisley to stay home after the birth of their first child in part due to the COVID-19 pandemic. Even though many school programs were remote, special education programs were in-person and they wanted to avoid unnecessary exposures. Their baby was born six weeks prematurely and spent a month in the NICU (Neonatal Intensive Care Unit), and their doctors advised being very cautious of COVID-19 exposure as their baby was prone to severe respiratory infections. Furthermore, the cost of childcare was only slightly less than what Paisley would earn working.
>
> Although Paisley adores William and feels a strong bond with him, she misses her career and feels a loss of identity. She is fearful of losing the intellectual dynamic with her husband and that he will not find her as interesting since her day consists of diaper changes, naps, and breastfeeding their son. She misses her coworkers and the sense of accomplishment she felt working with her former students. Due to COVID-19 concerns, she is not going to in-person "mommy and me" classes either and feels isolated. She had been diagnosed with generalized anxiety disorder previously and sought treatment before but stopped taking her medication when she became pregnant due to fears for her baby's wellbeing during pregnancy.
>
> Her anxiety increased with her baby's health issues and fears of COVID-19 exposure. She uses handwipes anytime she goes out, but is still fearful of bringing in germs. Her anxiety also centers on a fear of her baby dying from SIDS (sudden infant death syndrome) and it became more severe as she woke up several times a night worried that her baby might not be breathing.
>
> As a SAHM, she has experienced a loss of individuality and her baby has felt like an appendage. Most days, she cannot even get alone time to use the bathroom. The highlight of her day is taking William for a morning walk to a local park in his stroller. After lunch and his nap, the afternoons drag on. She tries to apply the common advice to "sleep when your baby sleeps" during his nap time and often lays down while he naps, but her mind races with worries about finances, housework, and health concerns, and she does not get any rest. Sometimes she feels unsure how to fill the hours and wishes she had a plan for the day like other

mothers seem to. Lately, when she starts to feel this way, she starts crying and then feels ashamed that she cries in front of William. When her husband gets home from work, she sometimes thrusts William into his arms and runs upstairs crying. Carl is concerned that she seemed overwhelmed and is crying more often. He tries to give her breaks when he gets home from work and time alone on weekends.

In addition to the day-to-day stressors, Paisley feels guilty that she is no longer contributing to the family's finances, even though it was a joint decision for her to stay home to care for their son. At a six-month pediatrician appointment, Paisley began crying when asked how things were going. Although Pasiley has a good relationship with William's pediatrician, she was reluctant to share about how bad her anxiety and crying spells were getting but did share that she was worried about SIDS. The pediatrician reassured her and provided information about SIDS and healthy sleep habits. The pediatrician also provided referral information to a local counselor who specialized in maternal mental health and offered telehealth appointments. Although she was scared to start counseling and concerned about the cost, after talking with Carl about it, Paisley decided to pursue counseling and schedule appointments for when her baby usually napped. The family does not have behavioral health coverage, so will pay out of pocket for the counseling sessions. Carl is hoping that counseling can help Paisley get a handle on her crying, feel happier during the day with William, and help her feel less anxious during the night.

Reflection Questions for Clinicians

- If you were Paisley's counselor, what aspects of Paisley's story and presenting concerns would you want to follow-up with during the assessment process?
- What aspects of Paisley's story may suggest a possible DSM-5-TR diagnosis?
- Do you personally relate to any aspect of Paisley's story or does this case study trigger you in any way? If so, what sort of support or supervision might you need to process your own reactions to Paisley's story?
- How could you apply the STRENGTHS model to develop a case conceptualization of Paisley and an effective treatment plan? What aspects of the STRENGTHS model seem especially salient in this case?

APPLYING THE STRENGTHS MODEL—THE CASE OF PAISLEY

Significant Individual, Infant, Family, Societal, and Cultural Factors

- Paisley became a SAHM after the birth of her son.

- Their baby was born six weeks premature, and their doctor advised them that he was prone to severe respiratory infections.
- Paisley became pregnant and gave birth during the COVID-19 pandemic.

Treatment Barriers

- Paisley has expressed fear about seeking treatment.
- Paisley does not have childcare available for self-care on weekdays or while she pursues treatment.
- The family has limited financial resources and are relying solely on the husband's income and do not have behavioral health insurance to cover counseling appointments.

Risk Factors

- Previous diagnosis of generalized anxiety disorder.
- Increased crying and feelings of guilt and shame.
- Disruption of sleep cycle due to anxiety about SIDS.

Enlisting Support from Family, the Community, and Medical Professionals

- Paisley's husband Carl is supportive and concerned about her wellbeing.
- Paisley's pediatrician checked in with Paisley about her own wellbeing and offered referral information for a local counselor.
- Paisley has made an appointment to meet with the counselor.

Noticeable Symptoms, Severity, & DSM-5-TR Diagnosis OR Needs Identified by Family & Treatment Team

- Paisley is experiencing anxiety that is interfering with her sleep.
- Paisley has a history of generalized anxiety disorder and stopped taking her medication during pregnancy.
- Paisley is experiencing more bouts of crying.

Goals Identified by Family

- Reduce feelings of distress during the day.
- Reduce anxiety at night, especially about SIDS.
- Increase overall wellbeing and happiness

Treatment Recommendations

- Although Paisley has not endorsed suicidal ideation, she presents with sleep disruption, crying, and anxiety as well as feelings of shame and guilt. Complete a suicide risk assessment as part of a thorough assessment process in addition to completing an anxiety assessment such as the Beck Anxiety Inventory.
- Implement Cognitive Behavioral Therapy to address Paisley's thoughts, feelings, and behaviors and increase her positive coping.
- Consider involving Carl in some joint sessions and/or recommending couples therapy to support both members of the couple and enhance their resilience.

Helpful, Protective, and Resilience Factors

- Paisley and Carl have a supportive relationship.
- Paisley is willing to seek help even though she is scared to do so.
- Paisley feels a strong bond with her baby.

Self-Care & Wellness

- Paisley currently takes a walk to the park with William on most days, getting exercise and time outside.
- Carl provides support on weekends for Paisley to have time alone.
- Paisley is proactive with healthcare appointments and has a good relationship with William's pediatrician.

Case Study: Myriel

Myriel is a 38-year-old Black first-time mother of a baby daughter, Jessica. Her partner Eileen is White and seven years older than Myriel. Myriel and Eileen identified a familial sperm donor (Eileen's first cousin), as they wanted their baby to share their genetic backgrounds, and proceeded with IVF. After one miscarriage (after the first implanting of an embryo) their second attempt at having an embryo implanted resulted in a successful pregnancy and the eventual birth of their daughter Jessica. Myriel took the loss of their first pregnancy very hard. It took several months before she agreed to try again. Myriel had a difficult pregnancy with Jessica as she experienced preeclampsia and had to be on bedrest for the last six weeks of the pregnancy. Due to COVID-19 restrictions, although Eileen was able to be present during the birth, Myriel's mother could not be present. Myriel experienced a difficult birth with labor lasting over 24 hours.

Eileen went back to work full-time two weeks after Jessica's birth. Myriel resumed her full-time employment after 12 weeks of FMLA. Her company provided six weeks of paid parental leave and the remaining six weeks she used some accrued vacation time to provide some pay, about half of her typical salary. Myriel and Eileen hired a childcare worker for the first six months after Myriel resumed her full-time employment as an executive at an insurance agency. Due to remote work options during the COVID-19 pandemic, Myriel was initially able to work from home and breastfeed Jessica. Now Myriel's company is expecting all employees to return to the office at least three days per week. Although Myriel and Eileen loved having Jessica at home, they found the childcare costs prohibitive and decided to pursue daycare. They finally found a daycare facility they felt comfortable with that had a slot for Jessica.

Myriel struggled emotionally with Jessica's transition to daycare and being back in the office more often. She misses checking on Jessica and being able to breastfeed her. Now she is adjusting to pumping at work. Myriel often feels a sense of guilt while working and wishes she could be with Jessica, yet when she picks up Jessica, she also feels guilty that she is ending the workday earlier than she used to. In prioritizing Jessica, she wonders if she is perceived as not having the same level of commitment as she used to and is fearful about an upcoming annual review. She sometimes has trouble focusing during meetings and often thinks about Jessica and what she might be doing.

She is having difficulty concentrating and is experiencing indecisiveness, which are new issues impacting her efficiency at work. Although Myriel is not trying to lose weight, she has lost a significant amount of weight in a short time, and she has almost no appetite. Myriel and Eileen take Jessica to a local park several times a week and play with her daily at home. Eileen is concerned that Myriel seems emotionally shut down and does not seem to enjoy playing with Jessica like she used to. Eileen is also concerned that Myriel no longer does yoga like she used to before Myriel was born.

Myriel decided to attend sessions with an online Executive Wellness Coach to help her with her efficiency and decision-making at work. Eileen wants Myriel to see a counselor or psychologist in addition, to make sure that Myriel gets the support she needs to feel better. Eileen is worried that Myriel may be more distressed than she is letting on. Myriel is willing to try counseling but is a little bit scared that her employer will find out that she is pursuing mental health treatment.

Reflection Questions for Clinicians

- If you were Myriel's counselor, what factors would you address first in treatment?
- Do you see evidence of a possible DSM-5-TR diagnosis for Myriel?

- Are any aspects of Myriel and Eileen's story triggering for you? If so, how could you address this in supervision/consultation/your own therapy?
- How could you demonstrate cultural humility working with Myriel?

APPLYING THE STRENGTHS MODEL—THE CASE OF MYRIEL

Significant Individual, Infant, Family, Societal, and Cultural Factors

- Myriel experienced preeclampsia and had to go on bedrest for the last six weeks of her pregnancy and experienced a difficult birth with a long labor.
- Myriel and Eileen are in a same-sex marriage and pursued pregnancy with a sperm donor and IVF.
- Myriel became pregnant during the COVID-19 pandemic.

Treatment Barriers

- Myriel already feels pressured for time as a working mother in an executive level position.
- Myriel is more comfortable pursuing services with an executive wellness coach than a counselor or psychologist.
- Fear of stigma by employer associated with pursuing treatment for mental health concerns.

Risk Factors

- History of prior miscarriage after first round of IVF.
- Myriel experienced the medical complication of preeclampsia during pregnancy and had to go on bedrest for the last six weeks of the pregnancy.
- Difficult birth lasting over 24 hours.

Enlisting Support from Family, the Community, and Medical Professionals

- Eileen is supportive of Myriel pursuing counseling.
- Collaborate with the executive wellness coach to communicate need for treatment beyond coaching.
- Work with a psychiatrist and primary care provider to ensure that Myriel has a complete physical and psychiatric assessment.

Noticeable Symptoms, Severity, & DSM-5-TR Diagnosis OR Needs Identified by Family & Treatment Team

- Seeking support to manage guilt about being a working mother.
- Myriel has experienced significant weight loss recently (not seeking to lose weight).
- Myriel is having trouble concentrating and is experiencing indecisiveness.

Goals Identified by Family

- Eileen wants Myriel to have counseling support to help her feel better.
- Reduce the guilt Myriel feels about being a working mother.
- Increase overall wellbeing and ability to enjoy time with Jessica.

Treatment Recommendations

- Start treatment with a counselor or other mental health professional.
- Implement CBT (Cognitive Behavioral Therapy) to address emotions of guilt, and related thoughts and feelings.
- Recommend full psychiatric assessment and referral to a primary care provider to assess for any general medical condition that could account for unwanted weight loss.

Helpful, Protective, and Resilience Factors

- Myriel and Eileen have a strong relationship.
- Myriel is willing to seek treatment.
- Myriel has self-awareness that she could benefit from treatment.

Self-Care & Wellness

- Commitment to playing and spending time with her daughter.
- Spending time at a local park.
- Increase self-care activities to support her own wellbeing.

REFERENCES

Addati, L., Cassirer, N., & Gilchrist, K. (2014). *Maternity and paternity at work: Law and practice across the world.* Geneva, Switzerland: International Labour Office.

Andres, E., Baird, S., Bingenheimer, J. B., & Markus, A. R. (2016). Maternity leave access and health: A systematic narrative review and conceptual framework development. *Maternal and Child Health Journal, 20,* 1178–1192. doi:10.1007/s10995-015-1905-9

Aslam, A., & Adams, T. L. (2022). "The workload is staggering": Changing working conditions of stay-at-home mothers under COVID-19 lockdowns. *Gender, Work & Organization 29*(6), 1764–1778. doi:10.1111/gwao.12870

Bell, E., Hunter, C., Benitez, T., Uysal, J., Walovich, C., McConnell, L., Vega, C., Cisneros, N., Hidalgo, L., Reyes Walton, J., & Wang, M. (2022). Intervention strategies and lessons learned from a student-led initiative to support lactating women in the university setting. *Health Promotion Practice, 23*(1), 154–165. doi:10.1177/15248399211004283

Brannon, G. E., & Wiant Cummins, M. (2022). "Never time to do anything well": Mothers' reported constraints during a pandemic. *Journal of Family Studies*, 1–20. doi:10.1080/13229400.2022.2057349

Burns, E., Gannon, S., Pierce, H., & Hugman, S. (2022). Corporeal generosity: Breastfeeding bodies and female-dominated workplaces. *Gender, Work & Organization, 29*(3), 778–799. doi:10.1111/gwao.12821

Crowley, J. E. (2013). Perceiving and responding to maternal workplace discrimination in the United States. *Women's Studies International Forum, 40*, 192–202.

Crowley, J. E. (2014). Staying at home or working for pay? Attachment to modern mothering identities. *Sociological Spectrum, 34*(2), 114–135. doi:10.1080/02732173.2014.878605

Dagher, R. K., Hofferth, S. L., & Lee, Y. (2014). Maternal depression, pregnancy intention, and return to paid work after childbirth. *Women's Health Issues, 24*(3), e297–e303. doi:10.1016/j.whi.2014.03.002

Dugan, A. G., & Barnes-Farrell, J. L. (2020). Working mothers' second shift, personal resources, and self-care. *Community, Work & Family, 23*(1), 62–79. doi:10.1080/13668803.2018.1449732

Forbes, L. K., Lamar, M. R., & Bornstein, R. S. (2021). Working mothers' experiences in an intensive mothering culture: A phenomenological qualitative study. *Journal of Feminist Family Therapy: An International Forum, 33*(3), 270–294. doi:10.1080/08952833.2020.1798200

Gladding, S. T., & Newsome, D. W. (2018). *Clinical mental health counseling in community and agency settings* (5th ed.). Pearson.

Holmes, E. K., Wikle, J., Thomas, C. R., Jorgensen, M. A., & Egginton, B. R. (2020). Social contact, time alone, and parental subjective well-being: A focus on stay-at-home fathers using the American Time Use Survey. *Psychology of Men & Masculinities, 22*(3), 488–499. doi:10.1037/men0000321

Hyde, J. S., Essex. M., Clark, R., & Klein, M. (2001). Maternity leave, women's employment, and marital incompatibility. *Journal of Family Psychology, 15*(3), 476–491. doi:10.1037/0893-3200.15.3.476

Internal Revenue Service (IRS). (2022). IRS Fact Sheet. *IRS updates the 2021 Child Tax Credit and Advance Child Tax Credit frequently asked questions.* https://www.irs.gov/pub/newsroom/fs-2022-03.pdf

Johnson, K. M., & Salpini, C. (2017). Working and nursing: Navigating job and breastfeeding demands at work. *Community, Work & Family, 20*(4), 479–496. doi:10.1080/13668803.2017.1303449

Julian, M., Le, H.-N., Coussons-Read, M., Hobel, C. J., & Dunkel Schetter, C. (2021). The moderating role of resilience resources in the association between stressful life events and symptoms of postpartum depression. *Journal of Affective Disorders, 293*, 261–267. doi:10.1016/j.jad.2021.05.082

Katz-Wise, S. L., Priess, H. A., & Hyde, J. S. (2010). Gender-role attitudes and behavior across the transition to parenthood. *Developmental Psychology, 46*(1), 18–28. doi:10.1037/a0017820

Kelland, J., Lewis, D., & Fisher, V. (2022). Viewed with suspicion, considered idle and mocked-working caregiving fathers and fatherhood forfeits. *Gender, Work & Organization, 29*(5), 1578–1593. doi:10.1111/gwao.12850

Lamar, M. R., Forbes, L. K., & Capasso, L. A. (2019). Helping working mothers face the challenges of an intensive mothering culture. *Journal of Mental Health Counseling, 41*(3), 203–220.

Lambermon, F., Vandenbussche, F., Dedding, C., & van Duijnhoven, N. (2020). Maternal self-care in the early postpartum period: An integrative review. *Midwifery, 90*, 102799. doi:10.1016/j.midw.2020.102799

Linde Leonard, M., & Stanley, T. D. (2020). The wages of mothers' labor: A meta-regression analysis. *Journal of Marriage and Family, 82*(5), 1534–1552. doi:10.1111/jomf.12693

Lutz, A., Lee, S., & Bokayev, B. (2022). Intensive mothering in the time of coronavirus. *Journal of Social Issues*, 1–25. doi:10.1111/josi.12515

Miller, K. E. (2021). The ethics of care and academic motherhood amid COVID-19. *Gender, Work & Organization, 28*(S1), 260–265. doi:10.1111/gwao.12547

National Career Development Association. (NCDA). (2009). Minimum competencies for multicultural career counseling and development. https://www.ncda.org/aws/NCDA/asset_manager/get_file/26627?ver=50664

Niles, S. G., & Harris-Bowlsbey, J. (2017). *Career development interventions in the 21st century* (5th ed.). Pearson.

Obama, M. (2018). *Becoming*. Crown Publishing.

Peterson Gloor, J. L., Okimoto, T. G., & King, E. B. (2021). "Maybe baby?" The employment risk of potential parenthood. *Journal of Applied Social Psychology, 52*, 623–642. doi:10.1111/jasp.12799

Plotka, R. (2012). *Maternity leave, mother–child interactions, and attachment*. UMI Number: 3512306. Doctoral dissertation. Fordham University. APA PsycInfo.

Roskam, I., & Mikolajczak, M. (2020). Gender differences in the nature, antecedents and consequences of parental burnout. *Sex Roles, 83*(7–8), 485–498. doi:10.1007/s11199-020-01121-5

Rubin, S. E., & Wooten, H. R. (2007). Highly educated stay-at-home mothers: A study of commitment and conflict. *The Family Journal, 15*(4), 336–345.

Schott, W. B. (2011). *Returning to the workforce: The effects of family policy, motherhood, and schooling on women in the workforce*. [Doctoral dissertation. University of Pennsylvania]. UMI 3475913. ProQuest, LLC.

Sterling, H. M., & Allan, B. A. (2020). Construction and validation of the Quality of Maternity Leave Scales (QMLS). *Journal of Career Assessment, 28*(2), 337–359.

U. S. Department of Health and Human Services. (HHS). (n.d.). Title IX of the Education Amendments of 1972. https://www.hhs.gov/civil-rights/for-individuals/sex-discrimination/title-ix-education-amendments/index.html

U.S. Department of Health and Human Services, Health Resources and Services Administration, Maternal and Child Health Bureau. (2011). Women's Health USA 2011.

United States Department of Labor [DOL]. (2010). Break time for nursing mothers. http://www.dol.gov/whd/nursingmothers/U. S. Equal Employment Opportunity Commission. *Pregnancy Discrimination Act*, 1978. https://www.eeoc.gov/statutes/pregnancy-discrimination-act-1978.

Vair, H. (2009). *Work and motherhood: Challenging or reinforcing gendered dualisms?* [Doctoral dissertation, The University of New Brunswick].

Wiens, D., Theule, J., Keates, J., Ward, M., & Yaholkoski, A. (2022). Work–family balance and job satisfaction: An analysis of Canadian psychologist mothers. *Canadian Psychology/Psychologie Canadienne*. (No pagination specified.)

Zagefka, H., Houston, D., Duff, L., & Moftizadeh, N. (2021). Combining motherhood and work: Effects of dual identity and identity conflict on well-being. *Journal of Child and Family Studies, 30*, 2452–2460. doi:10.1007/s10826-021-02070-7

11

Treatment Approaches for Peripartum Depression

Eric S. Thompson

with contributors Katlyn Bagarella and Tyler Elizabeth Hernandez

Personal Narrative

I was 26 when I had my first child, who is now 5 years old, Wow! I was healthy and had a relatively healthy pregnancy and enough medical care. My family is present and, overall, we have gotten along well. Having a child impacted my wellbeing in a big way. I thought I was prepared for the challenges, but when depression took over it got difficult. Being an African American woman has exposed me to feelings of isolation, mistrust of professionals, feeling like I am not being heard/misunderstood, little support from my partner, and an overwhelming feeling of needing to carry the burden on my own. I live in a crowded neighborhood and my family is close to me but when I started to become depressed … I don't know how to explain it, I began to feel so overwhelmed and isolated. I mean I am here with all of these people around me who are just trying to make it out of here alive. We only have public transportation, and I didn't really know anyone here, so I am just here mostly alone with my child, my new responsibilities, and all of these thoughts. I know I have old friends to call, but it felt like I couldn't reach out to them or that it would matter; I mean, even if I asked for help, I don't know what I would say.

My family tries to help but they have to work a lot and my partner's family became less welcoming after birth. It was weird, they would look away from me and would barely greet me so I didn't feel like I should talk to them, let alone ask for help. I couldn't sleep, and I didn't want to really be around anyone, and I just wanted to stay away from everyone. Even when I got a call from family, I just stare at the phone ringing, not sure what I should do; I was paralyzed with my emotions and the weight of the isolation.

Another problem is that I didn't feel like I could trust anyone. It was scary because I had a session with my counselor whom I've been talking to for a while. I told her that I needed help and that as a new mother I didn't think I had the ability to take care of my baby, that I was always scared, and worried, and so overwhelmed by the burden. I was just trying to tell her my fears so that I could get support and feel understood. Within 24 hours there were people knocking down my door saying that I am not fit to keep my baby and that I don't want them or can't cope with this new role. So I fought back and they realized eventually what I was saying and that I do have family support. I felt so betrayed. I just needed help with coping, not for them to try to take my baby away. People will judge you and they will even act like they are all open and nice and being confidential but they are taking down your history and they know how to work the system. It's not right.

Another time I was out at the store and my baby was being loud. They weren't listening so I raised my voice to get their attention and tell them to quiet down so they don't bother anyone. And some manager just walked up to me telling me that I'm too loud and that I gotta go. It's like I am always afraid of being misunderstood and being judged as a bad mother, when I am doing everything that I know how to take care of my baby.

The other problem is that my partner changed too. My partner just stopped helping. When he started to see me depressed it was like he didn't know how to handle it so he'd go out all the time; gym, clubs, anything but sit here with us. It starts to drive you crazy because you both wanted to have this baby then he stops being there. It makes me feel like I'm doing this all alone and that I don't want to do all of this by myself. Instead of worrying about connecting and building a family, I was worrying about my partner and if they'll stay. It like he didn't know how to be a father like this, like he was disappointed in how we built our family and didn't know how to get help. For a long time, I didn't think that I could ask him for help anyway.

The preceding personal narrative is integrated into a first-person narrative from the experiences of many women of color living in poverty, as illustrated by Keefe et al. (2021).

The purpose of this chapter is to describe the applications of evidence-based psychotherapeutic approaches to the treatment of perinatal depression (experiences of anxiety and or depression during or a year after the first-year postpartum). The chapter will revisit the STRENGTHS model for case conceptualization and will discuss relevant theoretical underpinnings for understanding PPD outcomes. The contents of this chapter will emphasize:

unique elements of existing treatments, predictors of peripartum depression (PPD) outcomes, the role of the therapeutic relationship, overview of current treatments and recommendations for integration into practice, behavioral therapies, interpersonal psychotherapy, solution-focused brief approaches, and complementary and alternative approaches to treatment.

PERINATAL DISTRESS

Perinatal depression, also known as postpartum depression, is a type of mood disorder that can occur during pregnancy or in the first year after childbirth. It is a serious condition that affects up to 20 percent of women who have given birth and can have significant impacts on the health and wellbeing of the caregivers and the child (Cena et al., 2020; Mughal et al., 2019). There are several factors that can contribute to the development of perinatal depression, including individual risk factors such as a history of depression or other mental health disorders, social factors such as a lack of social support or relationship stress, and contextual factors such as exposure to trauma or stress during pregnancy.

Depression in the postpartum period was not recognized until the fourth edition of the DSM. The time after birth has so many hopes for the future but the challenges of late nights of sleep deprivation, body image issues, and issues surrounding possibly birth trauma. Treatment for perinatal depression typically involves a combination of medication and therapy and may also include support from loved ones and community resources. This chapter will focus primarily on mental health treatment modalities of perinatal depression.

EFFICACY OF TREATMENT MODALITIES FOR PPD

Current treatment modalities for peripartum depression include medication, therapy, and additional support as needed. Most psychological therapies used for peripartum depression are short term and range between 6 and 20 sessions; 10–12 is most common. While there is no diagnosis of postpartum depression in the DSM-5-TR, clients typically experience a unipolar major depression that frequently develops within the first two months after birth (O'Hara & Engeldinger, 2018a). Peripartum depression is commonly treated with medication and in conjunction with other forms of treatment from a mental health professional (e.g., psychiatrist, clinical mental health counselor, social worker, case managers, and nurses). Effective and evidence-based non-pharmacological treatment modalities have been identified: cognitive behavioral therapy (CBT), interpersonal psychotherapy (IPT), and other treatments including Internet-based CBT and brief solution-focused therapies (Huang et al., 2022; Kaya & Guler, 2022; O'Hara & Engeldinger, 2018a).

COMMON EXISTING TREATMENTS

Horowitz and Goodman (2005) identified a number of psychotherapeutic approaches to treat PPD, including cognitive behavioral therapy (CBT), interpersonal therapy (IPT), supportive psychotherapy, and psychoeducation. Table 11.1 summarizes key aspects of these approaches to treating PPD.

Table 11.1

Common Existing Treatments for PPD

Cognitive-behavioral therapy (CBT) is a time-limited treatment approach that usually lasts 12 to 14 weeks. It focuses on how thoughts shape how a person feels and behaves. It aims to help individuals identify distorted perceptions of the world and themselves and replace them with thoughts that lead to more desirable outcomes (X. Li et al., 2022; Z. Li et al., 2020).

Interpersonal therapy is another time-limited treatment approach focusing on the individual's interpersonal relationships, role transitions, grief, and interpersonal challenges. In the context of treating postpartum depression, it may also focus on the individual's relationships with their infant and partner, as well as their transition back to work and other roles (Sockol, 2018; Tan, 2020).

Psychoeducation is a treatment approach that involves providing factual information to the client about their current problems and health status. In the context of treating postpartum depression, it may involve discussing problems related to infant care, relationships, role transitions, and other specific difficulties, and offering problem-oriented solutions. Psychoeducation is often combined with supportive psychotherapy (Janssen et al., 2018; Rowe et al., 2017).

Complementary and alternative treatments is an approach that can be used in conjunction with psychological and/or psychopharmacological treatments. Examples include self-compassion, supplements like Folic acid and Omega 3 Acids, self-care routines, etc. (Dubreucq et al., 2022; Văcăraş et al., 2017).

Source: Adapted from F. D. Horowitz, 1996.

SELECTING A TREATMENT MODALITY

The contents of this chapter focus on many of the empirically driven and widely accepted practices for treating peripartum depression. These include evidence-based therapies such as cognitive behavioral therapy (CBT), solution-focused/brief, and interpersonal psychotherapy (IPT). Many other theories can be integrated into a theoretical framework that is practical and works. The STRENGTHS model can be useful to help clinicians process the many factors that guide case conceptualization. Cognitive behavioral theory can help clinicians work with maladaptive automatic thoughts, dispute faulty beliefs, and set new goals and expectations. Interpersonal psychotherapy uses similar techniques to discuss how social roles shift during perinatal adjustment. Clinicians might find that an IPT approach alone does not fit the circumstances and that perhaps a more feminist perspective or multicultural approach would serve as a strong support to theory integration. Likewise, it is important to consider other perspectives such as a feminist or multicultural approach, or to incorporate motivational interviewing to support the CBT process in clients who struggle with help-seeking behavior. Table 11.2 details common theories and types of treatments.

Table 11.2
Description of Common Treatments

Theory	Description of treatments
Cognitive	Unrealistic expectations of childbirth and motherhood may lead to anxiety, perfectionism, and compulsive tendencies. Depressive mood is caused by thought disturbances, such as pessimism toward oneself and the future. Lack of suitable role models can lead to a lack of control and anxiety in caring for the infant (Güney et al., 2022; Muñoz et al., 2007).
Social and Interpersonal	Environmental factors and interpersonal struggles can affect mental health. Relationship uncertainties can lead to depression and anxiety. Insufficient social support and marital conflicts can contribute to postpartum disorders. Sudden psychosocial changes and stresses during motherhood may trigger PPD (Lenze & Potts, 2017; Tan, 2020).
Behavioral	Depressive episodes can result from major life events that disrupt normal support patterns. Stressors such as parental divorce, low parental emotional support, and self-esteem can predict PPD. Depression may be a result of decreased positive reinforced behavior or negative feedback from social reinforcement behaviors (Dimidjian et al., 2016; Le et al., 2011).
Feminist	Environmental factors, oppression, social role expectations impact mental health. Deal with the context to manage the possible trauma of giving birth, managing body image issues, anxiety, sleep deprivation, etc. (Krzemieniecki & Doughty Horn, 2022).

ROLE OF THE THERAPIST

The above-mentioned modalities all emphasize a strong therapist–client relationship. While these theories are all effective it can be more beneficial to use them in conjunction. The STRENGTHS model can be a useful tool for clinicians to process the variety of factors that drive case conceptualization. For instance, while the therapist should be actively involved in IPT, they should generally avoid giving frequent advice. However, the therapist should assist the client in developing their own problem-solving capabilities rather than relying solely on advice. However, in the case of IPT for PPD, the therapist may be more directive in certain areas. This may include helping the mother find resources for childcare, managing the role shift to becoming a mother, or offering practical advice on resources and support for issues like nursing or feeding.

Furthermore, some births may have complications like a peripartum hysterectomy where the infant survived but the mother was traumatized. Such delicate and often painful experiences require a unique combination of treatment skills and understanding of the mother's experience (De La Cruz et al., 2013). Thus, a feminist or multicultural perspective may serve as a strong support to integrate theory into these cases as well as the introduction of other practices like deep breathing and self-compassion.

COGNITIVE BEHAVIOR THERAPY

Below is a case study illustration of when a CBT approach would be helpful in addressing the client's presenting concerns and symptoms. This case will be used to demonstrate how to utilize the skills and activities taught in CBT.

> **Case Study: Carey**
>
> Carey has a lovely three-week-old child and has noticed anxiety and feelings of isolation setting in. Her partner works full-time and has become less emotionally available over the last month. This leads Carey to feel disappointed and she begins to ruminate on her sense of self-worth. Carey describes herself as a perfectionist and has a master's degree in accounting and in law. While financially stable, her career has taken a secondary role since giving birth. Carey describes her time spent working less as a necessary part of having a child but that she can't wait to get back to work soon.
>
> When Carey has moments of feeling alone, tired, and vulnerable she begins to ruminate into further irrational thinking that provides grounds for panic and anxiety. She becomes worried about her physical exercise and appearance (e.g., how does she keep on track with her career, and is she capable of keeping a child alive?). Carey also notices that there appears to be a hidden expectation that she does the housework, dishes, cleaning, etc. and it is starting to become unmanageable. When challenged in therapy about asking others for support, Carey explained how she could do this on her own, that it's not too bad, she just needs to do more earlier in the day, and that it feels like it would be a burden to ask others to help with such mundane and easy things.

The therapist can help Carey challenge her irrational thoughts by questioning the evidence supporting them and looking for alternative perspectives. For example:

- "I cannot take time to care for myself. I have to take care of the baby and all of the household activities now!" Carey could challenge this thought by asking herself, "Is it true that I can't take time to care for myself? What evidence do I have to support this belief? What if I said that I can work towards balance."
- "Exercise and good nutrition are exhausting and take too much time out of the day. I won't make any progress so I might as well give up now." Carey could challenge this thought by asking, "Are exercise and good nutrition always exhausting? Is it possible to make progress with small, manageable steps?"
- "I cannot ever burden others for help as I am not worthy of love like that." Carey could challenge this thought by asking herself, "When have I felt worthy of love?"

By questioning and reframing these negative thoughts, Carey could develop a more balanced and realistic perspective of her experiences.

> **Reflection Questions for Clinicians**
>
> - If you were working with Carey from a CBT approach, how would you develop a strong therapeutic alliance while also addressing her irrational preoccupations?
> - What aspects of Carey's story are most compelling for you? Do any aspects of her story trigger a personal reaction that you would need to seek supervision/consultation regarding?

THERAPEUTIC BENEFITS FOR PPD

In general, CBT was an effective treatment modality for perinatal maternal depression, anxiety, and stress in multiple time periods and modalities. The unique needs of someone experiencing perinatal depression need careful individual consideration; thus, the common CBT interventions developed to treat general depression may not be suitable interventions. Li et al. (2022) suggest that CBT interventions with the perinatal population must therefore be tailored to meet their specific needs. A new mother who is dealing with finding social meaning in her new role would likely benefit from IPT as a primary theoretical approach and integrate CBT as necessary. CBT approaches emphasize maternal beliefs and behavioral constraints present during pregnancy (O'Mahen et al., 2013; Shortis et al., 2020). In a meta-analysis of psychological treatments of perinatal depression, a significant effect was found and persisted for 6–12 months after treatment (Cuijpers et al., 2021; Stuart & Koleva, 2014).

Cognitive behavioral therapy is an effective treatment for depression and anxiety and has been used frequently to treat peripartum depression. The process typically occurs once per week over 12–16 weeks and entails helping clients become more active behaviorally and addresses maladaptive beliefs and thought processes (Corey et al., 2017). Problem solving, goal setting, and role plays are used frequently as well. Cognitive behavioral therapy has been used to treat peripartum depression by helping mothers develop bonding relationships with their babies, linking pleasant activities with positive moods, and to seek social support. Cognitive behavioral therapies have strong research support for the treatment of depression (Society of Clinical Psychology, 2021). Most CBT sessions are offered in group formats as opposed to individual sessions. Likewise, groups are a cost-effective method of providing this type of treatment and have statistically similar results as individual treatments (Kleiber et al., 2017; Slomian et al., 2019). Of the many techniques and approaches to the treatment of depression using CBT, the approaches and techniques highlighted below have been used in previous studies, recommended by medical agencies, or discussed in perinatal depression workbooks.

Challenging Automatic Thinking

When a challenge occurs, automatic thoughts or emotions emerge in response to the problem. These automatic responses can be useful in some situations like driving or a task requiring quick reactions, however when these automatic processes become maladaptive, they lead to negative outcomes. Thus, it is beneficial to learn how to challenge maladaptive automatic thinking to treat PPD.

For example, a new mother having a difficult time focusing on a big work project due to the timing of the childbirth and leave of absence may experience automatic thoughts of giving up or feelings of lower self-worth. Therapists can help clients refocus these automatic thoughts by first teaching them about the types of negative automatic thoughts or cognitive distortions that can occur. By doing so, the client can learn to identify these distortions and begin "restructuring" thoughts in a more adaptive way. Table 11.3 illustrates various types of negative thoughts and provides examples.

Table 11.3

Types of Negative Automatic Thoughts

Automatic Thought	Description	Example
All-or-Nothing (Black-and-White) Thinking	Thinking only of possible outcomes at either extreme (really good or really bad; black or white) and not seeing all the possible outcomes in between ("gray" area).	"If my baby does not sleep through the night, I am a bad mother, and they will be unhealthy."
Overgeneralization	Making judgments about ourselves or others based on limited experiences. These thoughts typically contain the words "always" or "never."	"I will never get back on track with my career." "He never listens to my concerns."
Fortune-Telling	Believing you can predict the future.	"I just know he is going to leave because we've been arguing since the baby was born."
Mind Reading	Believing you know what others are thinking, typically assuming it is negative, without any real evidence.	"My friends think I am irresponsible for having this child."
Catastrophizing	Imagining the worst-case scenario, no matter how unlikely the reality.	"Since birth, I have not felt romantic, so I am unlovable as a spouse."
Negative Brain Filter	Focusing only on the negative and discrediting the positives or things that are going well.	"I can't enjoy dinner because there will be to many judgmental people there without children."

Source: https://www.anxietycanada.com/articles/automatic-thoughts/Anxiety Canada, 2022.

AUTOMATIC THOUGHT RECORD

As a new mother, Casey has difficulty focusing on a big work project due to the timing of the childbirth and her leave of absence. This concern has led her to think about giving up and has created a sense of lower self-worth. Casey and her therapist have been working on challenging her automatic negative thoughts and have decided to use an Automatic Thought Record to apply the skills learned in session to Casey's everyday life and automatic thinking process. Table 11.4 is an example of one of Casey's five-column thought records relating to automatic thoughts, the emotions connected to it, and alternative more adaptive responses.

Table 11.4
Automatic Thought Record

Situation	1. What event is associated with unpleasant emotion?	Missing the deadline for big work project.
Automatic thought(s)	1. What thought(s)/and/or images went through your mind (before or after the event)? 2. How much did you believe in the thought(s) (1–100%)?	1. I can't believe I missed the deadline; I can never follow through with anything. 2. 90%.
Emotion(s)	1. What emotion(s) did you feel (before, during, or after the event)? 2. How intense was the emotion (1–100%)?	1. Anxious (40%). 2. Sad (20%). 3. Angry (40%).
Adaptive response	1. What cognitive distortion did you make? 2. Challenge negative automatic thought.	1. All or nothing thinking. 2. I missed the deadline for a big work project that I agreed to take on. I am angry with myself for not completing the project on time and I am feeling anxious about how my boss will react. I feel sad about not being able to work like I could pre-baby. This is the first time I have missed a deadline and having a baby has been a big life adjustment. My boss knows that I am a hard worker and that I am adjusting to motherhood. If my boss fires me, I can get a job that fits better for my new lifestyle. The best outcome would be that my boss doesn't realize that I missed the deadline. The most realistic outcome is that my boss asks me to communicate my needs next time to ensure I can set myself up for success in the future.

(Continued)

Table 11.4 **(Continued)**

Automatic Thought Record

Outcome	1. How much do you believe each automatic thought? 2. What emotions do you feel now? 3. What would be good to do?	1. 50%. 2. Anxious (20%), Sad (20%). 3. Ask my boss for an extension and ask my husband to watch the baby when I need to do work.
Questions to ask self to develop an adaptive response		What might go well in this situation? What could I do to accept myself and this situation? What would I say to a good friend who was struggling with a similar situation—having a new baby and a big deadline that they missed? What are alternative, realistic thoughts about myself and this situation that I could try?

INTEGRATING CBT AND MOTIVATIONAL INTERVIEWING FOR HELP-SEEKING BEHAVIORS

A powerful tool to help with CBT is motivational interviewing. Motivational interviewing has been used to treat depression and has also been used with perinatal populations. In one trial, Holt et al. (2017) utilized the Promoting, Motivation, Empowerment, and Readiness (PRIMER) intervention intended to capture the essence of motivational interviewing. The PRIMER intervention has four phases:

1. Elicit the story—The therapist listens and validates the patient's experiences, and discusses depression screening results.

2. Elicit change talk—The therapist assesses the patient's desire and confidence in making changes.

3. Provide information—The therapist provides information, resources, and services to the client. This is more psychoeducational in nature, intended to provide additional supports.

4. Elicit commitment talk—The therapist assesses the patient's commitment to change and works on increasing it if necessary.

In the study, Holt et al. (2017) delivered the above intervention to new mothers during routine health assessments during postnatal consultations. The goal was to increase help-seeking behavior over the 12 months after birth and other measures included depression, anxiety and stress, and barriers to seeking help. Approximately 27 percent of the participants experienced emotional distress post-birth. Those involved in the PRIMER intervention group were four times more likely than the control group to seek help. Of those who received help from a psychologist, almost half attended six or more sessions. The use of motivational interviewing in conjunction with CBT to treat PPD is a skillful way to help new mothers and family members assess their readiness to change and help provide methods to change.

Case of Carey Using the PRIMER Intervention

Therapist: So, Carey, one of our primary focuses during our sessions has been your hesitancy with asking for help. It sounds like you have been taking on all the responsibilities in the house but have not had time to take care of yourself. You are worried about your health and your career. You mentioned that you would like more support from others. What if we considered adding asking for help in your interpersonal communication skillset? How willing are you on a scale of 1–10 to change this scenario (elicit change talk), to ask others for help?

Casey: Whenever I accept help or ask for help from my husband, I automatically get this anxious feeling that I am a horrible mother and that I am lazy. The feeling is so overwhelming that I end up not even being able to relax or get work done. I have found that just doing things by myself is easier because it makes me feel less anxious.

Therapist: So, it sounds like although taking on all of this is physically and mentally taxing, you are hesitant to ask for help because there is this overwhelming feeling of anxiety and maybe even guilt that comes up for you when you accept it. Say we don't change anything about this situation, how do you think that decision would impact you six months from now (emphasizing importance of making change)?

Casey: Exactly, based on how I feel now both physically and mentally I am worried that if I don't change something I am going to lose my job from not being able to keep up with my work. I feel like my frustration towards myself not being able to complete my work has impacted my patience for my husband and baby. I worry that I will start to resent them if my situation continues this way.

Therapist: With these concerns in mind, on a scale of 1–10, "1" being not confident at all and "10" being very confident, how confident are you that you could ask your social support for help?

Casey: Hmmm… I would say a 7.

Therapist: Okay, that seems confident. What makes it a 7?

Casey: I think after having this conversation it has made me realize that although it is hard for me to ask for help because of the feelings I have as a result, I know that if this continues my situation will just become worse, which will continue to be detrimental to health and my ability to be there for my baby. My baby means everything to me.

Therapist: Okay, it sounds like you are aware of the problem and somewhat ready to make changes. What keeps your confidence from being a 10?

> *Casey:* I think it is because of my past experiences trying to work on asking for help. I always ended up feeling worse so I would give up and just do things myself.
>
> *Therapist:* That makes sense that you would be cautious with your level of confidence. It sounds like attempting to make this change in the past has hurt your self-esteem, so you are trying to protect yourself. I am proud of you for being open to trying this out, next week we can touch base to reflect on how it goes. Until then, can we keep working on our self-care behaviors and logging our activities?

Table 11.5

Behavioral Activation Log

Day:	Monday	Completed	Mood rating
Morning	5-min guided meditation	X	7
Afternoon	Eat lunch	X	4
Nighttime	Read story to Jack before bedtime	X	9

Behavior Activation (BA) is a specific CBT skill that helps clients understand how behaviors influence emotions. BA involves helping a client experiencing depression increase activities that can reduce their depressive symptoms. A symptom often seen in depression is a loss of interest in previously enjoyed activities. The goal is for a client to identify those activities once enjoyed and intentionally implement them into their life to improve mood (O'Mahen et al., 2013). A therapist can support a client in developing this skill by collaboratively working on a daily/weekly behavioral activation log. The client can choose two to three activities that are enjoyable and easily achievable. Casey created a behavioral activation log for Monday (Table 11.5). She chose three activities to do and was successful in completing her chosen tasks. Having Casey rate her mood between 1 and 10, with "0" indicating "low mood" and "10" indicating "good mood," allowed both therapist and client to reflect on the impact of the chosen activities on mood. Casey's mood improved significantly by starting her day with meditation and ending it with reading to her son. As Casey continues to complete her logs, the activities that have been shown to boost her mood the most can become more intentionally implemented into her daily life to promote a lifestyle surrounded by values, pleasure, goals, and worth.

Cognitive behavioral methods are cited numerous times as an effective treatment modality for peripartum depression. However, PPD is complex and can involve more than behavioral and thought shifts. When a child is born, a mother and family change their roles. Many mothers find that they need to cut back on work hours; they feel isolated from friends and other enjoyable activities that are typically easier to do without children. Interpersonal psychotherapy helps clients navigate role shifts like this in their interpersonal environment.

INTEGRATING FEMINIST THEORY INTO TREATMENT

Feminist theory posits that women's experiences are unique and heterogeneous. When working with a client, understandings should be based on the client's knowledge and context and therapists must have an authentic understanding of the client's personal experiences of social interactions and marginalization within society (Mollard, 2014). Women's experiences differ from men's and are not homogenous. Likewise in a feminist paradigm, feelings and intuition are considered valid sources of information and resources. A feminist view of PPD accounts for the variety of factors that women experience at multiple levels. The STRENGTHS model covers the multiple sources of valid information a counselor can explore while treating PPD. Feminist therapies can be used in interpersonal psychotherapy as both consider the shifts in the mother's roles and the gaps between the reality of these roles and their expectations. Feminist theory is also helpful to work with a mother to consider how many expectations for motherhood are based off of cultural experiences and societal backgrounds.

Feminist therapy is also used to treat the trauma that can be linked to PPD. A feminist trauma approach can be used to help treat the issues related to PTSD symptoms following childbirth. At times the experience of childbirth gives rise to fears of injury or death, intense pain, and high levels or inappropriate obstetric intervention, and these symptoms are commonly associated with postpartum depression (Krzemieniecki & Doughty Horn, 2022). While there are many treatment methods used for PPD, Krzemieniecki and Doughty Horn (2022) argue that these approaches do not address commonly reported experiences related to the "destruction of identity, disempowerment, lack of trust in the medical community, and social isolation" (p. 120).

A feminist trauma approach responds to the above concerns by focusing on empowerment, egalitarianism, analysis of power, and social location. The traumatic experiences are treated through taking the client as a whole and accounting for external causes of distress connected to their environment (Krzemieniecki & Doughty Horn, 2022). Likewise, trauma-informed practices are used to enhance the client–therapist relationship, minimize distress, and maximize autonomy and traumatic screening. The primary goal of the feminist trauma approach is empowerment through any process that helps, and the individual becoming aware of their power and gaining access to new power. Empowerment comes in many forms and a client's narrative can provide information about their sources of power and how to access them. Empowerment can vary from validating the unique issues of body image that arise from the changes in the body after birth, de-pathologizing understandable responses to extreme stress, like sleep deprivation, and trauma. Like the IPT approaches, an egalitarian relationship is helpful to empower clients to heal from birth-related traumas. Other approaches include gender role analysis and trauma reprocessing (Krzemieniecki & Doughty Horn, 2022).

INTERPERSONAL THERAPY

Interpersonal therapy (IPT) shows strong evidence of research support from the Society of Clinical Psychology (*Interpersonal Therapy for Depression | Society of Clinical*

Psychology, n.d.). In one instance, IPT had an even larger effect size than CBT (O'Hara & Engeldinger, 2018b). IPT is a form of therapy that is based on the assumption that depression is often caused by changes in one's interpersonal environment. The theory suggests that depression can lead to changes in how a person interacts with others, which can lead to more stressful events. The goal of IPT is to address these life stressors and increase social support, with the belief that if the interpersonal context is changed, the likelihood of depression will change as well. During therapy sessions, the focus is on improving relationships that may contribute to depression. IPT typically lasts 12–16 sessions, but as few as 3–8 sessions can be effective (Sockol, 2018; *Interpersonal Therapy for Depression | Society of Clinical Psychology*, n.d.).

The IPT process has four focus areas:

1. Grief
2. Interpersonal role disputes
3. Role transitions
4. Attachment styles

The major adaptations of IPT for women with PPD include an emphasis on the mother's relationships with her infant, partner, family, and friends/support network (Stuart & Koleva, 2014). While most techniques for IPT can be used to treat PPD, special focus is on the mother's issues, her validation, and including a stronger emphasis on psychoeducation regarding the perinatal period and how it impacts relationships (Stuart & Koleva, 2014). Figure 11.1 illustrates the complex treatment processes and factors.

Figure 11.1

Case Formulation for IPT—Areas of Role Stress and Change Diagram

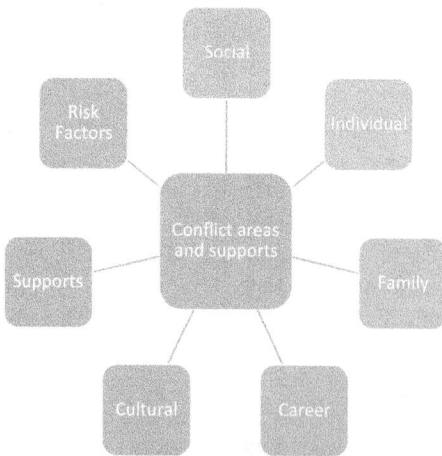

With IPT treatments for depression there are generally three phases of treatment. IPT uses a biomedical model and relies heavily on psychoeducation during the first few sessions to explore the impacts of PPD (Cuijpers et al., 2014; Zlotnick et al., 2016). Once the issues are discussed, the therapist and client negotiate a contract that will help focus treatment and stay focused on the selected problem areas. The second phase of treatment identifies and addresses approximately two of five problems associated with the depression that the mother experiences. The focus is on understanding how the problem is linked to depression. Finally, the termination phase focuses on the general termination process, lessons learned, transferring the skills, and discussion of progress.

The IPT process was modified to treat those with PPD with a partner (Carter et al., 2010; Stuart & Koleva, 2014). These sessions included:

1. *Providing psychoeducation about PPD*—The focus is to review the symptoms, diagnosis, and provide client with psychoeducation about PPD.

2. *Linking PPD to relationship distress*—The focus is to explore the quality of the relationship when PPD became present. The IPT theory emphasizes that the social roles are changing and are causing stress which is a source of relationship distress.

3. *Clarifying the therapeutic contract*—This is where the client and counselor determine the contract, including the roles in therapy, treatment focus, goals, and parameters of the sessions. If working with a couple, the goals and processes are agreed upon by the group, not the individuals.

4. *Assessing the mental health functioning of both the mother and her partner*—In this step, one assesses the symptoms and effects of the mental health functioning. Both partners are assessed, and help is offered to partners who are impacted by their partner's PPD.

5. *Conducting interpersonal inventories*—This process assesses the interpersonal worlds of both members of the relationship. This process focuses on the social supports of each partner. Here the clinician enquires about the impact of the postpartum environment on their relationship with others. They ask how the birth of the child has impacted relationships with others, what support have they expected compared with what has been received, and the relationship with the child.

6. *Exploring relationship models*—This section explores what partners learned from their relationships with their families and other significant members while growing up. This section explores attachment experiences and styles. A new parent might be triggered from the stress of having a new child and they are reminded of how their caretakers were neglectful; then overcompensate by becoming intrusive and overly preoccupied with the infant and become less responsive to the partner, which may destabilize the relationship.

7. *Exploring the history and current conflicts in the relationship*—This section focuses on the bond and the relationship of the two partners. Here the early stages of the relationship, romance, and how they solve conflicts successfully in the past are considered.

8. *Assigning homework to clarify each party's issues, "the dispute list."* This section asks each member to identify two or three issues in their relationship that they want to work on during the middle phase of treatment.

The middle phase of IPT for PPD is generally during session five through ten. The fifth session begins with a discussion of the dispute themes clients were asked to complete during the previous sessions. The skillset for IPT includes open-ended questioning, clarification techniques, positive regard, and specific uses of affect, communication analysis, role playing, decision analysis, and working toward change between sessions. The following example shows a dialogue of someone undergoing treatment for PPD using the IPT framework, specifically the skill of decision analysis.

> *Counselor:* You have missed this work deadline and you are anxious about how your boss will react. What are your options to manage this anxiety?
> *Carey:* Well, I could ask someone to watch the baby while I nap, I could try deep breathing, I could talk to my boss to what their reaction was.
> *Counselor:* Great ideas. Let's keep brainstorming more ideas. What else, what other options?
> *Carey:* I could talk to my husband. I could take a walk and try not to think about it.
> *Counselor:* OK, now that we have discussed some of the options, let's identify the positives and negatives about each option.
> (Counselor and Carey discuss positives and negatives about each option.)
> *Counselor:* OK, now that you have identified the positives and negatives, let's pick one or two options to try during the week.
> *Carey:* OK, I want to try asking someone to watch the baby while I take a nap, and talking to my husband.

The termination phase is typically two sessions and is intended to consolidate gains made in therapy, offering feedback, transferring skills to daily life, and focusing on how the couple has been responsible for these changes.

The IPT treatment process for PPD can help a client manage their new roles and role shifts. Another treatment method, dialectical behavioral therapy (DBT), uses techniques to manage emotional distress, tolerate distress, and increase interpersonal effectiveness. The IPT and DBT treatment methods can be integrated, and the combination may help treat changes and manage the emotional distress that comes from these larger changes.

DIALECTICAL BEHAVIORAL THERAPY

Dialectical behavioral therapy (DBT) is an evidence-based treatment for depression and anxiety and has clinical use for the treatment of perinatal depression (Nunnery et al., 2021). Dialectical behavioral therapy is an effective approach for the treatment of depression, trauma, and anxiety and has been used more recently in the treatment of perinatal depression (Agako et al., 2022; Kleiber et al., 2017; Nunnery et al., 2021). Specific skills trained in the use of DBT include mindfulness, emotion regulation, distress tolerance, and interpersonal effectiveness. It is used individually or in groups. Group sessions would meet approximately two hours per week to discuss attempts to utilize the new skills and reinforce new behaviors. Perinatal periods tend to be full of isolation and the group format may help with these feelings of isolation (Suwalska et al., 2021; Watson et al., 2019).

Dialectical behavioral therapy emphasizes validation as well as challenging clients to change through dialectical thinking. Mindfulness is used as a technique to help clients focus on emotional regulation, acceptance, and the development of loving-kindness for self and others. The mindfulness technique helps to develop the "Wise Mind," where practical and emotional needs are negotiated through a clear perspective full of choices. Mindfulness can be used in conjunction with distress tolerance techniques (Linehan & Wilks, 2015).

Figure 11.2
Types of Mind

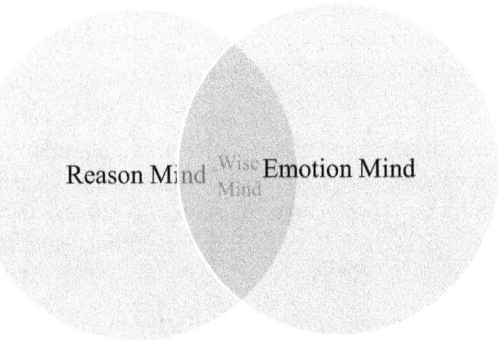

When in reasonable mind, you are driven by facts, reason, logic, and pragmatics. Values and feelings are not important.

When in wise mind, you are able to see the value of both reason and emotion. You are able to use these values to effectively interact and problem solve within your environment.

When in emotion mind you are ruled by your moods, feelings, and urges to do or say things. Facts, reason, and logic are not important.

Source: Adapted from Linehan and Wilks, 2015.

Distress tolerance techniques are methods used to cope with emotional distress. They include distraction, self-soothing, and emotional regulation skills, used during "emotional emergencies." Emotional emergencies are intense periods of emotional distress caused by various factors such as sleep deprivation, health complications, or fear-inducing events. In therapy, therapist and client identify practices to help soothe the client during a crisis, to manage distress and difficult emotions rather than eliminating them.

The therapist and client work to identify practices or activities that will help during an emotional crisis. The goal of distress tolerance skills is to help a client deal with distress and/or difficult and uncomfortable emotions, rather than trying to get rid of difficult emotions or to never have difficult emotions again (Eich, 2015). For example, if someone begins to fall into emotional distress from feeling isolated, they can call a friend, or practice deep breathing/relaxation exercises or the STOP technique to regain emotional regulation. Likewise, the STOP technique, or some other emotional regulation processes, can help with the challenging transition from a night of intermittent sleep and hours of managing a crying baby to being presentable for a conference work call.

The STOP technique is useful for when one is in distress. For example, when Carey gets distressed from work–life tension, she can attempt to regulate her emotions through using the STOP technique. In this case Carey can stop whatever she is doing and pause (S). The next step is to (T) take a breath and focus on the tactile sensations of the breath as it enters and leaves the body. Next, she observes (O) her surroundings and experiences inside and outside. Finally, she proceeds (P). Once she has paused, taken a breath, and observed, then it is time to move forward with the day peacefully. This technique helps one re-engage with the present moment and with reality while disengaging from habitual thought patterns.

Interpersonal effectiveness is useful because it helps clients clarify relationship goals, how to engage in individual and group contexts, and maintain relationships intimacy. One research study used DBT to treat PPD with adolescent mothers. The skills used included mindfulness, interpersonal effectiveness, emotion regulation, distress tolerance that focused on distractions, STOP, self-soothing, weighing pros and cons, and acceptance (Kleiber et al., 2017).

Another trial used a group approach to DBT for the treatment of PPD with seven sessions (Agako et al., 2022). The first session focused on introducing the group and mindfulness, psychoeducation during the perinatal period, and setting group goals. The second session focused on mindfulness skills and the difference between the "Emotion Mind" and accessing the "Wise Mind." Other sessions emphasized mindfulness and psychoeducation and "other skills," including self-soothing, learning to "STOP," and self-validate. The final session wrapped up the group and set new goals to prevent relapse. Each session included homework and additional activities. An outline of their sessions is included in Table 11.6.

Table 11.6
DBT Treatment Sessions

Session	Content		
Session 1	Introductions and group rules.	Overview of mindfulness and five senses.	Psychoeducation on emotion dysregulation during the perinatal period. Setting personal goals for group.
Session 2	Mindfulness psychoeducation and exercise: "What" skill.	Check-in and homework review: Emotion Mind and accessing Wise Mind.	"Other" skills review.
Session 3	Mindfulness psychoeducation and exercise: "How" skill.	Check-in STOP and TIPP (**T**emperature—**I**ntense Exercise—**P**aced breathing and—**P**aired muscle relaxation; https://dialecticalbehaviortherapy.com/distress-tolerance/tipp/)	"Additional" skills review.
Session 4	Mindfulness psychoeducation and exercise: Self-compassion.	Check-in Wise Mind and self-soothe.	"Additional" skills review.
Session 5	Mindfulness psychoeducation and exercise: Mindfulness of thought.	Check-in and homework review: Self-validation.	"Additional" skills review.
Session 6	Mindfulness psychoeducation and exercise: Mindfulness of emotion. Check-in and homework review: Reducing emotional vulnerability, PLEASE skill (https://www.behavioralhealthflorida.com/blog/please-skill-how-can-it-help/), "Other" skills review.		
Session 7	Check-in with personal goals and setting new goals. New teaching: relapse prevention and coping ahead. Debrief and homework assignment.		

SOLUTION-FOCUSED BRIEF THERAPY (SFBT) APPROACHES

With many possible responses to the changes and stressors of having a child, PPD can trigger painful emotional symptoms that are frequently the focus of treatment. Sometimes the emphasis on reducing painful symptoms or solving a problem makes it challenging to stay motivated and participate fully in treatment. Solution-focused brief therapy models (Huang et al., 2022) emphasize the positive aspects of treatment and using their unique strengths to achieve positive outcomes. In a recent study investigating a solution-focused model (SFM) to treat PPD, a five-part series was implemented which included a description of the problem, developing well-formed goals, exploring exceptions, feedback at the end of sessions, and evaluating the effect of the group. A total of 148 participants were divided into an intervention group (SFM) and a control group in a double-blind design. Both groups received routine pregnancy healthcare services without counseling while the SFM group received five sessions from weeks 30–39. Several measures were used to assess the effects of SFM on anxiety and PPD at 28 weeks of gestation, post-delivery, and post intervention. In each measure there were no differences in baseline, yet the treatment group significantly had lower post-delivery and post-intervention scores than the control group. Essentially only five sessions of SFM showed stronger results in the reduction of PPD, anxiety, and sleep disturbances in women from 28 weeks of gestation to six weeks postpartum.

The solution-focused model (SFM) was used to help pregnant women with depression and anxiety. The process involved the following steps:

1. *Describe the problem*: Encouraged pregnant women to express their problems and discus these problems with them and their families. Worked to increase their confidence in solving these issues. When similar problems arise in the future, they were prepared to manage them.

2. *Develop well-formed goals*: Pregnant women were encouraged to set specific and achievable goals based on their circumstances. They were assisted in finding solutions to problems.

3. *Explore for exceptions*: After establishing clear objectives, they continued to discuss exceptions to the problems, or similar problems were easily resolved. The process helped mothers realize that small changes can have an impact. Identifying exceptions was a key focus of the SFM, as it helped the pregnant women define their values, identify changes, and solve problems.

4. *End of session feedback*: Based on previous communication and understanding, they explored strengths, resources, and efforts of the pregnant women and provided positive feedback to enhance chances of achieving their goals. If the expected goals were not met, they discussed the reasons with the pregnant women and adjusted the goals as needed. They also shared the successful experiences of other pregnant women to improve their understanding of the method and increase confidence in solving future problems.

5. *Evaluation effect*: Throughout the intervention process, used graduated questions to emphasize the importance of change to the pregnant women, starting with small changes and gradually increasing the degree of change. Pregnant women were encouraged to build their confidence and realize the impact of their efforts in solving problems.

Relationship in SFBT

The therapeutic relationship is key in the SFBT process. A therapeutic alliance that includes trust and a positive attitude is helpful. The therapist's role of identifying and utilizing client strengths is essential. The process is also eclectic and uses a higher number of techniques than other theoretical orientations, so it is a challenge to stay focused on the client as a holistic person while also utilizing a variety of effective and compelling techniques. The therapeutic process is determined and driven by client goals and feedback.

Solution-focused brief therapy has been used to treat many psychological problems: alone and as a conjoint treatment. The authors found that 74 percent of studies reported significant positive effects from SFBT (Mousavi et al., 2021). Solution-focused brief therapy is useful for preventing PPD symptoms and for generating positive behaviors. A series of assumptions regarding SFBT include that solutions are uncovered through exceptions to them, people have strengths and rely on them to be successful, small achievements lead to hope, solutions have been created by others and can be modelled, there is no perfect solution, so each solution is special. Solutions occur through these positive attitudes, assumptions, and behaviors. The hope is that a client can learn to see that solutions to their issue exist, there are many solutions that can be created or already exist and can be built upon, counselors can use their own strengths to create solutions or model solutions from others. The SFBT approach is useful for time-limited interventions, is cost effective, and relevant for issues related to the treatment of PPD including decreased childbirth fear and increased self-efficacy (Huang et al., 2022; Kaya & Guler, 2022).

Basic Assumptions

The goals of SFBT utilize the abilities, resources, strengths and hopes of the clients. The therapist acts as a researcher who focuses on conditions and aspects of their stories that generate relevance and meaning in the client's life. This approach utilizes past, present, and future orientations.

The solution-focused model is based on several key assumptions about how individuals can find solutions to their problems. These assumptions include (Corey, 2015; Kaya & Guler, 2022; Lethem, 2002; Mousavi et al., 2021):

Exceptions reveal solutions: When an individual encounters a problem, they may think that it is a constant and unchangeable part of their life. However, the SFM posits that there are likely times when there are exceptions to the problem, that it does not occur or is less severe. For example, a therapist can ask a client: Was there a time when you felt more supported? Therapists can help clients by identifying and exploring these exceptions, and individuals can gain insight into how they might solve the problem to make positive life changes.

Small achievements lead to hope: Even small and seemingly insignificant achievements can give individuals a sense of hope and motivation to continue working toward their goals. Recognizing and celebrating these achievements is an important part of the SFM process. If Carey implements some of her self-care plan, that is a cause for celebration. Perfection is not necessary here.

People rely on their own abilities: SFM believes that people have the skills and abilities needed to perform successful behaviors. By focusing on these strengths, individuals can build confidence and find solutions that work best for them. By focusing on Carey's abilities and strengths, she will be able to gain the confidence to ask for help.

Each solution is unique: The SFM recognizes that there is no one-size-fits-all solution to every problem. Each individual's circumstances and needs are unique, and the solutions they develop will be tailored to their specific situation. This means that the SFM is flexible and adaptable, allowing individuals to find solutions that work best for them (Huang et al., 2022; Lethem, 2002; Mousavi et al., 2021).

Others have found solutions: When individuals are struggling to find solutions to their problems, they may feel like they are the only ones facing these challenges. The SFM acknowledges that others have likely faced similar problems and found solutions and encourages individuals to learn from these examples and apply them to their own situations.

Scaling questions: Scaling questions are helpful when observable change is difficult to determine. They can help to uncover various feelings, attitudes, level of confidence, and awareness of their successes. A simple scaling question asks a client to rate on a scale of 1–10 how they feel about their progress. The discussion can focus on the reasons for choosing the number and explore how to improve the experience from a 4 to a 7 over the next few months.

Changing the attitude by reframing: Reframing is a common cognitive technique and can be useful in SFBT as well. It is used to provide an alternative frame of reference (reframe). When Carey gets upset about having to take time away from work, the therapist uses a reframe to highlight how this is a special opportunity for Carey to bond with her child.

Highlighting exceptions: This approach to SFBT includes looking at a time or an experience when the problem did not occur; or when an exception happened. For example, "Was there a time when you did not feel overwhelmed about having the responsibility of a new child?" or "When are there times that you do not feel overwhelmed about xyz?" Exceptions can occur in the past to the time of the problem, unproblematic situations that have occurred recently, cases that occur periodically, and in the future when the problem will be resolved.

Miracle questions: These are among the most popular types of interventions in SFBT. They are used to help one better understand how the solution would appear if obstacles were removed. One simply asks the client something to the effect of, "Imagine that you went to sleep last night, and the problem was resolved while you slept. What is the first thing that you are aware of when you realize that the problem is resolved?" One example would be when a mother woke up later than usual feeling more rested because her partner took care of the child in the morning to let her sleep.

Table 11.7

Structure of Solution-Focused Counseling for Preventing Peripartum Depression during Pregnancy

Session	Issues
1	Welcome and introduction of group members, explanation of the number of sessions, and purpose of counseling sessions. Materials on depression and postpartum blues, including definitions, causes, and symptoms.
2	Precise definition of the problem by the client, setting of specific and achievable goals based on circumstances, and assistance in finding solutions to the problem using SFBT techniques. Assignment of homework.
3	Encouragement of pregnant women to express their problems, discussion of these problems with them and their families, and efforts to increase their confidence in solving these issues. Exploration of exceptions, or times when the problems did not occur or were easily resolved. Detection of exceptions to help pregnant women define their values, identify changes, and solve problems.
4	Assignment of homework and exploration of strengths, resources, and efforts of pregnant women, with positive feedback to enhance chances of achieving goals. Adjustment of goals as needed and sharing of successful experiences of other pregnant women to improve understanding and confidence.
5	Review of previous homework, exploration of exceptions in the lives of pregnant women, and emphasis on the importance of change through graduated questions. Encouragement of confidence and realization of the impact of efforts in solving problems. Summary of the meeting.

Source: Adapted and expanded from Mousavi et al., 2021; Singh & Gotlib, 2014.

SUPPORTIVE APPROACHES AND PSYCHOPHARMACOLOGICAL INTERVENTIONS

Postpartum depression has many treatment modalities and psychopharmacology is one of them. Many of the treatments for PPD are mood stabilizers or antidepressants (Bennett & Sylvester, n.d.). A counselor's role can be to help the client process risk factors to support the medical regimen prescribed to aid in compliance and provide psychoeducation about the normal effects and the effects that require medical attention. Hormonal treatment is also mentioned as a primary psychological intervention by mothers who do not breastfeed (Bennett & Sylvester, n.d.). While the efficacy of this treatment is mixed, counselors can listen and help the family make decisions regarding hormonal therapies and breastfeeding. A key decision point is whether medication will impact breastfeeding and if the benefits of medication outweigh the risks of not taking the medication.

Some patients will benefit from psychopharmacological treatments. Clients experiencing the following clinical factors are most likely to benefit from a combined treatment approach of psychopharmaceuticals and psychotherapy: chronic depression, childhood trauma, comorbid personality disorder, other comorbidity, high levels of suffering and functional impairment, interpersonal problems, psychosocial issues, suicide risk, poor compliance to psychopharmacological interventions (Deng et al., 2020).

COMPLEMENTARY TREATMENT MODALITIES

This section explores complementary approaches to the treatment of PPD. In addition to talk therapy and medication for the treatment of PPD, several complementary treatment modalities may be beneficial for mothers, including breastfeeding, infant massage, exercise, and pre and postnatal yoga. Breastfeeding, while not a treatment for PPD per se, has numerous benefits for both mother and baby as a health behavior.

Breastfeeding

Not all mothers can or are inclined to breastfeed their children for a variety of reasons. This is the choice of the mother and is to be respected. Many alternative health approaches are available to benefit women who do not breastfeed. For those who are able to breastfeed, or are inclined to do so, there are also benefits. Breastfeeding helps to regulate cortisol levels in the blood; cortisol regulation is important for decreasing mothers' stress levels (Figueiredo et al., 2014). In a study of lactating mothers without clinical depression, Mezzacappa (2004) reported that breastfeeding mothers had lower baseline sympathetic nervous system activity and a decreased stress response to a physical stressor when compared with non-breastfeeding mothers. These findings suggest that breastfeeding acts as a buffer for physiological stress responses. The potential of successful breastfeeding experiences to buffer PPD symptoms includes the positive impact of breastfeeding on the mother's physiological stress response.

Moreover, breastfeeding may improve sleep quality and duration in new mothers. Mothers who are well rested have more energy and are less irritable, which may also contribute to an effect of breastfeeding on depressive symptoms (Doan et al., 2007). For example, Doan and colleagues (2014) found that first time mothers who exclusively breastfed slept an average of 30 to 45 minutes more than mothers who supplemented with formula. Mothers of formula-fed infants self-reported more sleep disturbance than breastfeeding mothers (Doan et al., 2007).

While breastfeeding seems to be successful in reducing depressive symptomatology, it does prove to be challenging and detrimental if breastfeeding is perceived as particularly difficult or impossible. For this reason, breastfeeding education and support are imperative. Breastfeeding support groups empower women through education, support, and vicarious experience (Moore & Coty, 2006; Nash et al., 2014; Nolan et al., 2015; Romano, 2007; Sloan et al., 2006). Mothers can come together and discuss breastfeeding challenges they are experiencing and receive validation, understanding, solidarity, and practical advice. However, there is a gap in the literature in regard to treatment of PPD that targets breastfeeding and breastfeeding challenges as an important component in reducing depressive symptoms.

Infant Massage

Research has shown that mothers who utilize infant massage experience a rapid decline in depressive symptomatology when compared with mothers who did not practice infant massage (Holditch-Davis et al., 2014). The decline in maternal depressive symptoms and increased maternal–infant bond is associated with increased maternal sensitivity to infants' needs through infant massage (Kersten-Alvarez et al., 2011).

Exercise

Exercise is beneficial not only for our bodies, but our minds as well. The literature contends that exercise reduces depressive symptomatology and stress by increasing serotonin in the brain and releasing beta-endorphins, which are natural opioids, resulting in improved mood, improved sleep, and increased energy (Abdollahi et al., 2017; Stathopoulou et al., 2006).

Prenatal and Postnatal Yoga

Prenatal yoga can be a helpful complementary approach to managing stress during pregnancy. Postnatal yoga that incorporates baby can be an easy way to get exercise and stress relief. While yoga programs that allow mothers to bring baby with her are relatively rare, they can be especially beneficial for mothers who do not have regular childcare (Uebelacker et al., 2016).

OTHER COMPLEMENTARY AND ALTERNATIVE APPROACHES

A metanalysis of other complementary approaches found benefits for perinatal depression from a variety of approaches including dietary supplements (Deligiannidis & Freeman, 2014). Omega-3 fatty acids have proven benefit for those experiencing depression and the authors "recommend perinatal patients with depression should consume 1 gram EPA plus DHA daily" (Deligiannidis & Freeman, 2014, p. 87). Folate is recommended for pregnant women "to reduce the risk of neural tube birth defects" and it shows promise for reducing depression and supporting maternal mental health as well (Deligiannidis & Freeman, 2014, p. 88).

Bright light therapy involves the use of 7,000-plus lux light and has demonstrated efficacy for treating seasonal and non-seasonal forms of depression, as well as peripartum depression (Deligiannidis & Freeman, 2014). Deligiannidis and Freeman (2014) recommended that mothers experiencing symptoms of depression implement bright light therapy in the morning but should be monitored for any sign of manic or hypomanic episodes. Other promising treatments include exercise, massage, and acupuncture (Deligiannidis & Freeman, 2014).

CERTIFICATION IN PERINATAL MENTAL HEALTH

For clinicians who want to specialize in supporting birthing parents, the Certification in Perinatal Mental Health offered by Postpartum Support International (www.postpartum.net) consists of 14 hours of training about perinatal mood and anxiety disorders as well as six hours of training with a specialty. The three types of certification specialties are: 1) training for counseling/therapists, 2) psychopharmacology for professionals whose scope of practice includes prescribing medications, and 3) training for affiliated professions including occupational therapy and doulas (PSI, n. d.).

BRINGING BABY HOME TRAINING

Bringing Baby Home Training is an evidence-based course designed to teach helping professionals to work with clients on how to maintain healthy relationships during the postpartum period (*Bringing Baby Home Educators Training | The Gottman Institute*, n.d.). The program has 90 videos and offers a 10.5-hour CEU credit. The program covers strengthening friendships, increasing intimacy, managing conflict, and improving the overall wellbeing of selves and children. This program teaches facilitators how to teach a workshop related to the program for their clients.

MULTIPLE PERSPECTIVES: FATHER/PARTNER

While this chapter mainly focuses on maternal mental health, there is good information on paternal mental health. A family therapy approach described by Freitas and Fox (2015) for working with new fathers to support their mental health and address paternal peripartum depression (PPPD) includes eight considerations:

1. Build a strong therapeutic alliance with fathers and help them to develop a language to describe emotional experiences: "Many fathers simply lack the language needed to identify and share their emotional experience" (Freitas & Fox, 2015, p. 423).

2. Connect with the father's emotional experiences about their baby and the transition to fatherhood.

3. Explore fatherhood, and the role of fatherhood, and your client's personal goals as a father.

4. Examine how fatherhood is constructed socially and how this impacts your clients' experiences.

5. Support father–baby bonding and validate "good enough" fathering to support fathers with engaging directly with their babies.

6. Community building to help the father develop a sense of community with other fathers.
7. Collaborative treatment approach that includes other providers.
8. Self-reflection and examining gendered assumptions about fatherhood.

These eight considerations highlight the ways in which fathers need support around their emotional expression and mental health (Freitas & Fox, 2015). Emotional validation and exploring what it means to be a father and to connect with their babies are key aspects of this approach. Therapists' self-reflection is essential to avoid imposing gender-based assumptions and stereotypes on fathers.

MINDFULNESS-BASED INTERVENTIONS

Mindfulness-based interventions have gained prominence as effective interventions for numerous disorders, including depression and anxiety. For example, mindfulness-based cognitive therapy has shown promise as a relapse/recurrence prevention intervention among pregnant women with a history of depression (Dimidjian et al., 2017). There is a link between maternal psychological symptoms and parenting practices (Fernandes et al., 2022) where parents with more depressive and anxious symptoms exhibited more impaired bonding, maladaptive parenting behaviors, and lower levels of mindful parenting. Mindful parenting is the practice of directing complete attention and presence to the child during interactions. This includes a stance of non-judgmental awareness, acceptance of self, self and other regulation, and a compassionate stance toward a child.

Mindfulness of Breath

One simple method of regulating nervous system response and "clearing the mind" is through the soothing practice of attending to one's breath. There are many techniques to explore, but for the purpose of this chapter we will focus on relaxation through a body scan. In this practice one takes first steps toward simply accepting experiences. When meditating, one is encouraged to accept pleasant or unpleasant experiences and to avoid judging what is happening in the mind and body. During the practice, if the attention wanders, one realizes the wandering and recognizes how the mind drifts at times, and at times goes too lax, or too active. At this point one redirects one's mind back to the breath, the tactile sensations of the breath as air enters the lungs and the belly fills with air. Table 11.8 outlines steps to take to begin a relaxing mindfulness of breath practice.

Table 11.8

Mindfulness of Breath–Body Scan and Relaxation

1. Assume a comfortable posture.
2. Bring forth your highest aspirations to be of the greatest benefit to yourself and to others.
3. Bring awareness into field of tactile sensations and remain mindfully present with your tactile sensations.
4. With a witnessing mode of bare attention, without analysis or commentary, settle the body and mind by letting go of the breath and simultaneously letting go of your thoughts.
5. Settle in relaxation, stability, and vigilance.
6. With a vigilant posture of attention, straight spine, and soft abdominal muscles, release involuntary thoughts.
7. While inhaling, observe the sensation of breath throughout the body without preferring or influencing one experience over another.
8. If your mind wanders, come back to the sensations of the breath. Count up to ten at the beginning of the outbreath to refocus.
9. Release all aspirations, imagery, desires, and mental objects.
10. Conclude practice by bringing forth meaningful aspirations for own flourishing and fulfillment and wishes for the world around you.

Self-Compassion

Generally, the concept of compassion is characterized as an attitude or aspiration for one to be free of suffering and the causes of suffering, and self-compassion is included in the umbrella of self/other compassion. It is operationalized into three bipolar components: self-kindness vs self-judgement, mindfulness vs overidentification, and common humanity vs isolation. The process of self-compassion described by Neff (Neff et al., 2019) is an adaptive way of:

> self-to-self relating, characterized by an attitude of care, and understanding toward oneself, the capacity of being aware of one's painful experiences and the recognition that all human beings are imperfect and suffer, can be highly beneficial for mothers experiencing postpartum challenges.
>
> (Fernandes et al., 2022, p. 3)

Mothers who had a negative emotional impact from the COVID-19 pandemic presented lower levels of mindful parenting and self-compassion and had higher levels of PPD than those who did not report a negative impact from the pandemic. The lower levels of self-compassion are possibly attributed to increased threat levels because the pandemic, as an active threat system, prevented mothers from being able to feel calm compassionate toward themselves (Fernandes et al., 2022). Likewise, higher levels of self-compassion are linked to self-kindness, which enables mothers to be aware of their own experiences, be more accepting toward their own growth areas and sufferings, less critical toward their parenting behaviors, and have lower psychological symptoms, greater emotion regulation, and a sense of common humanity.

Simple self-compassion breaks are useful tools to begin practice. One can begin by sitting or lying down, placing hands on heart and taking a few slow, deep breaths. Following the relaxation steps above, begin to identify an area of pain or suffering. Note that this a moment of suffering and suffering is a common part of humanity. While thinking about that suffering say, "May I be free of suffering, may I be kind to myself, may I accept myself or this situation," and generate an aspirational phrase that connects with the client, for example, "May I be free of this suffering, may I be peaceful, may I be protected, may I accept what I cannot change, etc." (Rockman & Hurley, 2015). Once one generates these aspirations, one can extend the wish for others to be free of suffering or simply rest in the relaxed compassionate state, generally experienced in the heart. The Center for Mindfulness Studies has a practical self-compassion workbook to begin a self-compassion and mindfulness journey (Rockman & Hurley, 2015). After a general exploration of these techniques, it is possible to determine if they are appropriate for you; a qualified teacher is indispensable for progress and safety.

Lovingkindness

Lovingkindness is the process of removing the barrier of anger and maliciousness to happiness. Frequently, new mothers deal with negative self-talk, self-criticism, doubt, and being thwarted from self-care. The practice of lovingkindness and other mindfulness-related practices can help shift their focus from ruminating on the anger-inducing event to a genuine acknowledgment that they have loveable qualities, that they deserve to be happy and to flourish, and that cultivating a kind and loving heart leads to kinder behaviors, which lead to calming the nervous system and agitated minds. This can be practiced by simply taking a few deep breaths to relax, or follow the above relaxation steps, and contemplate the following questions (Wallace, 2006; B. A. Wallace, personal communication, 2007):

1. What would make you truly happy, a sense of complete fulfillment?

2. What would you love to receive from the world around you, from those near and far, so that you can find the happiness that you seek?

3. In order to realize the happiness that is your heart's desire from what qualities of behaviour, qualities of mind would you love to be free? And with what qualities would you love to be imbued? How would you love to transform and mature, spiritually evolve as a human being? In short, would kind of person would you love to become?

4. What would you most like to offer to the world around you? Drawing on your own unique background, your skills, your abilities, your aspirations, what is the greatest good that you can imagine?

CONCLUSION

While the peripartum period can be challenging for many mothers and families, there is hope and effective treatments to help mothers who are struggling. In this chapter, we discussed prominent evidence-based treatments for PPD that can help mothers recover and enjoy their experiences as mothers again. We included specific examples of how to apply these in the peripartum context. We also explored complementary approaches to augment traditional therapies and support mothers in their healing process.

APPLYING THE STRENGTHS MODEL—THE CASE OF CASEY

Significant Individual, Infant, Family, Societal, and Cultural Factors

- Partner is working full-time and is less available.
- Carey is career-oriented but struggling with the role shift of having a new baby.

Treatment Barriers

- She is pressed for time and does not think she has time for therapy.
- She can't take time to care for herself due to work and family demands.

Risk Factors

- She feels isolated from her partner.
- She is struggling with negative rumination.
- Difficulty reaching out for help from others.

Enlisting Support from Family, the Community, and Medical Professionals

- Family is supportive of Carey.

Noticeable Symptoms, Severity, & DSM-5-TR Diagnosis OR Needs Identified by Family & Treatment Team

- Negative rumination.
- Feels overwhelmed and overly responsible.

Goals Identified by Family

- Interpersonal communication skills to ask for help.
- Setting boundaries to reduce her stress level and manage parenting demands.

Treatment Recommendations

- CBT to address distorted thinking and challenging automatic thoughts.
- IPT to work with negotiating boundaries in relationships.
- Including relaxation exercises would be helpful.

Helpful, Protective, and Resilience Factors

- She is highly educated.
- She is financially stable.

Self-Care & Wellness

- Setting boundaries to create time for self-care.
- Develop self-care plan and log self-care activities and practices.
- Journaling about her experiences with self-care and impact on wellness.

REFERENCES

Abdollahi, A., LeBouthillier, D. M., Najafi, M., Asmundson, G. J. G., Hosseinian, S., Shahidi, S., Carlbring, P., Kalhori, A., Sadeghi, H., & Jalili, M. (2017). Effect of exercise augmentation of cognitive behavioural therapy for the treatment of suicidal ideation and depression. *Journal of Affective Disorders, 219*, 58–63. doi:10.1016/J.JAD.2017.05.012

Agako, A., Burckell, L., McCabe, R. E., Frey, B. N., Barrett, E., Silang, K., & Green, S. M. (2022). A pilot study examining the effectiveness of a short-term, DBT informed, skills group for emotion dysregulation during the perinatal period. *Psychological Services.* doi:10.1037/SER0000662

Bennett, E. D., & Sylvester, A. N. (n.d.). *Postpartum Depression: What Counselors Need to Know.* Retrieved January 26, 2023, from http://www.counseling.org/library/Article24

Bringing Baby Home Educators Training | The Gottman Institute. (n.d.). Retrieved January 26, 2023, from https://www.gottman.com/professionals/training/bringing-baby-home/

Carter, W., Grigoriadis, S., Ravitz, P., & Ross, L. E. (2010). Conjoint IPT for postpartum depression: Literature review and overview of a treatment manual. *American Journal of Psychotherapy, 64*(4), 373–392. doi:10.1176/APPI.PSYCHOTHERAPY.2010.64.4.373

Cena, L., Palumbo, G., Mirabella, F., Gigantesco, A., Stefana, A., Trainini, A., Tralli, N., & Imbasciati, A. (2020). Perspectives on early screening and prompt intervention to identify and treat maternal perinatal mental health. Protocol for a prospective multicenter study in Italy. *Frontiers in Psychology, 11.* doi:10.3389/fpsyg.2020.00365

Corey, G. (2015). *Theory and Practice of Counseling and Psychotherapy.* Cengage. doi:10.2307/583738

Corey, G., Nicholas, L. J., & Bawa, U. (2017). *Theory and practice of counselling and psychotherapy* (2nd SA ed.). Croatia: Zrinski DD Cengage Learning.

Cuijpers, P., Karyotaki, E., Weitz, E., Andersson, G., Hollon, S. D., & Van Straten, A. (2014). The effects of psychotherapies for major depression in adults on remission, recovery and improvement: A meta-analysis. *Journal of Affective Disorders, 159*, 118–126. doi:10.1016/j.jad.2014.02.026

Cuijpers, P., Franco, P., Ciharova, M., Miguel, C., Segre, L., Quero, S., & Karyotaki, E. (2021). *Psychological treatment of perinatal depression: a meta-analysis.* Psychological Medicine; Cambridge University Press. doi:10.1017/S0033291721004529

De La Cruz, C. Z., Coulter, M. L., O'Rourke, K., Alio, P. A., Daley, E. M., & Mahan, C. S. (2013). Women's experiences, emotional responses, and perceptions of care after emergency peripartum hysterectomy: A qualitative survey of women from 6 months to 3 years postpartum. *BIRTH, 40.*

Deligiannidis, K. M., & Freeman, M. P. (2014). Complementary and alternative medicine therapies for perinatal depression. *Best Practice & Research Clinical Obstetrics & Gynaecology, 28*(1), 85–95. doi:10.1016/J.BPOBGYN.2013.08.007

Deng, P., Yeshokumar, A., Ruzek, J. I., & Miller, B. (2020). *Integrating Psychotherapy and Psychopharmacology in the Treatment of Major Depressive Disorder* (Vol. 37). MJH Life Sciences. https://www.psychiatrictimes.com/view/integrating-psychotherapy-and-psychopharmacology-treatment-major-depressive-disorder

Dimidjian, S., Goodman, S. H., Felder, J. N., Gallop, R., Brown, A. P., & Beck, A. (2016). Staying well during pregnancy and the postpartum: A pilot randomized trial of mindfulness-based cognitive therapy for the prevention of depressive relapse/recurrence. *Journal of Consulting and Clinical Psychology, 84*(2), 134–145. doi:10.1037/ccp0000068

Dimidjian, S., Goodman, S. H., Sherwood, N. E., Simon, G. E., Ludman, E., Gallop, R., Welch, S. S., Boggs, J. M., Metcalf, C. A., Hubley, S., Powers, J. D., & Beck, A. (2017). A pragmatic randomized clinical trial of behavioral activation for depressed pregnant women. *Journal of Consulting and Clinical Psychology, 85*(1), 26–36. doi:10.1037/ccp0000151

Doan, T. H. (2007). *Breastfeeding increases sleep duration in new mothers and fathers* (Doctoral dissertation, UCSF).

Doan, T., Gay, C. L., Kennedy, H. P., Newman, J., & Lee, K. A. (2014). Nighttime breastfeeding behavior is associated with more nocturnal sleep among first-time mothers at one month postpartum. *Journal of Clinical Sleep Medicine, 10*(3), 313–319. doi:10.5664/jcsm.3538

Dubreucq, J., Kamperman, A. M., Al-Maach, N., Bramer, W. M., Pacheco, F., Ganho-Avila, A., & Lambregtse-van den Berg, M. (2022). Examining the evidence on complementary and alternative therapies to treat peripartum depression in pregnant or postpartum women: Study protocol for an umbrella review of systematic reviews and meta-analyses. *BMJ Open, 12*(11), e057327. doi:10.1136/BMJOPEN-2021-057327

Eich, J. (2015). *Dialectical behavior therapy skills training with adolescents: A practical workbook for therapists, teens & parents.* PESI Publishing and Media. https://books.google.com/books?hl=en&lr=&id=MJc7BgAAQBAJ&oi=fnd&pg=PR17&dq=eich+dbt+2015&ots=pBHpZ5PL_N&sig=y5iliMoUs46HzcmlkAexnX_hHC4#v=onepage&q=eich dbt 2015&f=false

Fernandes, D. V., Canavarro, M. C., & Moreira, H. (2022). Self-compassion and mindful parenting among postpartum mothers during the COVID-19 pandemic: The role of depressive and anxious symptoms. *Current Psychology, 1,* 1–13. doi:10.1007/S12144-022-02959-6/TABLES/3

Figueiredo, B., Canário, C., & Field, T. (2014). Breastfeeding is negatively affected by prenatal depression and reduces postpartum depression. *Psychological Medicine, 44*(5), 927–936. doi:10.1017/S0033291713001530

Freitas, C. J., & Fox, C. A. (2015). Fathers matter: Family therapy's role in the treatment of paternal peripartum depression. *Contemporary Family Therapy, 37*(4), 417–425. doi:10.1007/s10591-015-9347-5

Güney, E., Cengizhan, S. Ö., Karataş Okyay, E., Bal, Z., & Uçar, T. (2022). Effect of the Mindfulness-Based Stress Reduction program on stress, anxiety, and childbirth fear in pregnant women diagnosed with COVID-19. *Complementary Therapies in Clinical Practice, 47*, 101566. doi:10.1016/j.ctcp.2022.101566

Holditch-Davis, D., White-Traut, R. C., Levy, J. A., O'Shea, T. M., Geraldo, V., & David, R. J. (2014). Maternally administered interventions for preterm infants in the NICU: Effects on maternal psychological distress and mother–infant relationship. *Infant Behavior and Development, 37*(4), 695–710. doi:10.1016/J.INFBEH.2014.08.005

Holt, C., Milgrom, J., & Gemmill, A. W. (2017). Improving help-seeking for postnatal depression and anxiety: A cluster randomised controlled trial of motivational interviewing. *Archives of Women's Mental Health, 20*(6), 791–801. doi:10.1007/s00737-017-0767-0

Horowitz, F. D. (1996). Developmental perspectives on child and adolescent posttraumatic stress disorder. *Journal of School Psychology, 34*(2), 189–191. doi:10.1016/0022-4405(96)00007-6

Horowitz, J. A., & Goodman, J. H. (2005). Identifying and treating postpartum depression. *Journal of Obstetric, Gynecologic & Neonatal Nursing, 34*(2), 264–273. doi:10.1177/0884217505274583

Huang, C., Han, W., & Hu, S. (2022). The effects of the solution-focused model on anxiety and postpartum depression in nulliparous pregnant women. *Frontiers in Psychology, 13*, 1586. doi:10.3389/fpsyg.2022.814892

Interpersonal Therapy for Depression | Society of Clinical Psychology. (n.d.). Retrieved January 3, 2023, from https://div12.org/psychological-treatments/treatments/interpersonal-therapy-for-depression/

Janssen, L., Kan, C. C., Carpentier, P. J., Sizoo, B., Hepark, S., Schellekens, M. P. J., Donders, A. R. T., Buitelaar, J. K., & Speckens, A. E. M. (2018). Mindfulness-based cognitive therapy v. treatment as usual in adults with ADHD: A multicentre, single-blind, randomised controlled trial. *Psychological Medicine*, 1–11. doi:10.1017/S0033291718000429

Kaya, N., & Guler, H. (2022). Online solution-focused psychoeducation as a new intervention for treating severe fear of childbirth: A randomized controlled trial in the pandemic period. *Perspectives in Psychiatric Care.* doi:10.1111/ppc.13038

Keefe, R. H., Rouland, R., Lane, S. D., Howard, A., Brownstein-Evans, C., Wen, X., & Parks, L. (2021). "I gotta carry the burden by myself": Experiences of peripartum depression among low-income mothers of color. *Advances in Social Work, 21*(1), 176–198. doi:10.18060/23937

Kersten-Alvarez, L. E., Hosman, C. M. H., Riksen-Walraven, J. M., Van Doesum, K. T. M., & Hoefnagels, C. (2011). Which preventive interventions effectively enhance depressed mothers' sensitivity? A meta-analysis. *Infant Mental Health Journal, 32*(3), 362–376. doi:10.1002/IMHJ.20301

Kleiber, B. V., Felder, J. N., Ashby, B., Scott, S., Dean, J., & Dimidjian, S. (2017). Treating depression among adolescent perinatal women with a dialectical behavior therapy-informed skills group. *Cognitive and Behavioral Practice, 24*(4), 416–427. doi:10.1016/J.CBPRA.2016.12.002

Krzemieniecki, A. J., & Doughty Horn, E. A. (2022). Counseling clients with postpartum posttraumatic stress disorder: A feminist-trauma approach. *Journal of Mental Health Counseling, 44*(2), 117–132. doi:10.17744/mehc.44.2.02

Le, H. N., Perry, D. F., & Stuart, E. A. (2011). Randomized controlled trial of a preventive intervention for perinatal depression in high-risk latinas. *Journal of Consulting and Clinical Psychology, 79*(2), 135–141. doi:10.1037/a0022492

Lenze, S. N., & Potts, M. A. (2017). Brief interpersonal psychotherapy for depression during pregnancy in a low-income population: A randomized controlled trial. *Journal of Affective Disorders, 210*, 151–157. doi:10.1016/j.jad.2016.12.029

Lethem, J. (2002). Brief solution focused therapy. *Child and Adolescent Mental Health, 7*(4), 189–192. doi:10.1111/1475-3588.00033

Li, X., Laplante, D. P., Paquin, V., Lafortune, S., Elgbeili, G., & King, S. (2022). Effectiveness of cognitive behavioral therapy for perinatal maternal depression, anxiety and stress: A systematic review and meta-analysis of randomized controlled trials. *Clinical Psychology Review, 92*, 102129. doi:10.1016/J.CPR.2022.102129

Li, Z., Liu, Y., Wang, J., Liu, J., Zhang, C., & Liu, Y. (2020). Effectiveness of cognitive behavioural therapy for perinatal depression: A systematic review and meta-analysis. *Journal of Clinical Nursing, 29*(17–18), 3170–3182. doi:10.1111/jocn.15378

Linehan, M. M., & Wilks, C. R. (2015). The course and evolution of dialectical behavior therapy. *American Journal of Psychotherapy, 69*(2), 97–110. doi:10.1176/appi.psychotherapy.2015.69.2.97

Mezzacappa, E. S. (2004). Breastfeeding and maternal stress response and health. *Nutrition Reviews, 62*(7), 261–268.

Mollard, E. (2014). *Exploring Paradigms in Postpartum Depression Research: The Need for Feminist Pragmatism.* doi:10.1080/07399332.2014.903951

Moore, E. R., & Coty, M. B. (2006). Prenatal and postpartum focus groups with primiparas: Breastfeeding attitudes, support, barriers, self-efficacy, and intention. *Journal of Pediatric Health Care, 20*(1), 35–46. doi:10.1016/J.PEDHC.2005.08.007

Mousavi, S. A., Ramezani, S., & Khosravi, A. (2021). Solution-focused counseling and its use in postpartum depression. In *The Neuroscience of Depression: Features, Diagnosis, and Treatment* (pp. 443–446). Academic Press. doi:10.1016/B978-0-12-817933-8.00047-5

Mughal, M. K., Giallo, R., Arnold, P. D., Kehler, H., Bright, K., Benzies, K., Wajid, A., & Kingston, D. (2019). Trajectories of maternal distress and risk of child developmental delays: Findings from the All Our Families (AOF) pregnancy cohort. *Journal of Affective Disorders, 248*, 1–12. doi:10.1016/j.jad.2018.12.132

Muñoz, R. F., Le, H. N., Ippen, C. G., Diaz, M. A., Urizar, G. G., Soto, J., Mendelson, T., Delucchi, K., & Lieberman, A. F. (2007). Prevention of postpartum depression in low-income women: Development of the mamás y bebés/mothers and babies course. *Cognitive and Behavioral Practice, 14*(1), 70–83. doi:10.1016/j.cbpra.2006.04.021

Nash, Z., Mascarenhas, L., & Nathan, B. (2014). A re-evaluation of the role of rotational forceps: Retrospective comparison of maternal and perinatal outcomes following different methods of birth for malposition in the second stage of labour. *BJOG: an International Journal of Obstetrics and Gynaecology, 121*(5), 642–643.

Neff, K. D., Tóth-Király, I., Yarnell, L. M., Arimitsu, K., Castilho, P., Ghorbani, N., Guo, H. X., Hirsch, J. K., Hupfeld, J., Hutz, C. S., Kotsou, I., Lee, W. K., Montero-Marin, J., Sirois, F. M., De Souza, L. K., Svendsen, J. L., Wilkinson, R. B., & Mantzios, M. (2019). Examining the factor structure of the Self-Compassion Scale in 20 diverse samples: Support for use of a total score and six subscale scores. *Psychological Assessment, 31*(1), 27–45. doi:10.1037/PAS0000629

Nolan, A., Kennedy, S., O'Malley, A., Kirwan, M., Hughes, A., Barry, A., Goodwin, V., Cunningham, A. M., Coyne, H., & Nugent, L. (2015). Mothers' voices: Results of a survey of public health nurse-led breastfeeding support groups. *Primary Health Care, 25*(7), 26–31. doi:10.7748/PHC.25.7.26.E998

Nunnery, R., Fauser, M., Hatchuel, E., & Jones, M. (2021). The use of Dialectical Behavioral Therapy (DBT) techniques creatively in the treatment of perinatal mood and anxiety disorders. *Journal of Counseling Research and Practice, 6*(2). https://egrove.olemiss.edu/jcrp/vol6/iss2/3

O'Hara, M. W., & Engeldinger, J. (2018a). Treatment of postpartum depression: Recommendations for the clinician. *Clinical Obstetrics and Gynecology, 61*(3), 604–614. doi:10.1097/GRF.0000000000000353

O'Hara, M. W., & Engeldinger, J. (2018b). Treatment of postpartum depression: Recommendations for the clinician. *Clinical Obstetrics and Gynecology*, *61*(3), 604–614. doi:10.1097/GRF.0000000000000353

O'Mahen, H., Himle, J. A., Fedock, G., Henshaw, E., & Flynn, H. (2013). A pilot randomized controlled trial of cognitive behavioral therapy for perinatal depression adapted for women with low incomes. *Depression and Anxiety*, *30*(7), 679–687. doi:10.1002/DA.22050

Postpartum Support International (n.d.). Certification in Perinatal Mental Health. https://www.postpartum.net/professionals/certification/

Rockman, P., & Hurley, A. (2015). Discovering self-compassion. *Self-Compassion and Mindfulness*. The Centre for Mindfulness Studies. https://www.mindfulnessstudies.com/wp-content/uploads/2015/09/Self-Compassion_and_Mindfulness.pdf

Romano, A. M. (2007). A changing landscape: Implications of pregnant women's internet use for childbirth educators. *The Journal of Perinatal Education*, *16*(4), 18–24. doi:10.1624/105812407X244903

Rowe, H. J., Wynter, K. H., Burns, J. K., & Fisher, J. R. W. (2017). A complex postnatal mental health intervention: Australian translational formative evaluation. *Health Promotion International*, *32*(4), 610–623. doi:10.1093/heapro/dav110

Shortis, E., Warrington, D., & Whittaker, P. (2020). *The efficacy of cognitive behavioral therapy for the treatment of antenatal depression: A systematic review*. doi:10.1016/j.jad.2020.03.067

Singh, M. K., & Gotlib, I. H. (2014). The neuroscience of depression: Implications for assessment and intervention. *Behaviour Research and Therapy*, *62*, 60. doi:10.1016/J.BRAT.2014.08.008

Sloan, S., Sneddon, H., Stewart, M., & Iwaniec, D. (2006). Breast is best? Reasons why mothers decide to breastfeed or bottlefeed their babies and factors influencing the duration of breastfeeding. *Childcare in Practice*, *12*(3), 283–297. doi:10.1080/13575270600761743

Slomian, J., Honvo, G., Emonts, P., Reginster, J. Y., & Bruyère, O. (2019). Consequences of maternal postpartum depression: A systematic review of maternal and infant outcomes. *Women's Health*, *15*. doi:10.1177/1745506519844044

Society of Clinical Psychology. (2021). *Depression | Society of Clinical Psychology*. https://div12.org/psychological-treatments/disorders/depression/

Sockol, L. E. (2018). A systematic review and meta-analysis of interpersonal psychotherapy for perinatal women. *Journal of Affective Disorders*, *232*, 316–328. doi:10.1016/j.jad.2018.01.018

Stathopoulou, G., Powers, M. B., Berry, A. C., Smits, J. A. J., & Otto, M. W. (2006). Exercise interventions for mental health: A quantitative and qualitative review. *Clinical Psychology: Science and Practice*, *13*(2), 179–193. doi:10.1111/J.1468-2850.2006.00021.X

Stuart, S., & Koleva, H. (2014). Psychological treatments for perinatal depression. *Best Practice and Research: Clinical Obstetrics and Gynaecology*, *28*(1), 61–70. doi:10.1016/j.bpobgyn.2013.09.004

Suwalska, J., Napierała, M., Bogdański, P., Łojko, D., Wszołek, K., Suchowiak, S., & Suwalska, A. (2021). Perinatal mental health during Covid-19 pandemic: An integrative review and implications for clinical practice. *Journal of Clinical Medicine*, *10*(11), 2406. doi:10.3390/jcm10112406

Tan, H. J. R. (2020). An illustration of interpersonal psychotherapy for perinatal depression. *Case Reports in Psychiatry*, *2020*. doi:10.1155/2020/8820849

Uebelacker, L. A., Battle, C. L., Sutton, K. A., Magee, S. R., & Miller, I. W. (2016). A pilot randomized controlled trial comparing prenatal yoga to perinatal health education for antenatal depression. *Archives of Women's Mental Health*, *19*(3), 543–547. doi:10.1007/S00737-015-0571-7

Văcăraş, V., Vithoulkas, G., Buzoianu, A. D., Mărginean, I., Major, Z., Văcăraş, V., Dan Nicoară, R., & Oberbaum, M. (2017). Homeopathic treatment for postpartum depression: A case report. *Journal of Evidence-Based Complementary and Alternative Medicine, 22*(3), 381–384. doi:10.1177/2156587216682168

Wallace, B. A. (2006). *The attention revolution: Unlocking the power of the focused mind.* (1st ed.). Wisdom Publications.

Watson, H., Harrop, D., Walton, E., Young, A., & Soltani, H. (2019). A systematic review of ethnic minority women's experiences of perinatal mental health conditions and services in Europe. *PLoS ONE, 14*(1). doi:10.1371/journal.pone.0210587

Zlotnick, C., Tzilos, G., Miller, I., Seifer, R., & Stout, R. (2016). Randomized controlled trial to prevent postpartum depression in mothers on public assistance. *Journal of Affective Disorders, 189*(3), 263–268. doi:10.1016/j.jad.2015.09.059

Index

Note: Locators in *italic* indicate figures, in **bold** tables and in ***bold-italic*** boxes.

4Ps Plus 129–130

ableism 51
abortion 117
ACA Code of Ethics (2014) 188, 209
adoption: adoptive mothers 154, 160; counseling 160–161, 162–163; ethical/legal considerations 180; LGBTQ+ 163; multicultural considerations (racial, gender) 160; postadoption depression (PAD) 131–132, *132*; stressors 131; transracial 160
Ahrons, C. 162
Alcohol Use Disorders Identification Test-Concise (AUDIT-C) 129
American Association of Sexuality Educators, Counselors, and Therapists (AASECT) 188–189
American Rehabilitation Counseling Association (ARCA) 51
Americans with Disabilities Act (1990) 61
anxiety, peripartum, postpartum *71–72*; assessment, screening 127–128, **128**, 130; career return *219–220*; COVID-19 pandemic 61, 140; definition/criteria (DSM) 7, 34; first time fathers/partners 159; first time mothers 98, 151–152, 153; home / social support and 25, **34–35**, 80, 253; older siblings 114; perinatal loss, previous 132–133, 141–143, *141*; sexual difficulties 141–143; stepmothers 155; traumatic birth, previous 114; treatment **247**, 248, 249, 259, 262, 269
ARCA Task Force on Competencies for Counseling Persons with Disabilities 51
Asian Americans 164
Ask Suicide-Screening Questions (ASQ) Tool 127
Assess, Intervene and Monitor for Suicide Prevention (AIM-SP) model 136, **136**
assessment tools: Depression Screening Scale (PDSS) **128**; Edinburgh Postnatal Depression Scale (EPDS) *4*, 85, 127, **128**; Patient Health Questionnaire-9 (PHQ-9) *3*, 85, 127, **128**; Perinatal Anxiety Screening Scale (PASS) 127, **128**, 130; Postpartum Depression Screening Scale (PDSS) 127, **128**; Postpartum Distress Measure (PDM) 127, **128**, 131; PPSC Suicide Assessment (PPSC) **128**; PTSD Checklist for DSM-5 (PCL-5) *3*
assistive reproductive technology (ART) 117, 153
Association for Multicultural Counseling and Development 48
attachment: interpersonal therapy (IPT) 256, 257; LGBTQ+ parents 206; online support / COVID-19 pandemic 211–212, **212**; patterns and relationships 11–12, 133, 162; process 81, 154, 199, *199*, 200–201 (*see also* bonding); styles 186–188; theory 187, 200–201, 202
Attitudes toward Motherhood Scale (AToM) 152
automatic thinking 249–250
automatic thought record **250**, 251, **251–252**

"Baby Blues" 6–7, 23, *24*, 126, 140
Baur, K. 180–182
Beck Depression Inventory (BDI) 127
Becoming (Obama) 229
behavior activation (BA) 254, **254**
Biopsychosocial Theoretical Model 84
bipolar I / II disorder with peripartum onset 26, 129
birth trauma *149*; infant 20; mother 9, 73, 80, 108–109; racial/ethnic health disparities 46
Black communities, COVID-19 pandemic, impact 61
Black mothers, breastfeeding 21, 205
Black mothers, systemic risk factors, health access/outcomes 14–15, 44–45, 46–47, 110, 164, 230
Black working mothers, maternal leave 44–45
Bobst, Ryanna 3–4
bonding, father/family–infant 159, 205, 229
bonding, mother–infant 5, 82, 98, 198–202, **199**; breastfeeding 78–79, 201–202; counseling 206–209, *208*; COVID-19 pandemic, impact 119, 190; difficulties, disruption, postpartum anxiety 130, 204; interruptions 110; multicultural considerations 205–206; non-biological mothers 153–154; PPD coping strategies 204–205; PPD

impact (mother, baby) 198–204; PPD treatment barriers 209–211; sensitivity, parental 11; treatment approaches, recommendations 267; *see also* attachment
bonding, multicultural considerations 205–206
Breaktime for Nursing Mothers law 231–232
breastfeeding: *Breaktime for Nursing Mothers* law 231–232; Drugs and Lactation Database (LactMed) 208; mother–infant bonding 78–79, 201–202; societal judgement 74–75; support 84; working mothers 224
Brief Sexual Function Index for Women (BSFI-W) 176, **177**
bright light therapy 267
Bringing Baby Home Training 268

career and identity 219–234; academic career vs motherhood 226–227; counseling 230–231; COVID-19 pandemic, impact 227, 233; ethical/legal considerations 231–232; fathers, families 229; gender role socialization 229; gender-based discrimination, feminism and sexism 226–227, 228–229; maternal role and professional priorities 226–228; multicultural considerations 230; PPD treatment barriers 232–233; PPD: work and motherhood 220–221; stay-at-home mothers (SAHM) 220, 225, 230, **234–235**; women, identity, career 220–221; work-from-home mothers (WFHMs) 165, 225–226, **238**; working mothers 221–224 (*see also* FMLA leave; maternity leave; working mothers); case conceptualization; *see* STRENGTHS model of case conceptualization case examples; *see* STRENGTHS model application, case examples
Caesarean section / C-section **97**, **99**, 104, 106, 109, 110, **149**, **173**, **197**
City Birth Trauma Scale 130
cognitive behavioral therapy (CBT) 30, 245–246, **246–247**, 248–249, **248**, 252–253, 254–256
Competencies for Addressing Spiritual and Religious Issue in Counseling (ASERVIC) 55–57, **56**
Competencies for Counseling Military Populations (MGCA) 60
Competencies for Counseling with Lesbian, Gay, Bisexual, Queer, Questioning, Intersex, and Ally Individuals (ALGBTIC LGBQQIA Task Force) 57–58, **58–59**, 61, 160
Competencies for Counseling with Transgender Clients (ACA) 57, 59–60, 160
Competencies for Multicultural Career Counseling and Development 230
complementary treatment for childless stepmothers (CSMs) 163

conception 100; infertility 100, 116–117; LGBTQ+ couples 113–114; risk factors 101
coping skills, positive 31
couple dynamic, shifts after pregnancy/birth 173–190; couple counseling 185–188, **186**, **187–188**; ethical and legal considerations, counseling 188–189; father/partner 179–180; Imago therapy 184–185, **185**; multicultural considerations 180; parenting 178–179; parenting, role/responsibility sharing 177–178, 183–185; sexual/intimacy difficulties and dysfunctions 175–182, **177**, **182**
COVID-19 pandemic, impact: birth plan restrictions 117, 119, 164–165, **237–238**; gender-/race-based inequalities 61; health care access 125; isolation 86, 98, 98–**100**, 164–165, 213–214; maternal isolation 13–14; maternal mental health impact 140, 270; mental health 189–190, 213–214; online support, opportunities 14, 86, 98, 211–212; "ordinary" pregnancy rituals 55; parenthood stress 190; pregnancy and birth experiences 13; sexuality, couple 189–190; working mothers, fathers/partners, families 233
CRAFFT 129, 130
Crenshaw, K. E. 48
Crooks, R. 180–182
Crugnola, R. 153
cultural humility as counseling approach 48
cultural norms/expectations, pregnancy and birth 2; *see also* multicultural considerations

Deligiannidis, K. M. 267
Diagnostic and Statistical Manual of Mental Disorders (DSM-4, DSM-4-TR, DSM-5, DSM-5-TR): anxiety, postpartum/'with peripartum onset' 6, 34, 130; major depressive disorder 'with peripartum onset' 7, 26; peripartum depression (PPD) 5–6, 9, 26–27, 81, 128–129, 245; postpartum depression 98, 245; postpartum OCD (obsessive-compulsive disorder) 130; postpartum psychosis (PPP) 76; postpartum PTSD (post-traumatic stress disorder) 130; sexual dysfunctions 176–177, **177**; traumatic event, birth as 108
dialectical behavioral therapy (DBT) 259–260, *259*, **262**
dietary supplements 267
disability and pregnancy 51–53, **52**, **53**
Disability-Related Counseling Competencies (ARCA) 52, **53**
Drugs and Lactation Database (LactMed) 208
DSM-4, DSM-4-TR, DSM-5, DSM-5-TR; *see* Diagnostic and Statistical Manual of Mental Disorders

Ecological Systems Theory 19–20
Edinburgh Postnatal Depression Scale (EPDS) **4**, 85, 127, **128**
Emotionally Focused Therapy (EFT) 185, 187–188, *187–188*
Endicott, J. 152
ethical/legal considerations: abortion 117; adequacy of training 188–189, 209; cultural competence 61; disability 61; family situation/dynamic 163; pregnant women, working mothers/students, rights 231–232; sexual difficulties and dysfunctions 188–189; suicidality / maternal suicide 139–140
exercise as PPD treatment 267

Fair Play system 183
Family Medical Leave Act (FMLA, 1993) 10, 44, 74
female orgasmic disorder 176
Female Sexual Function Index (FSFI) 176–177, **177**
female sexual interest/arousal disorder 176
feminist multicultural perspective 2
feminist therapy 228, 255
feminist trauma approach 255
first time fathers/partners 9, 111–112, 159–160
Five Factor Wellness Inventory (5-WeL) 34, 83
FMLA leave 10, 44–45, 51, 74, 223, 227, 232, **238**
Fox, C. A. 138–139, 268–269
Freeman, M. P. 267
Freitas, C. J. 138–139, 268–269
Furrow, J. 162

gender: conception, non-binary, gay-couple discrimination 60–62, 113; gender-based inequalities, work/workload 61; LGBQQ (Lesbian, Gay, Bisexual, Queer, Questioning) **58–59**; LGBQQIA (Lesbian, Gay, Bisexual, Queer, Questioning, Intersex, and Ally) 58, 61; LGBTGEQIAP+ communities 57–60, **58–59**; LGBTQ+ couples/parents 113–114, 180, 206; nonbinary parents 10, 44; role expectations, gender-based stereotypes 43–44, 60–62, 112, 133, 157, 160, 177–178, 220, 221, 226–230; transgender parents 10, 43, 44, 59–60, 150, 230
Gender Expansive Identities (SAIGE) 57, 58
Generalized Anxiety Disorder **234**, 236
genito-pelvic pain/penetration disorder 176
Gliatto, M. E. 136
goals identified by family 28–29, **29–30**, 38; *see also under each STRENGTHS model application, case examples*
Golombok Rust Inventory of Sexual Satisfaction (GRISS) 177, **177**

Gottman, John 183, 185–187
Gottman method 185–186, ***186***, 187, 188

health disparities: maternal health 47; racial and ethnic 46–47
helpful, protective, and resilience factors 31–32; *see also under each STRENGTHS model application, case examples*
hemorrhage, postpartum 109
Hispanic mothers, family, culture ***34–35***, 35–36, 36–37, 46–47
Holt, C. 252

Imago therapy 184–185, **185**
infant mortality 2, 43, 45, 47, 232
infanticide 4, 5, 6, 76, 117, 126–127
infertility 100, 115, 116–117, 163
inner strengths, mother 31
interpersonal psychotherapy (IPT) 30, 245, 246–247, **247**, 254, 255, 255–258, *256*
intersectionality, intersectional identities 48, **53**, **58**, 61, 77, 230
intersectional nature of oppression 48
intimate partner violence (IPV) 77–78, 116

Jou, J. 44–45

Keefe, R. H. 244

Latina / Latinx mothers, treatment barriers/outcome disparities 22, 46, 164
Latina / Latinx families, role expectations 158
Laney, E. K. 150–151
legal consideration; *see* ethical/legal considerations
lesbian mothers 47, 157, 160, 206
LGBQQ (Lesbian, Gay, Bisexual, Queer, Questioning) **58–59**
LGBQQIA (Lesbian, Gay, Bisexual, Queer, Questioning, Intersex, and Ally) 58, 61
LGBTGEQIAP+ communities 57–60, **58–59**
LGBTQ+ couples/parents 113–114, 180, 206
lovingkindness 259, 271

macrosystem, mother/family 19–20, 21, 116–117, 209, 210–211
major depressive disorder (MDD) 129
maternal health outcomes 14–15
maternal mortality 14–15, 109–110; defining 46; postpartum hemorrhage 109; racial and ethnic health disparities 43, 46–47, **50**; rates 43, 46–47, 110; social factors 43
maternal suicide: age 76; ethical/legal considerations 139–140; female veterans 60; peripartum 60; PPD

8, 26–27, 118, 125–126; PPP 76; risk factors 4–5, 76; screening, prevention 4–5, 126–128, **128**, 136–137, **137**, *137*, 139–140, 141
maternity leave 9–10, 44–46, 73–74, 126, 220, 222–223, 224, 232
medical complications, pregnancy 102
mental health history, personal 24, *24*, 73, 75
Mezzacappa, E. S. 152, 266
microsystem, mother/family 19–21, 22–23, 77, 117
military service personal, veterans, families 60
Miller, K. E. 226–227
mindfulness psychoeducation **262**
mindfulness-based interventions 269–271, **270**
mood disorders 6–7; common stressors 8–11, *24*; impact 11–12; mother-child separation during treatment 5; scope 7–8; screening, prevention risk factors, 12–13
mortality: infant 2, 43, 45, 47, 232; maternal 14–15, 46–47, 109–110; *see also* suicidality / maternal suicide
mother–baby bond; *see* bonding, mother–infant
motherhood: adjustment to 3, 150–151; Attitudes toward Motherhood Scale (AToM) 152; counseling 160–163, 206–209, *208*; COVID-19 pandemic, impact 164–165; ethical and legal considerations 163; family dynamics/relationships, impact 157–158; fathers/partners, extended family 9, 111–112, 159–160, 161–162; first-time biological mothers 151–152; friendships, impact 158–159; lesbian mothers 47, 157, 160, 206; mothers of multiples 152–153; multicultural considerations 160, 164; non-biological mothers (adoptive/stepparents) 113, 153–154, 155–157, 159, 160, 162, 163; PPD coping strategies 204–205; PPD impact (mother, baby) 198–204; PPD treatment barriers 209–211; PPD: work and motherhood 220–221; role expectation, gender-based stereotypes 43–44, 133, 157, 160, 177–178, 220, 221, 226–230; surrogacy 113, 152; treatment barriers 163; *see also* career and identity
motherhood needs 27–28, *28*
motivational interviewing 252–253
Multicultural and Social Justice Counseling Competencies (MSJCC) 48–49, **49–50**, *49*
multicultural considerations 60; breastfeeding differences 205; *Competencies for Multicultural Career Counseling and Development* 230; COVID-19 pandemic, impact 61; cultural birth narratives, understanding 112–113; gendered and heteronormative role expectation 160, 230; institutionalized racism 205; intersectional identities 230; LGBTQ+ parents 113–114, 180, 206; *Multicultural and Social Justice Counseling Competencies* (MSJCC) 48–50, **49–50**, *49*; non-birth parents 160; parental bonding, cultural impact 205; perinatal loss 135; peripartum experience, societal, cultural, subcultural impact 81–82; racial/ethnic health disparities 43, 46–50; societal norms and pregnancy perception 113; socioeconomic status (SES) 82; transracial adoptions 160

Nadeem, E. 22
Neff, K. D. 270
negative automatic thoughts **250**
neonatal intensive care 54–55, 109, ***234***
non-pharmacological treatments, PPD 30
noticeable PPD symptoms, severity, DSM-5-TR diagnosis / needs identified by family & treatment team; *see under each STRENGTHS model application, case examples*

obstetric violence 175–176
obstetrical complications 46, 102, 108–110
OCD, postpartum 130–131, 140–141

parental leave 44–46, 73–74, 117, 220, 232
parental postadoption depression (PAD) 131–132, *132*
parenthood adjustments, role shifts 3
parenting, role/responsibility sharing 177–179, 183–185
paternal depression (father, partner): risk factors, peripartum depression 112; treating 138–139
paternal peripartum depression, treatment 138–139, 268–269
Patient Health Questionnaire-9 (PHQ-9) *3*, 85, 127, **128**
Perinatal Anxiety Screening Scale (PASS) 127, **128**, 130
perinatal loss 132–136; bereaved parent support 135, **135**; cultural implications 135; definition 132–133; family, siblings, impact 134–135; isolation after 133; paternal PPD 134; physiological impact 133; psychological impact 132–135
peripartum anxiety 7, 34
peripartum depression (PPD): common stressors 8–11, *24* (*see also* stressors); counseling 136–139; definition/criteria (DSM-4-TR and DSM-5-TR) 5–6, 26–27, 245; diagnosis 126–128; diagnosis, screening, criteria (DSM) 5–6, 9, 26–27, 81, 128–130, **128**, 245; impact 11–12; infant development, impact 202–204; motherhood and PPD, coping strategies 204–205; mother–infant bonding, impact 198–201; prevalence 245;

protective factors 72–73, 78, 82, 86, 87; risk factors (*see* risk factors, peripartum depression); scope 7–8; screening, prevention 12–13; screening, suicide prevention 126–128; social and cultural factors 43; strengths-based perspective, STRENGTHS model 14; suicidality screening, prevention 4–5, 126–128, **128**, 136–138, **136**, **138**, *137, 138,* 139–140, 141; symptoms, severity, diagnosis 5–6, 26–28; treatment recommendations, approaches 30–31, 243–272 (*see also under own heading*); peripartum period, defining 2

personal history, mental illness 24, 73, 75–76, 245

persons with disabilities (PWDs); *see* disability and pregnancy

pharmacological treatments, PPD 30–31

postadoption depression (PAD) 131–132, *132*

postpartum anxiety (PPA) 7, 130

postpartum depression: diagnostic definition (DSM) 5–6, 98, 245; health disparities 47; screening tools **128**; treatment 245–246, **246**, 265

Postpartum Depression Screening Scale (PDSS) 127, **128**

Postpartum Distress Measure (PDM), assessments 127, **128**, 131

postpartum hemorrhage (PPH) 109

postpartum OCD (obsessive-compulsive disorder) 130–131, 140–141

postpartum psychosis (PPP): infanticide 5, 6, 76, 117, 127; risk factors 23, 76

Postpartum Support International (PSI) 72, 73, 79, **164**, **212**, 268

post-traumatic growth 14, 108–109

post-traumatic stress disorder (PTSD); *see* PTSD

pregnancy: abortion 117; adjustments of 101–102; barriers to treatment 117–118; biopsychosocial theoretical model 116–117; COVID-19 pandemic, impact 119; disability 51–53, **52**, **53**; LGBTQ+ couples 113–114; maternal age 76–78; medical complications 102; screening and intervention 119–120; sexual violence, history/during 115–116; substance use 115–116; treatment barriers 117–118; treatment birth narratives 114–115

Pregnancy Discrimination Act (1978) **53**, 228, 231

preterm birth 13, 109

PRIMER (Promoting, Motivation, Empowerment, and Readiness) intervention 252–253, **253**–**254**

protective factors, peripartum depression 78, 82, 86, 87

psychoeducation **246**, **262**

PTSD **3**, 9, 98, 108, 130, 133, *149*, 255

Quality of Maternity Leave Scales (QMLS) 223

racial/ethnic disparities: health disparities 46–47; maternal health, working with marginalized mothers 47–49

Rai, A. K. 136

resilience factors 31, 38, 108–109, 131; *see also under each STRENGTHS model application, case examples*

rhythm as mother, finding 197–212; *see also* bonding, mother-infant

risk factors, peripartum depression 72–73; conception-related 101; IPT case formulation *256*; life stressors (*see* stressors); maternal age 76–77; maternal life stressors 24, *24*, 36, 87, 192; maternal suicide attempts (SA) 76, 133, **136**, 140; mental health symptoms, history of 23; partner support 73; paternal depression (father, partner) 112; perinatal loss 133; personal history, mental illness 23–24, *24*, 73, 75–76, 245; postadoption depression (PAD) 131–132, *132*; postpartum psychosis (PPP) 76; psychosocial 77–78; racial/ethnic health disparities 47; research 23; screening 86; sexual difficulties, pregnancy-related 174–175; socioeconomic status (SES), societal support 73–74, 82, 245; suicidality (*see* suicidality / maternal suicide); *see also under each STRENGTHS model application, case examples*

Rodsky, E. 183

Roe V. Wade 117

SAIGE 57, 58

Scale for Suicidal Ideation (SSI) 127

self-care 32–34, 38–39, 79–80, 81–82, 83, 223; *see also under each STRENGTHS model application, case examples*

self-compassion 32–33, 161, 270–271

self-love 32–33

Self-Rating Depression Scale (SDS) 127

sensitivity, parental 11, 223, 267

Severe maternal morbidity (SMM) 46

sexual difficulties and dysfunctions: clinical assessment tools 176–177, **177**; DSM classification 176; obstetric violence 175–176; treatment guidelines (Crooks, Bauer) 180–182, **182**

Sexual Function Questionnaire (SFQ) 177, **177**

SIDS (sudden infant death syndrome) **234**–**235**, 236

significant individual, infant, family, societal, and cultural factors 19–21, 35–36; *see also under each STRENGTHS model application, case examples*

Slopen, M. 44–45

SMART goals 28–29, **29**–**30**, 38

social support 25, 31, 80–81; *see also under each STRENGTHS model application, case examples*
societal judgement 74–75
Society for Sexual, Affectional, Intersex, and Gender Expansive Identities (SAIGE) 57, 58
socioeconomic status, barriers 23, 24, 47, 51, 82, 210
solution-focused brief therapy (SFBT) approaches 261, 262–264, **265**
solution-focused model (SFM) 261–262, 263–264
spirituality, religious diversity 53–57, **56**
Standards of care for the health of transsexual, transgender, and gender-nonconforming people (WPATH) 59
Stanley-Brown Safety Plan 136–137, *137*
State-Trait Anxiety Inventory for Adults (STAI-AD) 127
stay-at-home father (SAHF) 229
stay-at-home mother (SAHM) 220, 225, 230, ***234–235***
stepparents, stepmothers, stepfamilies 113, 154, 155–157, 159, 162, 163
stillbirth; *see* perinatal loss
STRENGTHS model application, case examples: Casey 251–252, **251–252**, ***253–254***, 254, 272–273; Ceci ***165–166***, 167–168; Christina **62**, 63–65; Jaelyn ***88–89***, 91–93; Jesse ***98–99***, 120–121; Johanna 141–143, ***141***; Juliette ***87–88***, 89–91; Kennedy 213–215, ***213***; Leila *20*, ***34–35***, 35–39; Marisela 99–100; Myriel ***237–238***, 239–240; Paisley ***234–235***, 235–237; Roberta *191*, 192–193
STRENGTHS model, elements: enlisting social support (family, community, medical professionals) 25–26; goals identified by family 28–29, **29–30**; helpful, protective, and resilience factors 31–32; noticeable symptoms, severity, DSM-5-TR diagnosis / needs identified by family & treatment team 26–28; self-care and wellness 32–34, 38–39, 79–80, 81–82, 83, 161, 223; significant individual, infant, family, societal, and cultural factors 19–21, 35–36; treatment barriers (*see under own heading*); treatment recommendations 30–31
STRENGTHS model of case conceptualization 19–39, 87, 246, 247; maternal life stressors (*see* stressors); motherhood needs 27–28, *28*; mother's macrosystem factors 19–20, 21, 116–117, 209, 210–211; mother's microsystem factors 19–21, 22–23, 77, 117; PPD symptoms, severity, diagnosis 26–28; risk factors (*see* risk factors, peripartum depression); social environment / Ecological Systems Theory 19–20
stressors: adoptive mothers 131; breastfeeding as stress decrease 247; case study: Leila 35–36, 38;

COVID-19 pandemic 13, 164, 190, 214, 233; life stressors 24, *24*; marginalization-related 47; maternal life 23–24, *24*, 36, 87; medical complication, pregnancy 102; military families, military culture 60; multiple children birth 150, 153; parental divorce 247; peripartum period 8–11, 24, *24*; psychological, psychosocial 77–78, 82; returning to work 223, 229, 232; social support, lack 73–74; socioeconomic status (SES) 47, 83, 210, 235; stepmothers 157
Substance Abuse and Mental Health Services Administration 129
substance use / substance-related disorders 115–116, 129–130, 190
suicidality / maternal suicide: age 76; Ask Suicide-Screening Questions (ASQ) Tool 127; Assess, Intervene and Monitor for Suicide Prevention (AIM-SP) model 136, **136**; ethical/legal considerations 139–140; female veterans 60; peripartum 60; PPD 8, 26–27, 118, 125–126; PPP 76; risk factors 4–5, 76; screening, prevention 4–5, 126–128, **128**, 136–138, **136**, **138**, *137*, 139–140, 141
surrogacy 113, 152

Torabi, F. 183–184
transgender individuals 59–60, 113, 150, 160, 230
trauma: adopted children 154, 162; birth 8, 20, 46, 73, 80, 108–109; obstetric violence 175–176; sexual abuse 60, 116; Traumatic Event Scale 130; treatment, Feminist therapy 255; treatment, narrative counseling approach 115, 130
treatment barriers 22–23, 36, 232; cultural 22, 23, 36; family support, lack of 22; gender role expectation 232; individual 22; mental health stigma / shame 232; parental knowledge, lack 36, 232; social support, lack 24–25, 73–74; societal, systemic 22–23, 36, 232; *see also under each STRENGTHS model application, case examples*
treatment birth narratives 114–115
treatment recommendations, approaches 30–31, 121; Bringing Baby Home Training 268; certification 268; fathers/partners; partner, social support, enhancing 83–84; psychopharmacological interventions 30–31, 265–266; self-care, wellness 83; sexual difficulties and dysfunctions 176–177, **177**, 180–183; solution-focused brief therapy (SFBT) approaches 261, 262–264, **265**; treatment length 245; *see also under each STRENGTHS model application*
treatment recommendations, approaches, complementary/alternative **246**, 266–268;

breastfeeding 266–267; bright light therapy 267; exercise 267; infant massage 267; prenatal and postnatal yoga 79, 114, 118, 267

treatment recommendations, approaches, psychotherapeutic 30, 245–246, **246**, **247**; cognitive behavioral therapy (CBT) / Internet-based CBT 30, 245–246, **246**–**247**, 248–249, ***248***, 252–253, 254–256; dialectical behavioral therapy (DBT) 259–260, *259*, **262**; feminist therapy 228, 255; interpersonal psychotherapy (IPT) 30, 245, 246–247, **247**, 254, 255, 255–258, *256*; mindfulness-based interventions 269–271, **270**; motivational interviewing 246, 252–253; PRIMER (Promoting, Motivation, Empowerment, and Readiness) intervention 252–253, ***253***–***254***; psychoeducation **246**, **262**; selecting 246–247; therapist, role 247–248

TWEAK assessment 129

U.S. Department of Health and Human Service 231

violence: intimate partner violence (IPV) 77–78, 116; obstetric 175–176; racialized 61; sexual abuse/assault 60, 116

wellness 32–34, 38–39, 80, 83, 161; *see also under each STRENGTHS model application, case examples*

work-from-home mothers (WFHMs) 165, 225–226, ***238***

working mothers 222–224; COVID-19 pandemic, impact 233; gender-based double-bind pressure 222; maternity/parental leave 9–10, 44–46, 73–74, 126, 220, 222–223, 224, 232; paid employment, benefits 224; paid maternity leave, lack 222–223; PPD treatment barriers 232–233; primary responsibility, family/home 222; workplace discrimination 222

World Professional Association of Transgender Health (WPATH) 59

yoga, prenatal and postnatal 79, 114, 118, 267

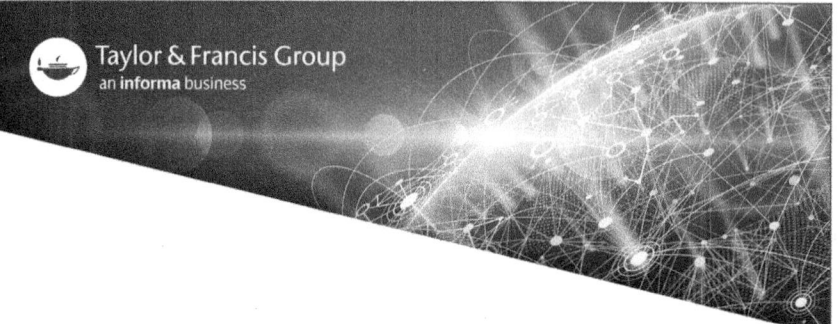